# MUSCULOSKELETAL
# ULTRASOUND

### in Physical and
### Rehabilitation Medicine

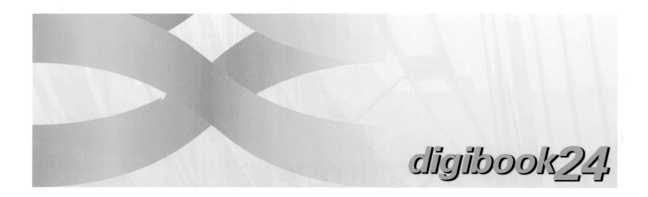

## Simple steps to get your digital edition:

**Levent Özçakar - Martine De Muynck (Editors)**

**MUSCULOSKELETAL ULTRASOUND in Physical and Rehabilitation Medicine - 1st edition**

1.  Go to the website **http://coupon.digibook24.com**
2.  Register at the *digibook24* portal (first time only) to obtain username and password (instructions also on the web page)
3.  Log in using your username and password
4.  Once you are logged in you enter your personal access code in the field in the web page. This code can be found (in this page) under the protection and can be removed by scraping with slight pressure from a coin.

EE4339010593

5.  Download the APP for your device
6.  Log in to the APP and download the digital book

**Technical Help Desk**: Technical help is available by email at *mths@digibook24.com*.

LEVENT ÖZÇAKAR
MARTINE DE MUYNCK

Editors

# MUSCULOSKELETAL
# ULTRASOUND

## in Physical and
## Rehabilitation Medicine

FRANCO FRANCHIGNONI
**Project Manager**

MAURO ZAMPOLINI
Associate Project Manager

Under the auspices of

## edi·ermes

**MUSCULOSKELETAL ULTRASOUND**
**in Physical and Rehabilitation Medicine**
by Levent Özçakar - Martine De Muynck (Editors)
Franco Franchignoni (Project Manager)- Mauro Zampolini (Associate Project Manager)

Copyright 2014 Edi.Ermes - Milan (Italy)

ISBN 978-88-7051-420-9 - Paper edition
ISBN 978-88-7051-433-9 - Digital edition

*Notices*

Knowledge and best practice in this field are constantly changing. As new research and experience broaden our understanding, changes in research methods, professional practices, or medical treatment may become necessary.

Practitioners and researchers must always rely on their own experience and knowledge in evaluating and using any information, methods, compounds, or experiments described herein. In using such information or methods they should be mindful of their own safety and the safety of others, including parties for whom they have a professional responsibility.

With respect to any drug or pharmaceutical products identified, readers are advised to check the most current information provided (i) on procedures featured or (ii) by the manufacturer of each product to be administered, to verify the recommended dose or formula, the method and duration of administration, and contraindications.

It lies within the responsibility of practitioners, relying on their own experience and knowledge of their patients, to make diagnoses, to determine dosages and the best treatment for each individual patient and to take all appropriate safety precautions. To the fullest extent of the law, neither the Publisher nor the authors, contributors, or editors, assume any liability for any injury and/or damage to persons or property as a matter of products liability, or arising from negligence or otherwise, or from any use or operation of any methods, products, instructions, or ideas contained in the material herein.

A book is the final product of a very complex series of operations that requires numerous tests on texts and images. It is almost impossible to publish a book with no errors. We will be grateful to those who find them and notify us. For enquiries or suggestions about this volume, please use the following address:

External relations - Edi.Ermes srl - Viale Enrico Forlanini, 65 - 20134 Milan (Italy)
Voice +39.02.70.21.121 - Fax +39.02.70.21.12.83

The Publisher is available for intellectual property owners with whom it was not possible to communicate, as well as for any inadvertent omissions and inaccuracies in the quotation of sources reproduced in this volume.

Paper edition printed in December 2014 by Arti Grafiche Colombo - Milan, Italy
for Edi.Ermes - viale Enrico Forlanini, 65 - 20134 Milan, Italy
http://www.ediermes.it - Tel. +39 02 7021121 - Fax +39 02 70211283

# Forewords

**Physical and Rehabilitation Medicine Board
of the European Union of Medical Specialists**

It is a great pleasure for me to write this preface on behalf of the European Board of Physical and Rehabilitation Medicine. "Musculoskeletal Ultrasound in Physical and Rehabilitation Medicine" is the first book sponsored by our Board aiming at promoting knowledge and skills within our medical speciality. The Board intends to sponsor regularly such books in the future and provide our community timely with learning material on important issues of our specialist practice. We are also very grateful to the European Society of Physical and Rehabilitation Medicine to share the sponsorship of this book with us. It is a token of the longstanding collaboration between our two professional bodies to promote a high level of professional competence within our medical specialty all over Europe.

Ultrasound imaging is used to explore the musculoskeletal system for almost 40 years. The technological progress during these 4 decades made ultrasound imaging a convenient diagnostic tool for soft tissue pathologies. Joints, muscles, tendons, ligaments, blood vessels and surrounding soft tissues can be explored easily, also dynamically. There is no exposure to radiation and the examination can be repeated for follow-up as many times as needed. High resolution diagnostic ultrasound allows now to explore anatomical details of large peripheral nerves. The possibility to explore structure and function immediately following history taking and physical examination or to carry out therapeutic interventions under the guidance of ultrasound make this tool extremely precious in all fields of Physical and Rehabilitation Medicine.

In near future mastery of diagnostic musculoskeletal ultrasound might well become a must for all specialists practising Physical and Rehabilitation Medicine. The challenge will be to train all these specialists for a high standard of practice and allow them to use the tool routinely and accurately. This future is already prepared by the European Musculoskeletal Ultrasonography Study Group Euro-Musculus, a group of European medical specialists in Physical and Rehabilitation Medicine founded in 2010. The aim of this group is to promote high standards of teaching and practice of diagnostic musculoskeletal ultrasound taking into account the specific needs specialists in Physical and Rehabilitation Medicine. The teaching of this group has a tremendous success worldwide and it might be extended to World-Musculus in the near future.

The European Board of Physical and Rehabilitation Medicine is very grateful that two of the leaders of Euro-Musculus, Professor Martine de Muynck and Professor Levent Özçakar, agreed to take on this book as scientific editors. We thank Professor Franco Franchignoni and Professor Mauro Zampolini for their work as managing editors. Last but not least we would also like to express our gratitude to all the Authors for their highly appreciated contribution.

*Rolf Frischknecht*

President

It is my distinct honor to have been asked to write a foreword on behalf of the European Society of Physical and Rehabilitation Medicine for this excellent book "Musculoskeletal Ultrasound in Physical and Rehabilitation Medicine", which is an enormous and distinctive contribution to the evolving field of musculoskeletal ultrasonography, inspired by the two main leaders of Euro-Musculus group (founded in 2010), Professor Martine de Muynck and Professor Levent Özçakar, internationally renowned in their field.

During the last five years, they have spent time lecturing in teaching seminars on musculoskeletal ultrasound and organizing International Musculoskeletal Ultrasonography Courses Euro-Musculus (I-V), having thus acquired an exceptional expertise, whilst in parallel they have numerous and outstanding contributions to the literature based on their relevant academic research. Euro-Musculus is a study group of European academic physiatrists (Physical and Rehabilitation Medicine physicians) who actively use musculoskeletal ultrasonography in their clinical practice and academic studies.

Among the aims of this remarkable team are to increase awareness concerning the role of musculoskeletal ultrasonography in the realm of Physical and Rehabilitation Medicine, to expedite European-wide the education process, to standardize its education and application, and to organize multi-country studies that will facilitate the formation of databases with respect to several components of the musculoskeletal system.

As ultrasound technology improves, its use to clinical diagnose and guide treatments of musculoskeletal conditions (through ultrasound-guided techniques), is an evolving and developing medical skill, providing diagnostic and therapeutic benefits to patients, whilst it remains an office-based technology. In recent years, PRM physicians, have been overwhelmed with the crescendo use of musculoskeletal ultrasonography due to its myriad advantages.

This book provides a better understanding of how to interpret and perform the procedures presented in a more efficient and safer way. Therefore, I am sure it will have a profound impact on the education of PRM specialists, residents and fellows, as well as to all physicians devoted to the diagnosis and treatment of musculoskeletal disorders.

We owe a great deal of gratitude to all the Authors for their valuable contribution, to Professor Martine de Muynck and Professor Levent Özçakar for taking on this book as scientific editors, as well as to Professor Franco Franchignoni and Professor Mauro Zampolini for their significant contribution as managing editors.

*Xanthi Michail*
President

**International Society
of Physical and Rehabilitation Medicine**

ISPRM

On behalf of the International Society of Physical and Rehabilitation Medicine (ISPRM) we are pleased to write this foreword for the book "*Musculoskeletal Ultrasound in Physical and Rehabilitation Medicine*". ISPRM is also proud to share the sponsorship of this publication with the European Society of Physical and Rehabilitation Medicine and the European Board of Physical and Rehabilitation Medicine.

The PRM specialist is *responsible for the prevention, diagnosis, treatment, and rehabilitation of people with disabling medical conditions and co-morbidities across all ages* [1]. As part of the clinical activities, the PRM specialist routinely deals with acute, sub-acute, and chronic conditions of the musculoskeletal system. Ultrasonography is becoming the *stethoscope of the physiatrist* dedicated to the musculoskeletal system. Advances in technology have contributed to the enhancement of the quality of ultrasound images making musculoskeletal ultrasonography a real option for the appropriate diagnosis of soft tissues and articular injuries. Furthermore, real time ultrasonography can be used in the treatment of musculoskeletal disorders by guiding the injection of various pharmacologic agents. This technique, in combination with a thorough clinical history and physical examination, and the physiatrist's knowledge of anatomy and biomechanics has the potential to enhance the quality of the clinical services provided to the patient. However, it must be recognized that the usefulness of ultrasonography in the exploration of the musculoskeletal system is dependent of the expertise and experience of the examiner. Thus, it is essential that the PRM specialists learn the theory and practice of musculoskeletal ultrasonography.

Two important aims of ISPRM encourage us to support this project. The ISPRM is interested in helping physicians and researchers active in physical and rehabilitation medicine to develop and apply optimal care [2]. In addition, ISPRM must collaborate on disseminating new knowledge, among the specialists and residents in training, from the basic to the clinical applications of research [3].

We congratulate and thanks Professors Levent Özçakar and Martine de Muynck, editors, and Professors Franco Franchignoni and Mauro Zampolini, managing editors, for an excellent contribution to the specialty of Physical and Rehabilitation Medicine, particularly in the area of musculoskeletal conditions.

*Jianan Li*
President

*Jorge Lains*
President-elect

*Walter Frontera*
Vice President

1. White Book on physical and rehabilitation medicine in Europe. Eur Medicophys. 2006; 42: 292-332.
2. ISPRM - The International Society of Physical Medicine and Rehabilitation. Mission& Goals. http://www.isprm.org/discover/mission-goals/Acceded August, 2014.
3. Stucki G, Grimby G. Organizing human functioning and rehabilitation research into distinct scientific fields. Part I: Developing a comprehensive structure from the cell to society. J Rehabil Med. 2007; 39: 293-8.

While magnetic resonance imaging has revolutionized imaging of the musculoskeletal system and become an established imaging modality since its introduction in 1980s, another imaging technique was quietly on rise – ultrasonography (US). US is gaining its ascendancy by numerous reasons: almost every patient can undergo US, it allows real-time dynamic examination and you can check exactly where it hurts, bilateral comparison is possible, it has the advantage in guiding a wide range of musculoskeletal interventions and is relatively inexpensive. By all means, I certainly believe that specialists who are dealing with musculoskeletal problems should implement US in their practices as their 6th finger. Although US is highly dependent on the skill of the examiner, there now exists a comprehensive guidance book to which we all can refer in order to perform US and interpret the findings.

Edited by two leaders in this area – Dr. Özçakar and Dr. De Muynck, with the help of two experts Dr. Franchignoni and Dr. Zampolini as Project Managers – this text "Musculoskeletal Ultrasound in Physical and Medicine Rehabilitation" leads us on an extensive trip around human body with specific emphasis on most frequent problems in adults as well as in children. The Editors have aimed this book for the practicing physiatrist, whether experienced or novice. So to those of you who have ignored US maybe for years and to those of you who would like to enhance their expertise in this area, I strongly recommend this book both as a place to start and as a text to refer.

Once again, I congratulate the Editors Drs. Özçakar and De Muynck and the Project Managers Drs. Franchignoni and Zampolini for this excellent work and finally thank them for giving me the honor and privilege of writing this foreword. I strongly believe that this valuable text in an important and expanding field will become a favorite.

*Ayşen Akıncı Tan*

President

# Ultrasound Physics

Abdullah Ruhi SOYLU, Bayram KAYMAK

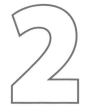

## 2.1 INTRODUCTION

Medical ultrasonography (US) is a tool for visualization of tissues in real time. Images are acquired by recording the reflections or echoes of ultrasonic pulses directed into the tissues. US is one of the most widely used imaging techniques in the world [1, 2] and it is generally accepted as a "safe imaging technique" because it uses high frequency sound waves rather than electromagnetic waves.

A basic US device has at least one transducer (Figures 2.1, 2.2) for sound production and detection and, a compact computer for data processing

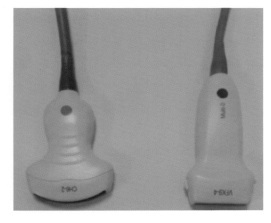

**Figure 2.2**    Convex and linear transducers.

and control of imaging modes, and a monitor for visualization (Figure 2.1). In this chapter we will provide an introduction to the complicated concepts of ultrasound physics. Interested readers can refer to the cited publications [3-7] for detailed information.

## 2.2 SOUND PHYSICS

Sound is a longitudinal (i.e. oscillation and propagation directions are the same), mechanical wave, which travels through a medium [4]. Sound wave is a periodic pressure disturbance that radiates from a vibrating source in the form of compression and rarefaction regions (Figure 2.3). In compression areas, particles are close together and there is high pressure while in rarefactions areas, particles are far apart and there is low pressure (Figure 2.3). Although these areas move forward and propagate, particles only oscillate back and forth along the direction of propagation [4].

The *wavelength* ($\lambda$) of a periodic sound wave is

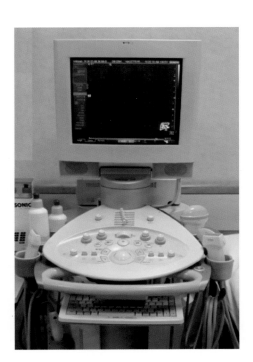

**Figure 2.1**    An ultrasound system with four transducers.

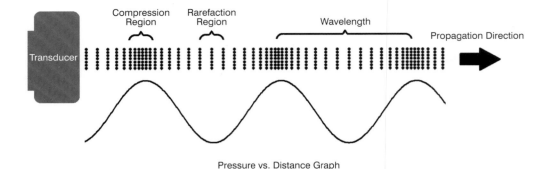

**Figure 2.3** Production of sound waves in a medium (top) and corresponding "pressure vs. distance" graph (bottom).

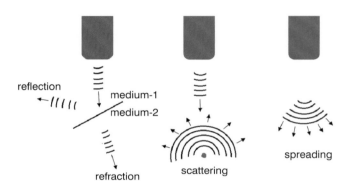

**Figure 2.4** The interaction of ultrasound waves with tissues.

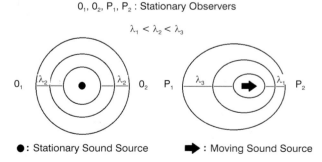

**Figure 2.5** Doppler Effect for stationary (left) and moving (right) sound sources. $P_2$ hears an increase in pitch compared to $O_2$. Similarly, $P_1$ hears a decrease in pitch compared to $O_1$. Note that only wavelengths ($\lambda_1, \lambda_2, \lambda_3$) are shown on the figures (wavelength and frequency are inversely related, $v = \lambda \times f$).

the distance between successive compressions or the distance between successive rarefactions (Figure 2.3). The *frequency* (*f*) of a periodic sound wave is the number of cycles produced by the source in one second, or the number of cycles that pass through a particular point in the medium each second. The unit for frequency is Hertz (Hz). US devices use sound waves in the range of approximately 1 MHz to 20 MHz (M - mega = 1 million), which is much higher than the frequency range of speech sounds [1]. There is a relation between wavelength and frequency:

$$v = \lambda \times f$$

where *v* is velocity of sound in the propagation medium. Speed of sound depends on stiffness (*s*) and density (*d*) of the medium (*v* = square root of *s*/*d*). It is higher in stiffer and low-density media. While speed of sound in soft tissue is ~1540 m/s, it is ~340 and ~4000 m/s in air and bone, respectively.

The interaction of ultrasound waves with tissues (Figure 2.4) during propagation can be described in terms of attenuation, absorption, scattering, reflection, refraction, and spreading [5]. The energy loss due to the transfer of energy into tissues as heat is called *absorption*. Absorption, spreading, scattering, and reflections cause attenuation. *Attenuation* is exponential decay of sound energy during propagation in a medium and it is a function of distance and frequency. As an example if the sound intensity is reduced by 50% for every one cm (assuming that the tissue is homogenous), at 20 cm depth, the reduction will be ~99.999905% (= 100% - $0.5^{20} \times 100\%$). If the wave frequency increases, penetration (the ability to image deep structures) decreases and vice versa. While 20 MHz sound waves can image up to a few cm, 2 MHz waves can image deep structures (up to ~20 cm). A *reflection* occurs at the boundary between two media when the acoustic impedances of the two media are different. The reflection of the beam is called echo and production/detection of echoes forms the basis of ultrasound imaging. Acoustic impedance (**Z**) is the product of mass density (**d**) of the medium and speed of sound (**Z = d × v**) in that medium [5]. Acoustic impedance is of vital importance for 2D imaging as the relative acoustic impedance differences produce sound reflections. Therefore, there will be no tissue texture in the image if there are no reflections since only the reflected echoes are detected and displayed. When ultrasound waves pass through an interface between two different tissues at an oblique angle, both *reflection* and *refraction* occur. If wavelength of ultrasound is comparable or smaller than tissue parts, *scattering* in various directions occurs. The scattered sound waves that can be detected by the transducer provide information on the tissue texture and therefore, are useful to distinguish different tissues (muscle, liver, spleen etc).

*Spreading* (i.e. divergence or diffusion) of sound waves decreases image quality since spreading causes unwanted echoes from surroundings. The echoes coming from the outside of the area of interest will create noise.

*Doppler Effect* is the change in the frequency of a wave for an observer moving relative to its source [4] (Figure 2.5). A typical example is a moving ambulance: its siren is heard as high-pitched as it comes towards the observer, and then becomes low-pitched as it moves away. Doppler modes of US make use of the Doppler Effect to determine and display blood flow velocity.

## 2.3 PRODUCTION AND DETECTION OF SOUND PULSES

### 2.3.1 B-mode or Gray Scale Imaging (2D mode)

Transducer is a device for sound pulse production and detection by converting electrical transmission pulses into ultrasound pulses and ultrasonic echo pulses into electrical signals [4, 5]. Piezoelectric crystals are used for both sound production and echo detection. A specialized computer controls the transducer during imaging. Immediately after the transmission of the pulse, the transducer is used as a receiver to detect reflected echoes. The reflected waves are recorded as a function of time. Each wave corresponds to a thin sound propagation line called scan-line (Figure 2.6). A 2D image is formed from consecutively acquired scan-lines (Figure 2.7). To get thin scan-lines, width of the transmitted sound pulses should be narrow enough to avoid echoes outside the scan-line, which would otherwise add noise to the image. Modern transducers usually use wideband waves rather than a single frequency. For example, a 5 to 10 MHz transducer sends and detects 5 to 10 MHz sound frequencies. The benefit of using a frequency range is to optimize penetration (5 MHz has higher penetration than 10 MHz) and resolution (10 MHz's resolution is higher than 5 MHz) simultaneously.

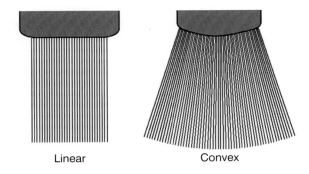

Linear                    Convex

**Figure 2.6** Scan lines of convex and linear transducers. Scanning usually starts from one side and continues in a stepwise fashion.

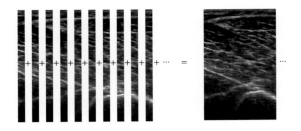

**Figure 2.7** Image strips from scan lines of a linear transducer.

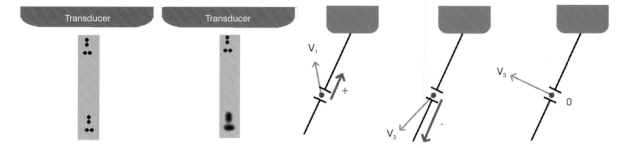

**Figure 2.8** Axial and lateral resolution examples from two transducers that scan the same medium. Both near and far field axial and lateral resolutions are good on the left but far field axial and lateral resolutions are very poor on the right. *See text for definitions.*

**Figure 2.9** Schematic drawing for three blood particles ($v_1$, $v_2$, $v_3$). PW Doppler can detect only projected velocities (blue colored vectors) not actual velocities (red colored vectors). While projected velocities on the left and middle are positive and negative, respectively; it is zero on the right because $v_3$ is perpendicular to the propagation direction of transmitted sound.

2D-mode displays relative acoustic impedance differences in the imaging plane. *Axial and lateral resolutions* (Figure 2.8) are the abilities to differentiate axial (along the ultrasound beam) and lateral (perpendicular to axial) structures, respectively [3]. *Contrast resolution* is the ability to differentiate the variations in intensity. Axial resolution and penetration are directly affected by the frequency as described previously. *M-mode* is a variant of the 2D-mode: the same line is continuously scanned and displayed in a sliding window. This mode is mainly used for moving structures.

### 2.3.2 Pulsed Wave Doppler Mode

*Pulsed Wave (PW) Doppler* measures blood flow velocities within a space window called sample window or sample gate, whereby location and size are user adjustable. PW Doppler calculates the projected velocity distribution of a blood sample in the sample gate, where the projection axis is the propagation direction of the transmitted sound waves (Figure 2.9). Projected velocity spectra are continuously calculated and vertically displayed in a sliding window (velocity histogram vs. time) in grey scale tones (Figure 2.10). Plus and minus signs on vertical axis usually correspond to blood velocity towards and away from the transducer, respectively.

In PW Doppler mode, echo pulses are transmitted along a user selected line through the tissue at a constant *pulse repetition frequency* (PRF) but echo acquisition and image formation

processes are different from 2D imaging [3].

A major drawback of PW Doppler is that velocity detection deteriorates for high velocities. There is a correctly detectable high velocity limit, which depends on PRF and depth of sample gate [3]. *Continuous Wave Doppler* (CW) mode has no high velocity limit [5] but it has another drawback: the sample gate includes all scan-line. Accordingly, CW is mainly used in cardiology to quantify high velocity blood flows. Similar to 2D mode, increasing frequency in Doppler modes increases sensitivity but decreases penetration and vice versa.

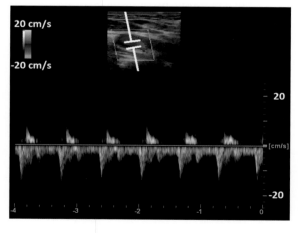

**Figure 2.10** An exemplary PW Doppler image. Velocity distribution vs. time graph is seen at the bottom; sample gate is drawn on color flow and 2D images on the top-middle, and top-left shows the color scale of velocity.

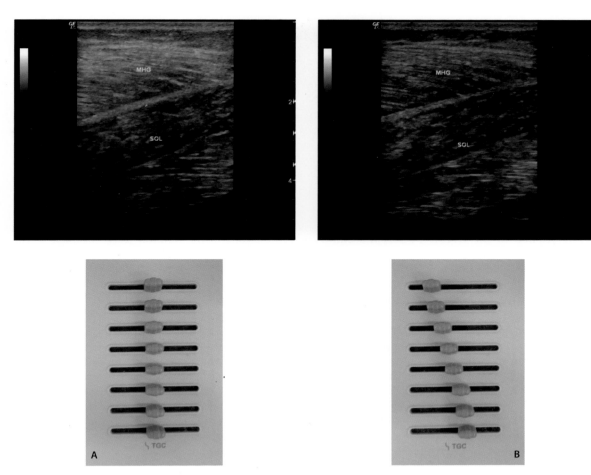

**Figure 3.2** Longitudinal scans of calf mucles. A - TGC sliders at neutral position. Superficial structures appear more hyperechoic in comparison with deeper ones and the normal echotexture is lost. B - TGC sliders adjustment results in a uniform distribution of echoes. MHG, medial head of gastrocnemius muscle; SOL, soleus muscle.

caused by tissues at increasing depths. Due to attenuation, weaker signals are received from structures that lie deeper than those which lie closer to the transducer. The TGC adjusts gain in specific depths of the image and can compensate for this loss of signal strength. This is achieved by applying a variable gain to the received signals so that signals returning later are amplified more than those previously received. TGC balances the image in order to obtain the same density of echoes throughout the image [5, 6].

The TGC control is presented as a series of sliders arranged in a vertical fashion on the control panel. Each of the sliders adjusts the amplification of the returning US signals at a specific image depth. Depending on the US machine, TGC is preset to a large degree and the

operator can make fine adjustments if necessary (Figure 3.2).

### 3.1.6 Depth

The depth control adjusts the maximum scanning range viewed on screen. Depth influences spatial resolution, pulse repetition frequency and frame rate. A depth greater than necessary should not be chosen because this reduces the frame rate and resolution of the image [5].

### 3.1.7 Focus

Focal zone is the region where the lateral resolution is the best. The focus of the ultrasound signal occurs at a point at which the beam is at its narrowest width. In order to obtain the best possible resolution the ultrasound beam should be focused at the depth at which the pertinent anatomic structures are located [6]. In modern linear-array transducers, focusing is currently not obtained by means of a fixed lens as in the old mechanical sector probes. Focusing is now produced electronically by activating a series of elements in the array with appropriate delays, so that the trigger pulses to the inner elements are delayed with respect to the pulses to the outer ones. In this way a curved wavefront results from constructive interference bringing the US beam toward a focus. By adjusting the values of the delays applied to the trigger pulses, the curvature of the wavefront and, therefore, the focal depth can be changed dynamically [3]. Focus optimizes the image by increasing the resolution for a specific area. The focal zone should be positioned at or just below the level of interest within the image. A graphic mark corresponding to the focal zone position(s) appears on the edge of the image.

The examiner can select more than one focal zone. However, as the number of focal zones is increased the number of frames per second is reduced, resulting in a slower frame rate [5]. This effect has to be taken in consideration when dynamic examination is performed or when ultrasound imaging is used to guide interventional procedures.

### 3.1.8 Freeze

The "freeze" function allows the operator to display a static image on the monitor. A number of frames can also simultaneously be stored in the image memory. The operator can navigate through these frames and select the appropriate still image for review, annotation, documentation or storage. This function is usually referred to as cineloop [5].

### 3.1.9 Zoom

Zoom is used to magnify a region of interest. There are two forms of zoom, read zoom and write zoom. Read zoom simply magnifies the image, without improving its quality. It is similar to digital zoom on modern digital cameras. Write zoom, also known as real zoom, increases the ultrasound information content within the image. Write zoom improves image resolution by increasing the scan line density and the number of pixels per square centimeter [5].

### 3.1.10 Measurements

A number of measurements can be taken with ultrasound equipment and are essential part for the interpretation of ultrasound scans and differentiation of normal anatomy from pathology. Measurements that can be obtained from frozen static B-mode (Brightness-mode) images include: distance, circumference, area and volume [5]. Ultrasound equipment can also perform measurements of angles according to Graf's technique and calculations of the femoral head coverage in the case of pediatric hip examination [7].

## 3.2 ADVANCED SETTINGS

The image optimization settings discussed in this section are usually preconfigured as "presets" according to the examination protocol the operator selects. Most of the times the preconfigured settings are adequate and no adjustments are required. However, the operator should understand the principles of these settings and be competent to apply appropriate adjustments whenever needed.

### 3.2.1 Dynamic Range

Dynamic range controls how echo intensities are converted to shades of gray, thereby increasing the adjustable range of contrast. A broader dynamic range yields more shades of gray, while a narrower dynamic range results in a more black and white appearance of the image (Figure 3.3).

The dynamic range is expressed in decibels (dB) and represents the ratio of the largest to the smallest signal that can be visualized [5]. Dynamic range is useful for optimizing tissue texture for different anatomy. If we do not need to differentiate between a wide range of gray levels, as for example in case of fluid collections or vessels, a lower dynamic range setting can be selected. For the musculoskeletal system we usually need to visualize subtle differences within and between tissues, therefore it is advisable to increase the dynamic range. However, in the presence of a large quantity of low-level noise, an increased dynamic range can compromise the quality of the image. As a principle, dynamic range should be

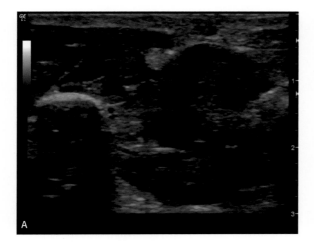

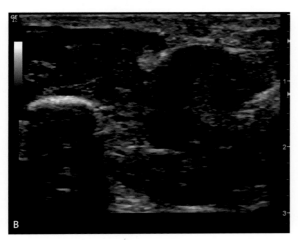

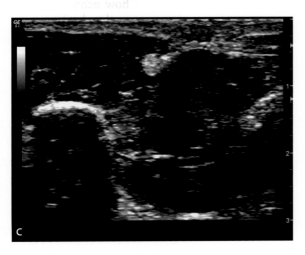

**Figure 3.3** The effect of dynamic range settings on the contrast of the image. A - Dynamic range set at 90 dB, which is considered a suitable value for the examination of the musculoskeletal system. B - Dynamic range set at 60 dB. C - Dynamic range set at 30 dB.

adjusted so that the highest amplitude edges appear as white while lowest levels (such as blood) are just visible.

### 3.2.2 Frame Rate

Frame rate refers to image update frequency. The frame rate determines the temporal resolution potential of the system and is therefore important when assessing moving interfaces. As focal zones are added, or imaging depth increased, the rate at which the ultrasound machine can produce complete, updated B-mode images is reduced. The examiner should adjust frame rates based on the clinical situation. Higher frame rates (typically more than 20 frames/s) are necessary to detect rapidly occurring events such as a snapping iliopsoas tendon or to track needle movement and injectate flow during an ultrasound guided injection [8]. At frame rates less than 16 frames per second, the displayed image degrades, and real-time capabilities are significantly compromised [9].

### 3.2.3 Sector width – Scan area

The sector width, also referred to as the sector angle, is important in determining the frame rate at a given depth. Reducing the sector width means that fewer scan lines are required to form an image. This reduces the time needed to build up an image, resulting in higher frame rates [5]. The examiner should increase the sector angle to see a wide field of view and decrease the sector angle when a faster frame rate is needed.

### 3.2.4 Rejection

Selects a level below which echoes will not be amplified (an echo must have a certain minimum amplitude before it will be processed). Appropriate adjustment allows for the elimination from the display of low level echoes caused by noise.

### 3.2.5 Extended Field-of-view Imaging

The field-of-view (FOV) of a real-time sonogram is limited by the probe width, which is typically 4 to 6 cm. The extended-FOV imaging technique provides high-quality panoramic B-mode images in real time by free-hand scanning with standard probes. While the operator moves the transducer slowly in the lateral direction over the region of interest, a programmable image processor integrated into the sonographic scanner estimates probe motion from sequentially acquired frames and reconstructs a large panoramic compound image in real time. Using the global motion information from each frame, the software smoothly blends the individual frames in a successive manner to generate the composite panoramic image. The in-process panoramic image has two portions: a real-time portion, which advances with the probe motion, and a static portion, which is the blended compound image from previous probe locations. When the scanning process is finished, the real-time portion is frozen and blended with the static portion to generate the total composite image. The algorithm allows the operator to halt during forward transducer movement or to move backward to correct part of the acquired composite image [10].

### 3.2.6 Steering-Based Imaging

The beam steering function has been applied to B-mode imaging to obtain a parallelogram format with lateral sides parallel but oblique instead of a rectangular field-of-view. In musculoskeletal US, this function seems to be useful when anisotropic structures, such as tendons or ligaments (for example the calcaneo-fibular ligament and the lateral collateral ligament of the knee), are examined with an incidence angle far from 90° due to their oblique course from surface to depth. Beam steering may optimize depiction of the fibrillar echotexture in an otherwise hypoechoic tendon area, thus helping to avoid confusion between artifact and disease [3].

### 3.2.7 Harmonic Imaging

The aim of the method is to produce a cleaner image with higher contrast resolution. In harmonic imaging the transducer transmits ultrasound at the fundamental frequency and detect echoes at both the fundamental and second harmonic frequencies. The signals produced by the fundamental frequency are filtered out. The principle of this method of imaging is that the second harmonic frequency contains the high amplitude echoes whereas the fundamental frequency,

which is filtered out, contains the low amplitude artifactual echoes [11]. The technique enhances near field resolution for improved imaging of small parts as well as far field penetration. According to Choudhry et al. the improved image quality with harmonic imaging is most apparent in obese patients and in lesions that are cystic or contain highly reflective tissues such as calcium, gas or fat [12].

### 3.2.8 Elastographic Imaging

Elastography techniques may be divided into those that measure strain and those that measure shear wave velocity. Most common commercial elastography techniques are based on strain methods. Strain elastography involves deformation of the tissue followed by imaging of the degree of compression or extension of the tissue. Strain elastography does not estimate tissue stiffness but the strain ratio may be used as a surrogate index of stiffness. It should be noted that strain elastography techniques are not quantitative as they measure strain, not elastic modulus. Shear wave elastography provides true quantitative information on elastic modulus. The recent introduction of shear wave techniques, especially shear wave imaging, is considered to present a great potential in offering quantitative measurements of elastic modulus and it could eventually over time become the industry standard [13].

Strain elastography measures in real-time the axial displacement of tissue caused by mechanical stress. The stress is either applied externally with the transducer by the operator or by physiological shifts inside the patient. Transducer stress is applied by continuously compressing and decompressing the skin of the patient. A gentle axial transducer movement suffices. The elastogram is derived from data of the change of radio frequency signals before and after compression. The elastogram is displayed in a split-screen mode with the conventional B-mode image and the elastogram on the monitor. The elastogram may be displayed as a color-overlay on the B-mode picture. Most strain elastography systems display tissue stiffness in a range of colors from red to blue, depending on the magnitude of tissue strain. However, there is no color standard for strain elastography imaging. There are several ways of providing a semi-quantifiable elastographic measure applicable in a clinical setting [14].

Shear wave elastography relies on the production and detection of shear waves. From the practical point of view the technique comprises three steps: induction of shear waves, tracking shear wave propagation through the tissues and finally the estimation of Young's modulus using the relevant equation [13].

Preliminary experience in the musculoskeletal system indicates that elasticity assessment may be promising to separate structures (i.e. degenerated from partially torn tendons) that are indistinguishable on gray-scale US imaging, as well as to disclose occult disease in otherwise normal appearing tissue. It is expected that elastography will become an important tool for the diagnosis of musculoskeletal disorders in selected clinical settings [3].

### 3.2.9 Three-Dimensional Imaging

Three-dimensional (3D) imaging can be obtained using either conventional transducers equipped with a positional sensor or special 3D-Volume transducers. Dedicated 3D transducers provide better quality data acquisition but are larger than conventional probes and harder to handle. 3D transducers in the frequency range suitable for the examination of the musculoskeletal system are available, offering promising perspectives for the evaluation of specific disorders of the musculoskeletal system [3]. Furthermore, 3D vascular images of the musculoskeletal sys-

tem can be obtained using dedicated systems and software for 3D rendering of power Doppler images [15].

### 3.3 DOPPLER ULTRASOUND

Three different types of Doppler imaging will be presented:
1. Color flow (CF)
2. Power Doppler (PD)
3. Spectral Doppler or pulsed wave Doppler (PW).

**1. Color flow imaging** is a Doppler mode intended to add color-coded qualitative information concerning the relative velocity and direction of blood flow. The CF imaging is used in conjunction with B-mode imaging. It should be noted that, as with any Doppler technique the angle of insonation is very important. When taking measurements of blood flow, a Doppler beam angle between 30° and 60° is important to ensure reliable Doppler shifted signals. Angles greater than 60° should be avoided while at 90° no Doppler shifted signals are generated [16].

**2. Power Doppler imaging** is a color flow technique used to map the strength of the Doppler signal coming from the flow rather than the frequency shift of the signal. Using this technique, the ultrasound system plots color flow based on the number of blood cells that are moving, regardless of their velocity. Because it does not map velocity, it is not subject to the aliasing. PD is a sensi-

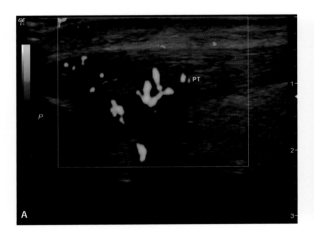 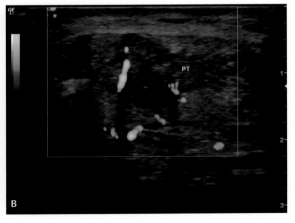

**Figure 3.4**  Power Doppler examination: neovascularization in a swollen patellar tendon in tendinopathy/tendinosis. A - Longitudinal scan. B - Transverse scan. P, patella, PT, patellar tendon.

**Table 3.1** Doppler imaging controls and settings

| | |
|---|---|
| Scan area | The color flow window is positioned with the use of the trackball on the region of interest. It should be remembered that the smaller the color window, the faster the frame rate and vice versa. |
| Angle steer | Steers the region of interest without moving the probe. The setting is applicable to linear probes. |
| Gain | Amplifies the overall strength of echoes processed in the color flow window or spectral Doppler timeline and is measured in decibels. |
| Pulse repetition frequency | Adjusts the sampling rate so as to eliminate aliasing. Imaging of higher velocity flow requires increased values to avoid aliasing. |
| Wall filter | Hides unusable motion by filtering out low flow velocity signals. It helps avoid motion artifacts caused from breathing and other patient motion. |
| Packet size | Controls the number of samples gathered for a single color flow vector. Decreasing the packet size, we increase the frame rate and lower the image quality. When we increase the packet size, we improve image quality and reduce the frame rate. |
| Threshold | Threshold adjusts the gray scale level at which color information stops. |

tive technique to detect low flows and explore small vessels (Figure 3.4). A significant disadvantage is that PD is extremely sensitive to motion [16]. Herewith, adjustments of the pertinent setting of the machine is paramount (Table 3.1).

**3. Spectral Doppler**, which is also referred to as pulsed wave Doppler, is combined with B-mode and color flow imaging techniques. It allows the assessment and evaluation of the blood flow selectively from a small region called the sample volume [16]. A detailed presentation of PW technique is beyond the scope of this book.

# REFERENCES

1) Finnoff JT, Smith J, Nutz DJ, Crogg BE. A musculoskeletal ultrasound course for physical medicine and rehabilitation residents. Am J Phys Med Rehabil. 2010; 89: 56-69.

2) Gibbs V, Cole D, Sassano A. Ultrasound physics and technology: how, why and when. 1st ed. Edinburgh: Churchill Livingstone; 2009. Chapter 6, Transducers; p. 27-37.

3) Derchi EL, Rizzatto G. Technical requirements. In: Bianchi S, Martinoli C, editors. Ultrasound of the musculoskeletal system. Berlin: Springer; 2007. p. 3-16.

4) Smith J, Finnoff JT. Diagnostic and interventional musculoskeletal ultrasound: part 1. Fundamentals. PM R. 2009; 1: 64-75.

5) Gibbs V, Cole D, Sassano A. Ultrasound physics and technology: how, why and when. 1st ed. Edinburgh: Churchill Livingstone; 2009. Chapter 10, Instrumentation and controls; p. 63-72.

6) Karmakar MK, Wing KH. Ultrasound guided regional anesthesia. In: Coté C, Lerman J, Anderson B, editors. Coté' and Lerman's a Practice of anesthesia for infants and children. 5th ed. Philadelphia, PA: Elsevier; 2013. p. 880-908.

7) Graf R. Guide to sonography of the infant hip. Stuttgart: Georg Thieme Verlag; 1987.

8) Pelsser V, Cardinal E, Hobden R, Aubin B, Lafortune M. Extra-articular snapping hip: sonographic findings. AJR Am J Roentgenol. 2001; 176: 67-73.

9) Kremkau F. Diagnostic ultrasound: principles and instruments. 6th ed. Philadelphia, PA: WB Saunders; 2002.

10) Weng L, Tirumalai A, Lowery C, Nock L, Gustafson D, Von Behren P, et al. US extended-field-of-view imaging technology. Radiology. 1997; 203: 877-80.

11) Gibbs V, Cole D, Sassano A. Ultrasound physics and technology: how, why and when. Edinburgh: Churchill Livingstone; 1st ed. 2009. Chapter 14, New technology and recent advances in ultrasound imaging; p. 111-9.

12) Choudhry S, Gorman B, Charboneau WJ, Tradup DJ, Beck RJ, Kofler JJ, et al. Comparison of tissue harmonic imaging with conventional US in abdominal disease. RadioGraphics. 2000; 20: 1127-35.

13) Hoskins PR. Principles of ultrasound elastography. Ultrasound. 2012; 20: 8-15.

14) Carlsen J, Ewertsen C, Lönn L, Nielsen M. Strain elastography ultrasound: an overview with emphasis on breast cancer diagnosis. Diagnostics. 2013; 3: 117-25.

15) Doria AS, Guarniero R, Molnar LJ, Modena M, Cunha FG, de Godoy Jr RM, et al. Three-dimensional (3D) contrast-enhanced power Doppler imaging in Legg-Calve-Perthes disease. Pediatr Radiol. 2000; 30: 871-4.

16) Gibbs V, Cole D, Sassano A. Ultrasound physics and technology: how, why and when. 1st ed. Edinburgh: Churchill Livingstone; 2009. Chapter 11, Physical principles of Doppler ultrasound; p. 73-89.

# Artifacts in Musculoskeletal Ultrasound

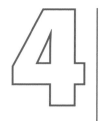

Levent TEKİN

The word "artifact" refers, in brief, to image errors. Various conditions may lead to artifacts, including those observed during the passage of the ultrasound (US) beam through biological tissues. Additionally, artifacts may result from erroneous scanning techniques [1]. Artifacts may mislead the physician in interpreting the images and making a prompt diagnosis. Therefore, recognition of these artifacts is crucial in clinical practice; the sonographer might observe and ignore them or, in certain conditions, they (anisotropy, posterior acoustic enhancement, acoustic shadowing, comet tail, ring down and rain artifacts) may aid the sonographer to better detect/visualize the relevant structure/pathology [2, 3]. For instance, while it

may be quite difficult to initially detect a very small foreign object within heterogenous echogenicities (or even during open surgery), its related artifact throughout the whole US screen would eventually make it almost impossible for the sonographer to miss the pathology.

## 4.1 ARTIFACTS ASSOCIATED WITH ATTENUATION ERRORS

### 4.1.1 Anisotropy

Anisotropy refers to the hypo-/hyper-echoic images (Figure 4.1 A) observed when the ultrasound

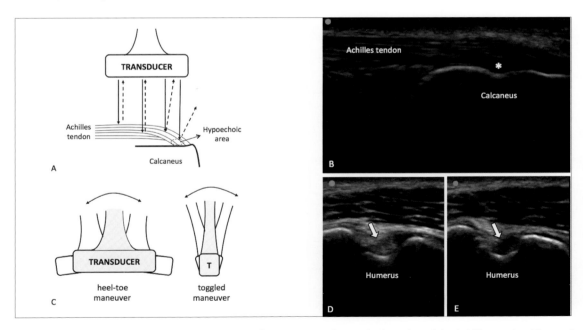

**Figure 4.1**   A - Schematic presentation. B - US image of anisotropy artifact at the insertion of the Achilles tendon. The tendon appears hyperechoic where the ultrasound beam is perpendicular to the tendon and hypoechoic (asterisk) when it is not. C - Schematic presentation of the toggle and hill-toe maneuver. D - Short axis of the biceps tendon (white arrow) is observed within the bicipital groove. E - With a small change in the angle of the probe, it becomes hypoechoic.

beam hits the structure at a non-perpendicular angle [4]. Although anisotropy is more commonly observed during the imaging of structures with an oblique course (tendons and ligaments), it may also be observed (to a certain extent) with muscles and nerves. At a perpendicular angle to the ultrasound beam, a tendon -due to its low water content- normally displays a hyperechoic appearance [5]. However, as the angle between the tendon's long axis and the US beam becomes non-perpendicular, the image gradually becomes hypo-/an-echoic (Figure 4.1 B, D). As such, anisotropy can easily be misinterpreted as tendinopathy (tendinosis, tendinitis or tear) [6]. On the other hand, using simple heel-toe and/or toggle maneuvers (Figure 4.1 C) with the transducer, one may take advantage of this artifact to distinguish tendons wherever difficult.

### 4.1.2 Posterior Acoustic Shadowing

Shadowing defines a hypoechoic or anechoic band observed deep to a reflecting or attenuating structure. These structures, such as gas collections (high absorption of the beam), bone surfaces (high reduction of the beam) or calcifications, act like barriers to the ultrasound beam and lead to a dark or hypoechoic band due to the weaker return of the signals [4] (Figure 4.2).

Three different forms of shadowing have been described so far. Clean shadowing is seen during imaging of concrete structures such as stones, bones and calcification. Since most of the sound is absorbed, a uniform anechoic signal occurs behind these structures. Partial shadowing usually occurs behind highly attenuating soft tissues as a hypoechoic signal. Although less likely, calcifications and stones may also be the cause. Dirty shadowing can be observed during imaging of a structure hidden behind a gas formation which causes a high degree of reflection at gas/tissue interfaces, eventually leading to a low-level echo.

### 4.1.3 Posterior Acoustic Enhancement (Increased Through-transmission)

In contrast to the shadowing artifacts, enhancement artifacts refer to hyperechoic areas behind the structures [4]. Relatively lower attenuation of the sound beam through the adjacent layers is the main reason of enhancement (brightness) [7] (Figure 4.3).

This artifact should prompt the physician to consider the presence of fluid filled lesions such as effusion, cyst and occasionally solid hypoechoic lesions superficial to it. On the other hand, if the fluid collection is small or spread over a large area, this artifact may not be observed.

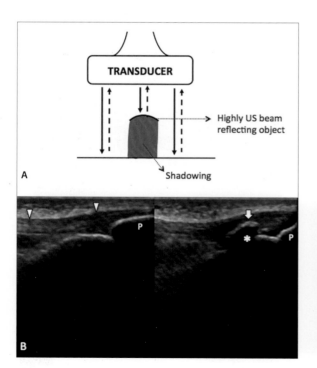

**Figure 4.2** A - Schematic presentation of posterior acoustic shadowing. B - US image of the patellar tendon (arrowheads) in long axis shows posterior acoustic shadowing (asterisk) behind a hyperechoic calcific structure (arrow). P, patella.

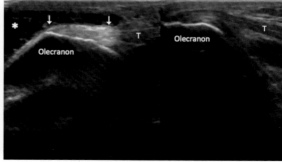

**Figure 4.3** Posterior acoustic enhancement/increased through-transmission (arrows) seen posterior to the olecranon bursitis (asterisk). T, triceps tendon.

### 4.1.4 Attenuation Artifact

This artifact causes non-visualization of deep structures [4]. The attenuation coefficient and the frequency of the US waves are the principle determinants i.e. tissues with great attenuation coefficients (e.g. fat) significantly hinder the underlying structures, eventually leading to complete attenuation. To overcome this artifact and optimize penetration, one should select a transducer with appropriate frequency.

## 4.2 ARTIFACTS ASSOCIATED WITH MULTIPLE ECHOES

### 4.2.1 Reverberation Artifact

Frequently observed at soft tissue-to-gas/bone / metal interfaces, this artifacts occurs when the ultrasound beam causes multiple back & forth reflections between two parallel nearby highly reflective surfaces [9] (Figure 4.4).

This condition is briefly described as multiple equidistantly spaced linear reflection [4].

### 4.2.2 Comet-tail Artifact (Posterior Reverberation Artifact)

This is actually a form of reverberation artifact (Figure 4.5) that appears in specific conditions where the acoustic impedance differences between an object and the surrounding tissues are significant [9-11].

Any metal, plastic, or air may be the cause of a comet-tail artifact.

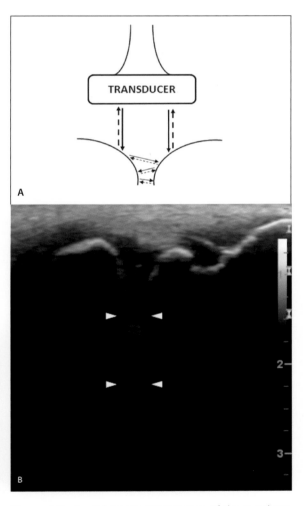

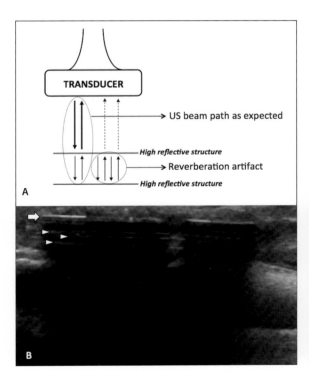

**Figure 4.4** A - Schematic representation of the reverberation artifact. B - Reverberations (arrowheads) arising from the highly reflective structure (arrow).

**Figure 4.5** A - Schematic presentation of the reverberation artifact. B - Axial US image shows echoes being repeatedly reflected (arrowheads) between radius and humerus (two highly reflective interfaces).

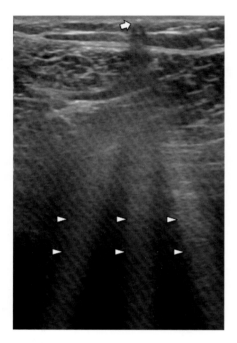

Figure 4.6 Comet-tail artifacts (arrow heads) generated by a piece of metal (arrow) -a strong reflector- usually seen in a form of reverberation artifact.

It appears as a dense tapering trail of echoes deep to a strongly reflecting structure (Figure 4.6).

### 4.2.3 Ring Down Artifact

This artifact -a line or series of parallel bands-ensues almost always posterior to a gas collection,

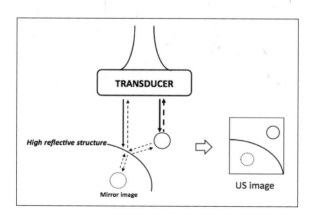

Figure 4.7 Mirror-image artifacts produced when an object is located in front of a highly reflective surface at which almost total reflection takes place.

especially in the presence of water entrapment in between the air bubbles [12]. Due to its similar appearance with the comet-tail artifact, it has been previously thought to be a variant of it.

### 4.2.4 Mirror-Image Artifact

Usually observed when scanning for a structure adjacent to highly reflective surface, the mirror-image artifact is described as a "duplicated structure equidistant from but deep to a strongly reflective interface" [4] (Figure 4.7).

### 4.2.5 Rain Effect

This artifact occurs when scanning any soft tissue overlying a fluid collection and appears as a band of low-to-medium echoes lying parallel to the transducer.

## 4.3 ARTIFACTS ASSOCIATED WITH ULTRASOUND BEAM CHARACTERISTICS

### 4.3.1 Side-lobe Artifact

US beams become narrower as they get closer to the focal zone and then diverge. Side lobes are actually multiple beams with low amplitude US energy projecting radially from the main beam, generally experienced with linear transducers [13].

When this low-energy encounters strong reflectors in the pathway, radially projecting beams create echoes detectable by the transducer. These echoes are displayed as originating from the main beam, presenting as the side-lobe artifact (Figure 4.8 A).

This artifact mostly arises from the extraneous echoes present within an expected anechoic structure such as the bladder, cysts, and fluid-filled structures, similar with the beam-width artifact [9].

### 4.3.2 Beam-width Artifact

If the scanned structure is smaller than the US beam, there may be extra echoes that seem to be inside the narrow beam -actually coming from the widened beam [10].

For instance, a highly reflective object located

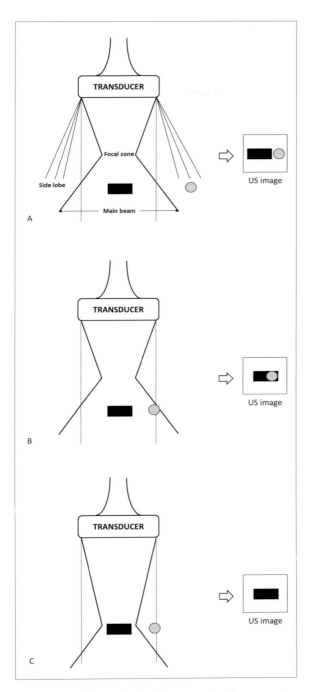

within the widened beam may generate such detectable echoes. To overcome this artifact, one must adjust the focal zone at the level of the target structure and centralize the probe over the structure (Figure 4.8 B, C).

## 4.4 ARTIFACTS ASSOCIATED WITH VELOCITY ERRORS

Usually referred as speed displacement artifact, this particular condition occurs when the sonographer screens tissues with differing densities. Because the speed of sound within a structure is dependent on its density and elastic properties, US beams travel at different speeds through different tissues (soft tissue at ~ 1540 m/s, fat at ~ 1450 m/s, bone at ~ 4080 m/s, air at ~ 330 m/s) [10]. Depending on the density of the structure(s), the returning echoes may reach the transducer in a shorter/longer time period and misinform regarding the true anatomical depth of the assessed structure.

## 4.5 DOPPLER ARTIFACTS

Pulse repetition frequency (PRF), which is defined as the Doppler sampling frequency of the transducer, should be higher than the twice of the maximum velocity of blood to obtain an accurate and alias-free imaging of the blood flow, a condition termed as the Nyquist limit [14]. A reverse flow, literally an artifact, occurs if the velocity of blood exceeds the Nyquist limit (aliasing) (Figure 4.9). To avoid this artifact; PRF should be increased and/or adjusted accordingly. Because PRF is also dependent on the Doppler angle, aliasing may also be removed by a change in the baseline Doppler position [14-16]..

Transducer pressure, if excessive, may block the flow in small vessels and diminish the flow in larger vessels during Doppler imaging (Figure 4.10). To avoid this artifact, care should be taken not to apply too much pressure [15].

Background noise is seen when the gain is increased too much (Figure 4.11). To achieve maximum image quality and avoid background noise, the gain setting should be decreased until almost all noise disappears [14, 15].

Twinkling artifact is seen behind a strongly reflecting interface such as urinary tract stones,

**Figure 4.8** Schematic drawing illustrates the narrowing and widening of the main US beam. A - Sometimes US beam is not solely concentrated in the main beam but also radiates towards the sides. As seen in the figure, these side lobes may also cause artifacts. B - The US beam narrows as it approaches to the focal zone and then widens. This situation results in an overlapping view of the objects in the periphery. C - To minimize or eliminate this artifact, one needs to adjust the focus, placing the object of interest within the center of the focal zone.

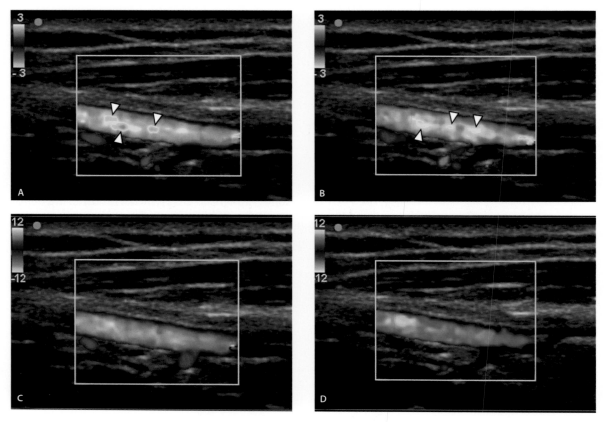

**Figure 4.9** Long-axis color Doppler US image of the radial artery at the wrist, manifested as reversed blue (aliased flow - white arrow heads) and red colors (non-aliased flow) (A) and as reversed yellow (aliased flow - white arrow heads) and blue colors (non-aliased flow) (B). Note the disappearing of the aliased flow after increasing the Pulse Repetition Frequency (C, D).

parenchymal calcifications, bones, or foreign bodies. This artifact imitates turbulent flow and appears as a color signal but without asso- ciated real flow [15, 17].

Mirror image occurs when a vessel resides close to a highly reflective bony surface. Doppler sig-

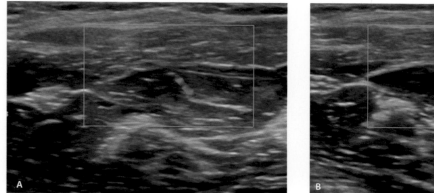
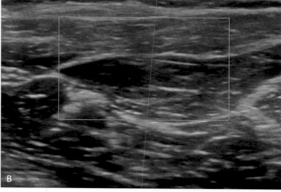

**Figure 4.10** A - Power Doppler US image of the forehand (axial view) showing a small vessel within the flexor muscles. B - Following extensive pressure, the vessel is not visualized.

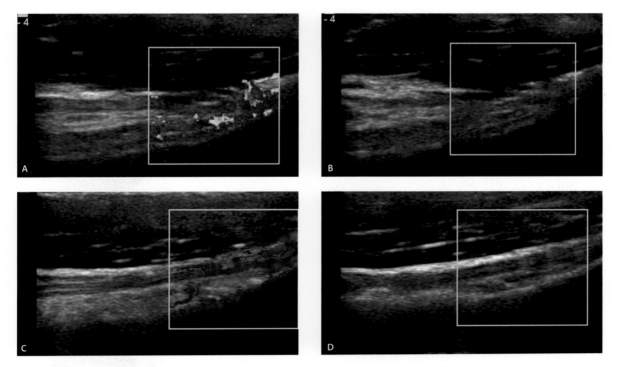

**Figure 4.11**  A - US image (long axis view along the bicipital tendon) with increased noise and degraded appearance due to increased gain on color Doppler. The noise displays a random frequency shift which causes a random direction of flow (reversed colors) in the Doppler box B. The color Doppler gain setting is adequately decreased to avoid noise whereby only the anterior humeral circumflex artery is seen. C - Increased power Doppler gain in the same region causes a uniformly colored background in the Doppler box with an enhanced signal from true flow. D - Likewise, the power Doppler gain setting is adequately decreased to avoid noise.

nals may generate a false mirror image inside the bone [15, 16] (Figure 4.12).

Blooming artifact appears as color outside of a vessel, making them seemingly larger (Figure 4.13]. This is a simple artifact caused by the gain settings and can be adjusted by the sonographer [18].

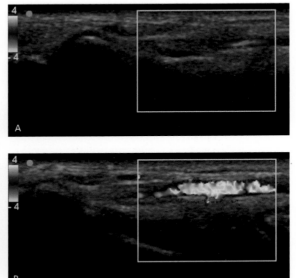

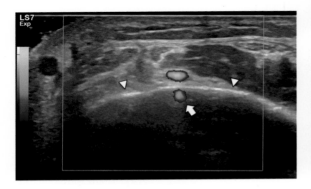

**Figure 4.12**  A false mirror image (arrow) occurs as a duplicated structure equidistant from but inside the bone (arrowheads).

**Figure 4.13**  A - Color Doppler image of the long axis of a small vessel.  B - Increased color Doppler gain erroneously leading to a larger appearance of the same vessel at the same location.

# REFERENCES

1) Martino F, Silvestri E, Grassi W, Garlaschi G, editors. Musculoskeletal sonography: technique, anatomy, semeiotics and pathological findings in rheumatic diseases. Milan: Springer, 2007. p. 4-6.

2) Teefey SA, Middleton WD, Yamaguchi K. Shoulder sonography: state of the art. Radiol Clin North Am. 1999; 37: 767-85.

3) Rumack CM, Wilson SR, Charboneau JW, Johnson J., editors. Diagnostic ultrasound. 3rd ed. St Louis: Mosby; 2004.

4) Hindi A, Peterson C, Barr RG. Artifacts in diagnostic ultrasound. Rep Med Imaging. 2013; 6: 29-48.

5 Crass JR, van de Vegte GL, Harkavy LA. Tendon echogenicity: ex vivo study. Radiology. 1988; 167: 499-501.

6 Jacobson JA. Fundamentals of musculoskeletal ultrasound. 2nd ed. Philadelphia, PA: Elsevier Saunders; 2013.

7 Scanlan KA. Sonographic artifacts and their origins. AJR Am J Roentgenol. 1991; 156: 1267-72.

8) Kremkau FW, Taylor KJ. Artifacts in ultrasound imaging. J Ultrasound Med. 1986; 5: 227-37.

9) Feldman MK, Katyal S, Blackwood MS. US artifacts. Radiographics. 2009; 29: 1179-89.

10) Middleton WD, Kurtz AB, Hertzberg BS. Ultrasound: the requisites. 2nd ed. St Louis: Mosby; 2004.

11) Ziskin MC, Thickman DI, Goldenberg NJ, Lapayowker MS, Becker JM. The comet tail artifact. J Ultrasound Med. 1982; 1: 1-7.

12) Avruch L, Cooperberg PL. The ring-down artifact. J Ultrasound Med. 1985; 4: 21-8.

13) Laing FC, Kurtz AB. The importance of ultrasonic side-lobe artifacts. Radiology. 1982; 145: 763-8.

14) Jansson T, Persson HW, Lindstrom K. Movement artefact suppression in blood perfusion measurements using a multifrequency technique. Ultrasound Med Biol. 2002; 28: 69-79.

15) Taljanovic MS, Melville DM, Scalcione LR, Gimber LH, Lorenz EJ, Witte RS. Artifacts in musculoskeletal ultrasonography. Semin Musculoskelet Radiol. 2014; 18: 3-11.

16) Pozniak MA, Zagzebski JA, Scanlan KA. Spectral and color Doppler artifacts. Radiographics. 1992; 12: 35-44.

17) Rahmouni A, Bargoin R, Herment A, Herment A, Bargoin N, Vasile N. Color Doppler twinkling artifact in hyperechoic regions. Radiology. 1996; 199: 269-71.

# Section 2
# Joint Evaluations and Common Pathologies

# Ultrasound Evaluation of the Shoulder

Martine DE MUYNCK, Wouter SABBE

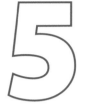

## 5.1 INTRODUCTION

In 1979, ultrasound (US) was introduced as an imaging technique for the shoulder joint, in particular for detecting fluid accumulations [1, 2]. Very soon, standardized examination protocols were proposed [3-6]. Sonographic criteria for diagnosing rotator cuff (RC) ruptures were already devised in the eighties [4, 7, 8]. Ultrasound allows immediate evaluation of periarticular soft tissues, both in a static and dynamic way. Particularly for the shoulder this is very interesting. The technique is non-invasive, safe, painless and relatively inexpensive. A drawback is that visualization and interpretation strongly depend on the anatomical knowledge and experience of the examiner.

## 5.2 EXAMINATION TECHNIQUE

As in all sonographic examinations, bony contours (echogenic lines with acoustic shadowing behind) are identified for orientation purposes. Soft tissues can be evaluated if not covered by bony structures. As in all sonographic examinations, the protocols were designed to start where there is the biggest chance to see minimal amounts of fluid. For the shoulder this is on the anterior side (intra-articular fluid will be visible around the long biceps tendon; fluid in the bursa will be like a little crescent in front of biceps and subscapularis).

A state of the art exam requires a right/left comparison of both shoulders, with a ventral, cranial and dorsal visualization, every time with two perpendicular views. Preferably, pathology is only affirmed if it is reproducible in two perpendicular planes, seen the problems with artifacts [9]. Since there is an important variation in the normal anatomical aspect (according to age, sex, constitution) and since there are many asymptomatic abnormalities (certainly above the age of 65), it is advocated to start the exam at the asymptomatic side and to look for right/left differences. The pa-

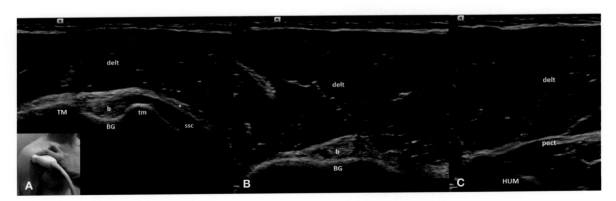

**Figure 5.1** Right shoulder, ventral horizontal view. A - Bicipital groove (BG), greater tubercle (tuberculum majus, TM), lesser tubercle (tuberculum minus, tm), tendon of the long head of the biceps (b), subscapularis (ssc), deltoid muscle (delt), subacromio-subdeltoid bursa (*). B - More distally, under the subscapularis muscle and tendon. Bicipital groove (BG), tendon of the long head of the biceps (b), deltoid muscle (delt). C - Still more distally, at the level of the pectoralis major tendon (pect). Humerus (HUM), deltoid muscle (delt).

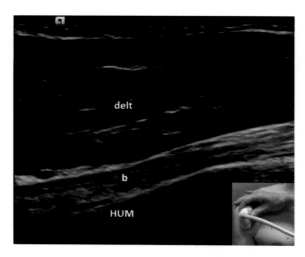

**Figure 5.2** Right shoulder, ventral vertical view. Humerus (HUM), tendon of the long head of the biceps (b), deltoid muscle (delt).

tient is sitting, the arms in a neutral position, elbow bent in 90° and in supination, hands resting on the upper legs.

### 5.2.1 Ventral Horizontal and Vertical View

The humerus with its bicipital groove and the coracoid process are the most important bony landmarks, above which the long biceps tendon and subscapularis tendon are located. The deltoid muscle covers these tendons. Moving the arm into external rotation allows better visuali-zation of the subscapular tendon and muscle. The subacromial-subdeltoid bursa is located in between biceps-subscapularis and deltoid; in young people it can be hardly visible; in older asymptomatic people it can be filled (Figures 5.1 and 5.2).

### 5.2.2 Coronal and Lateral View

The acromion and the greater tuberosity are identified with the supraspinatus tendon in between. This classical frontal or coronal view (long-axis view of the tendon) shows the image of a "birds beak", the lateral view (short-axis view of the tendon) a "tire". Following the Crass and Middleton techniques, the tendon is also evaluated with the arm in retroversion and internal and external rotation [10, 11]. The tendon, being uncovered from beneath the acromion, can be inspected over a wider surface (internal rotation for the middle part of the tendon; external rotation for the anterior part). The probe should be moved anteriorly and posteriorly to have a complete exam of the tendon (Figures 5.3 and 5.4).

In "modern" protocols the classical frontal image is not used anymore, still it offers a very interesting idea of the subacromial (SA) space (being narrowed in complete supraspinatus rupture, being widened in case of axillary nerve lesion or in

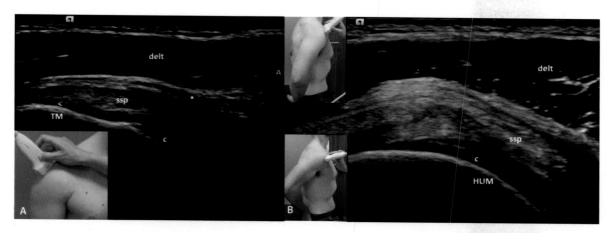

**Figure 5.3** A - Right shoulder, coronal view. Acromion (A), greater tubercle (TM), supraspinatus tendon (ssp), deltoid muscle (delt), cartilage (c) covering the humeral head (which has a slightly irregular cortex), normal hypoechoic insertion (<) of the supraspinatus tendon, subacromio-subdeltoid bursa (*). B - To have a better visualization of the supraspinatus tendon (ssp), the patient can be asked to put the arm in retroversion/adduction. Humerus (HUM), with cartilage (c) covering it, deltoid muscle (delt). When the palm of the hand is put on the iliac wing, as in the smaller picture, the anterior side of the supraspinatus tendon and the biceps tendon will become better visible (no corresponding ultrasound image shown).

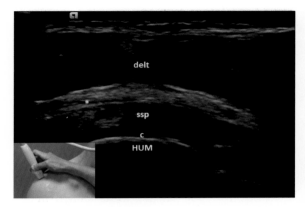

**Figure 5.4** Right shoulder, lateral view, immediately lateral to the acromion. "Tire image". Humerus (HUM), cartilage (c), supraspinatus tendon (ssp), deltoid muscle (delt), bursa (*).

glenohumeral subluxation in hemiplegic patients).

It is important to check the compressibility of the tendon (a muscle is compressible, a tendon is not; compressibility is a sign of a tear).

### 5.2.3 Dorsal Horizontal and Vertical View

Humeral head, glenoid rim with triangular hyperechoic labrum and acromion are identified.

The infraspinatus and teres minor tendon and muscle, covered by the deltoid, are visualized (Figures 5.5 and 5.6).

### 5.2.4 Coraco-acromial View

The probe is put in an oblique position; coracoid process, coraco-acromial ligament and acromion are visualized. Then the probe is tilted caudally and automatically supraspinatus, long biceps tendon and subscapularis are seen (Figure 5.7).

With a high quality probe the coracohumeral ligament (on top of the biceps) and the superior glenohumeral ligament (medial and parallel with the biceps tendon) can be seen ("the RC interval"). The latter is interesting in the study of frozen shoulder.

### 5.2.5 Acromio-clavicular Joint

On the apex of the shoulder, with coronal positioning of the probe (Figure 5.8). In addition the sterno-clavicular joint (ventral horizontal positioning) can be evaluated. Eventually, the suprascapular notch and the spinoglenoid notch can be visualized (Figure 5.9), and muscle examination in the fossa supra- and infraspinata can be done [mainly examination of supraspinatus muscle to look for atrophy (fatty degeneration) after rupture of the tendon, or in case of neuropathy].

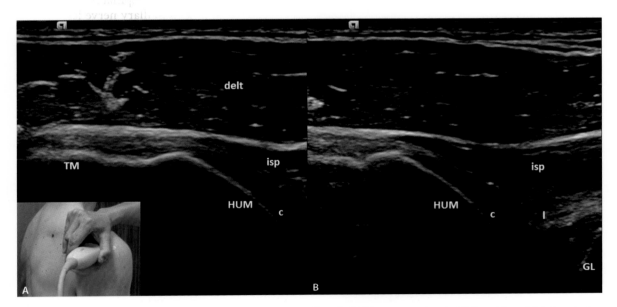

**Figure 5.5** Right shoulder, dorsal horizontal view. A - Humeral head (HUM), greater tubercle (TM), cartilage (c), infraspinatus (isp), deltoid muscle (delt). B - More medially. Glenoid (GL) and fibrocartilaginous labrum (l) now become visible. Humeral head (HUM), cartilage (c), infraspinatus (isp).

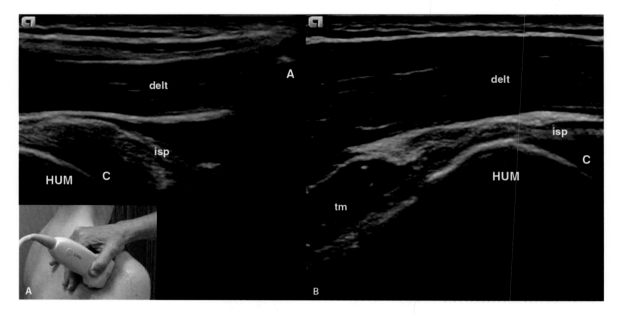

**Figure 5.6** Right shoulder, dorsal vertical view. A - Acromion (A), humerus (HUM), cartilage (c), infraspinatus (isp), deltoid muscle (delt). B - More distally. Teres minor (tm) is now becoming visible. Humerus (HUM), cartilage (c), infraspinatus (isp), deltoid muscle (delt).

It is usually suggested that "3 rules of 3" is followed when performing an US examination. Initially:
1.1. position the patient;
1.2. choose a probe;
1.3. check the settings (depth, focus, etc.).

After putting the probe in a chosen plane:
2.1. look at the bony edges: are they regular? (trauma, degeneration, inflammation can cause cortical irregularities);
2.2. look for fluid;
2.3. look at the soft tissues.

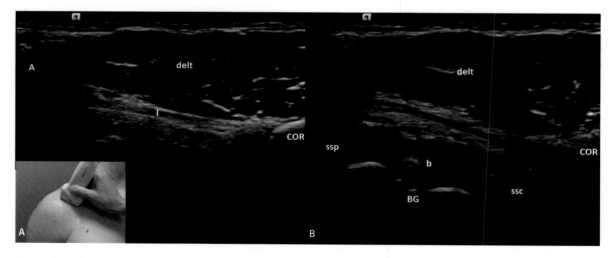

**Figure 5.7** Coraco-acromial view. A - Coracoid (COR), acromion (A), coraco-acromial ligament (l), deltoid muscle (delt). B - Tilting the probe makes the biceps tendon (b), between subscapularis (ssc) and supraspinatus (ssp) visible. Coracoid (COR), bicipital groove (BG), deltoid muscle (delt).

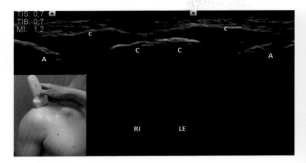

**Figure 5.8** Comparison of right (RI) and left (LE) acromio-clavicular joint. Acromion (A), clavicle (C), capsule (c).

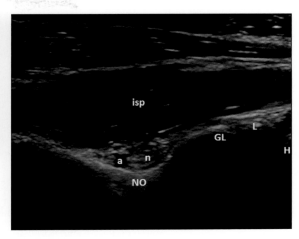

**Figure 5.9** Left shoulder, dorsal horizontal view, with detail of the spinoglenoid notch (NO), suprascapular nerve (n), artery (a). Glenoid (GL), humerus (H), labrum (L), infraspinatus (isp).

Examining a chosen tendon:

3.1. is the tendon present?
3.2. how is its shape? (is there swelling? global or focal thinning?) changes in shape are easier to evaluate for beginners than changes in echogenicity;
3.3. how is its echogenicity? (is it hypo- or hyperechoic? (in)homogeneous?).

In general, depending on the complaint and the clinical problem, a complete sonographic assessment of a joint can be done or focus can be put on a specific structure (for example only look at the patellar tendon or the Achilles tendon in case of suspicion of a tendinosis). For the shoulder joint, since fluid will sag down because of gravity and since there are many indirect signs of pathology, we tend to do a complete examination every time.

## 5.2.6 Additional Dynamic Testing

1. *Change positioning to have better visibility:*
   - to have a better view of the bone of the humeral head in the dorsal horizontal view: do internal rotation;
   - to have better visualization of fluid in the dorsal horizontal view: do external rotation;
   - to have better visualization of tendons: for the subscapularis and the pectoralis major: look at it in external rotation; for the supraspinatus: use the Crass and Middleton techniques.
2. *Check compressibility to look for fluid and to check the quality of the tendons.*
3. *Ask for active elevation and abduction in case of impingement.*
4. *Do passive testing to look for instabilities:*
   - of the biceps tendon: do sudden passive external rotation: does the tendon (sub)luxate medially?

- if there is a Hill-Sachs-lesion: do external rotation: does the erosion disappear in the glenoid fossa?
- give inferior stress and measure the SA space or give anteroposterior stress and measure the position of the humeral head in relation to the glenoid.
- put a burden in the hand of the patient and measure the AC distance in case of AC (sub) luxation.

## 5.2.7 Additional Use of Color Doppler/ Power Doppler

To look for hyperemia (in the synovia of the bicipital recess; in the bursa; in the tendon, around calcifications; in the RC interval).

## 5.2.8 Measurements

Comparing both sides, it is important to measure:
- the thickness of the bursa (less than 2 mm) [12];
- the thickness of biceps tendon (average 4.3 mm) and supraspinatus tendon (average 6 mm) [3, 4];
- the width of a rupture;
- the SA space [13].

Protocols and guidelines of international scientific societies (for example the European Society of Musculoskeletal Radiology, ESSR; and the

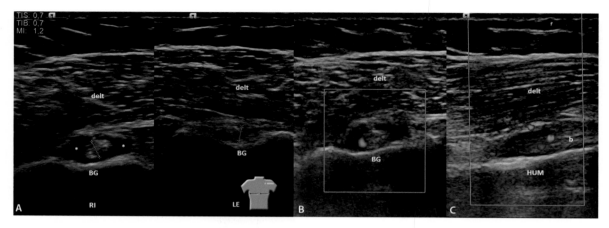

**Figure 5.10** Right (RI) and left (LE) shoulder. BG, bicipital groove; delt, deltoid muscle. A - Ventral horizontal view. Fluid (*) surrounding a slightly swollen right biceps tendon (3.4 mm on the right side, 3.0 mm left). B and C - Horizontal and vertical view left side: hyperemia in and around the biceps tendon (b): tenosynovitis of the biceps. HUM, humerus.

American Institute of Ultrasound in Medicine, AIUM) are preferably used [14-16].

## 5.3 SHOULDER PATHOLOGIES

### 5.3.1 Fluid Accumulation

In general, US is useful to detect and to localize fluid collections: in a joint and/or in a bursa, in a tendon sheath. Fluid will be anechoic or hypoechoic. It is not possible to differentiate the type of fluid (non-inflammatory, inflammatory, with or without crystals, infectious or blood). For this

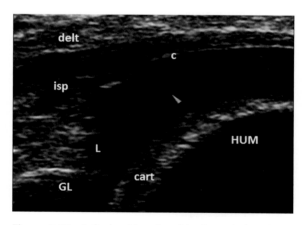

**Figure 5.11** Left shoulder, dorsal horizontal view. Intra-articular fluid (arrowhead). Humerus (HUM), glenoid (GL), labrum (L), hyaline cartilage covering the head (cart), capsule (c), infraspinatus (isp), deltoid muscle (delt).

purpose the fluid must be aspirated and sent to the laboratory for analysis (cell count, presence of crystals, culture). Ultrasound can help to differentiate between synovial swelling and fluid and visualize septa in a collection, thus helping to avoid dry taps when planning an aspiration. Compressing/releasing pressure and using color/power Doppler imaging can help to differentiate between synovial swelling and fluid.

Ultrasound admits to identify the presence of fluid in each of the 3 (4, including sternoclavicular joint) compartments of the shoulder. The finding of fluid post trauma necessitates a meticulous examination: an associated lesion was found in 94% of shoulders that contained fluid. Presence of fluid in two compartments (intra-articular and bursa) post trauma is indicative of a full thickness rupture of the RC [3, 11].

Since the synovial sheath of the long biceps tendon is in continuity with the glenohumeral joint, intra-articular fluid will accumulate around the biceps tendon (either as a little crescent behind the tendon, either as a halo around the tendon on a horizontal view) (Figure 5.10). Because of gravity, fluid will accumulate caudally, so it is important to move the probe downwards (towards the pectoralis major tendon). As always, it is important not to push with the probe, in order not to push the fluid away. If there is more fluid, it can also be seen on the dorsal views (best on the horizontal view, while moving into external rotation) (Figure 5.11).

The subacromial and subdeltoid bursae are almost always connected. This one subacromio-

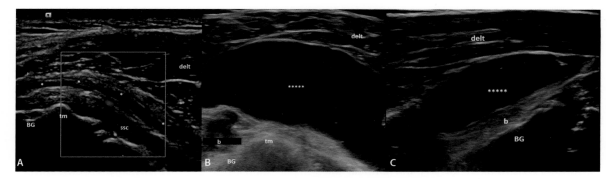

**Figure 5.12**   Right shoulder. A - Ventral horizontal view: crescent shaped, thickened, filled bursa (*), with hyperemia; ssc, subscapularis. B and C - Horizontal and vertical view: bigger amount of fluid (*****) in the bursa; b, biceps tendon (b). BG, bicipital groove; tm, tuberculum minus (lesser tubercle); delt, deltoid muscle.

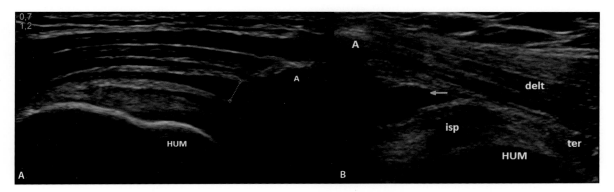

**Figure 5.13**   Filled bursa, coronal (A, filling 2.6 mm) and dorsal vertical view (B, arrow). Humeral head (HUM), acromion (A), infraspinatus (isp), teres minor (ter), deltoid muscle (delt).

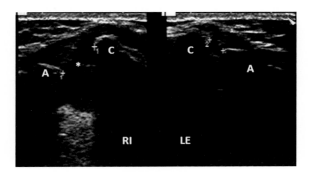

**Figure 5.14**   Subluxation of the right (RI) and normal left (LE) AC joint (10.2 mm versus 4.2 mm distance between the bony rims) with fluid (*). Acromion (A), clavicula (C).

subdeltoid bursa is visible on the frontal view, as a hypoechoic line between supraspinatus tendon and deltoid [12]. When there is fluid, because of gravity it will often sag down and be visible as a crescent between biceps/subscapularis and deltoid (Figure 5.12). Also on a coronal view, a swollen and fluid-filled bursa can be seen distally to the insertion of the supraspinatus tendon on the greater tubercle, between the humerus and the deltoid muscle (Figures 5.13 and 5.14).

### 5.3.2 Tendon Pathology

*Tenosynovitis/tendinosis of the long biceps tendon*

Isolated tenosynovitis (an inflammation of the fluid-filled sheath) or tendinosis (a process of degeneration) of the biceps is rare. Secondary tenosynovitis or tendinosis can be present in case of antero-superior impingement or RC rupture. Very soon, this common pitfall was described: fluid around the biceps does not automatically mean tenosynovitis of the biceps! Most of the times it is articular fluid, accumulating caudally. In the case of tenosynovitis/tendinosis, there should be changes in shape (the tendon becomes rounded instead of oval), blurring or changes in echogenicity of the tendon itself (see figure 5.10).

## Calcifying tendinitis (tendonitis/tendinosis) of the rotator cuff

To elucidate the pathogenesis of calcifying "tendinitis", Uhthoff et al. [17] did clinical and morphological investigations on surgically treated cases in 1976. Contrary to the concept of dystrophic calcification, they found no evidence for an active or a healed degenerative process. The affected tendon was transformed into fibrocartilage. The formative phase of calcification was followed by a resorptive phase, during which the hydroxyapatite deposits were surrounded by phagocytosing cells, with proliferation of vascular channels. They found a significant correlation between severe pain and resorption.

The "natural" stages of calcifying "tendinitis" are thus:
1. the pre-calcific stage: metaplasia of tenocytes into chondrocytes (fibrocartilagineous metaplasia);
2. the calcific stage: formative phase; resting phase; resorptive phase: neovascularisation, macrophage reaction;
3. the post-calcific stage: collagen production.

This cell mediated, rather than degenerative process, mainly in the supraspinatus tendon, is often asymptomatic. Symptoms are more frequent in female patients, in their forties and rare above the age of seventy. 90% of the calcifications disappear within three years. There is still discussion about the terminology: should we use tendinitis/tendonitis or tendinosis?

In the diagnosis, the radiological classification of Gärtner and Heyer is often used:
- type I:    clearly circumscribed and dense- formative, resting;
- type II:   mixed characteristics of type I and type III (where it is not possible to designate the specific radiological morphology to a given deposit);
- type III:  no clear circumscription, cloudy and translucent-resorptive [18].

The French Arthroscopy Society adds one type:

- type A: dense, homogeneous, sharp borders;
- type B: polylobular, more heterogeneous;
- type C: inhomogeneous, unsharp borders;
- type D: calcification of the enthesis (rather an enthesopathy due to overuse?) [19].

Gärtner and Heyer recommended that radiographs be taken at least in anteroposterior projections with the shoulder in internal and external rotation to demonstrate the deposits without super-imposition [18]. During the chronic initial phase, a calcific deposit is formed in the tendon of the RC. In the radiograph, it is clearly circumscribed and has a dense appearance (type I). Pain is inconsistent and may exist for years. In the acute phase, the deposit undergoes spontaneous resolution. Now it takes on a translucent and cloudy appearance without clear circumscription (type III). Patients experience severe pain for two-three weeks. Finally, a normally functioning shoulder joint will result [18].

Ultrasound can show concomitant bursitis and is useful for the differential diagnosis of rupture of the RC [18] (Figure 5.15). A sonographic classification was proposed by French sonographers:
- type 1: dense, with complete shadow;
- type 2: echogenic, incomplete shadow;
- type 3: without shadow [20].

During the resting phase, the calcification is dense; during construction and during resorption there is less density [21]. When do calcifications become painful? Courthaliac et al. [21] described that the acute painful shoulder corresponds to the resorption phase. Hydroxyapatite calcification is migrating into the bursa (sometimes remaining inside the tendon or even migrating into the bone, creating a bony erosion) (Figures 5.16 and 5.17 A, B). This often corresponds to radiographic type C (or B) and sonographic type 2-3. Sometimes a hypoechoic liquified area is visible inside this calcification on ultrasound. In the subacute and chronic painful shoulder, we should check for a dynamic conflict with the coraco-acromial ligament or the acromion and look for additional RC ruptures.

Courthaliac et al. [21] concluded that in acute shoulder pain a calcification of faint density with an impure shadow in the presence of hyperemic bursitis is definitely symptomatic; in chronic pain, a dense calcification with a complete shadow which deforms the tendon and is sometimes ac-

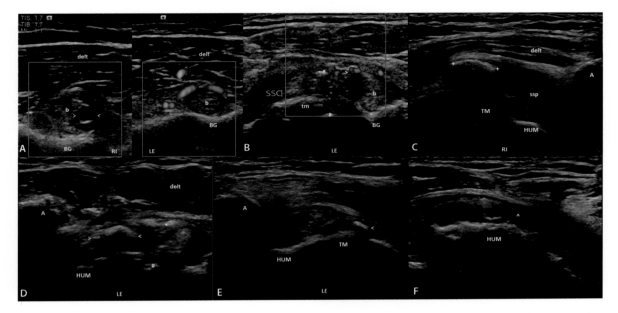

**Figure 5.15** Calcifying tendinitis: images of right (RI) (non painful) and left (LE) (painful) shoulder in an 80 year-old patient. A - The right shoulder shows a longitudinal anechoic zone (cleft) (><) in the long biceps tendon (b) (partial rupture); the left shoulder shows hyperemia in the bicipital tendon sheath. B and C - In subscapularis (SSC) and supraspinatus (ssp) there are multiple calcifications. On the right side there is a big calcification (++) with complete shadow. D - On the left side there are as well calcifications with incomplete shadow (><) as calcifications without shadow (*). There is hyperemia on the left side. E - There is also a calcification in the left supraspinatus insertion (15 mm). E and F - There are erosions on greater and lesser tubercles (#) and a focal hypo- /an-echoic zone (^) in the supraspinatus tendon, which is compressible, sign of a full-thickness tear. Bicipital groove (BG), lesser tubercle (tm), greater tubercle (TM), humeral head (HUM), acromion (A), deltoid muscle (delt).

companied by bursitis, is probably the cause of pain. Chiou et al. [22] found an excellent correlation between color Doppler findings and symptoms. The hyperemia corresponds to the neovascularization in the tendon described in the resorptive phase. They suggested that US with color

Doppler could differentiate between the formative and resorptive phases of the calcification.

For the French Arthroscopy Society, Clavert et al. [23] reviewed retrospectively 450 patients treated by arthroscopic excision for calcifying tendinitis with a minimum follow-up of five years, except for sub-

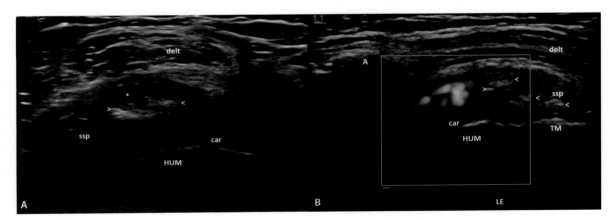

**Figure 5.16** Left shoulder, coronal view, calcifying tendinitis. Calcifications (><) without shadow in the supraspinatus tendon (ssp). A - Image of liquefaction (*). B - Doppler signal within the tendon. Humerus (HUM), greater tubercle (TM), acromion (A), cartilage (car), deltoid muscle (delt).

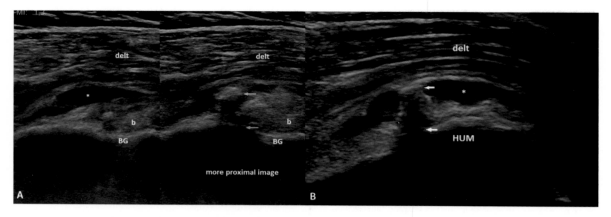

**Figure 5.17**  Right shoulder, calcifying tendinitis. Ventral horizontal (A) and vertical view (B): migration of calcification into the bursa (*). Calcification with impure shadow behind (arrows). Humerus (HUM), bicipital groove (BG), biceps tendon (b), deltoid muscle (delt).

scapularis and infraspinatus calcification (minimum two years). At the same time, they led a prospective study evaluating the prevalence of the calcifications in 1276 asymptomatic shoulders. The prevalence of RC calcification was 7.3%, with a female predominance. The subscapularis calcifications were rare (6% of the calcifications) and were associated with further deposit on the RC. Infraspinatus calcifications were more frequent (20%). The inter- and intraobserver agreement for the A-B-C classification was poor, specially to differentiate the type A and B calcifications. The long-term follow-up allowed to state that the calcifying tendinitis is temporary without any relation with RC rupture (the rate of full thickness tears was 3.9% at an average of nine years follow-up). However, preoperative associated partial tear of the RC affected significantly the results and increased the rate of full thickness tear at follow-up. Functional results were also lower after removing a type C calcification [23].

In the consensus paper of the ESSR, the indication for US in "calcific tendonitis" (so here the term tendonitis is used) is grated as "first choice level technique, other techniques rarely provide more information" [24].

### Rotator cuff ruptures

Very soon several authors presented different criteria to identify a RC rupture.
1. Changes in shape:
   – sonographic absence of a tendon (Figure 5.18);
   – focal thinning of a tendon, with the image of

a "flat tire" (Figure 5.19).
2. Changes in echogenicity:
   – hypoechoic focus;
   – central echogenic band [4, 7, 8].

Changes in shape were found to predict ruptures at 100%, whereas changes in echogenicity constituted a less reliable criterion. Other authors found that the sensitivity of the examination did not improve if, in addition to changes in shape, changes in echogenicity were used as signs of RC tears; the specificity was found to become lower. In comparison with arthrography, sensitivity of 70-95% and specificity of 90-98% were described [6-8, 25, 26]. The predictive value of negative sonography was found to be very high (95%) [7].

For less experienced examiners and/or older machines and probes of less quality, changes in shape are still technically easier to reproduce and interpret than irregularities in echogenicity (slight tilting of the transducer affects the echogenicity of the evaluated structure (anisotropism); a change in echogenicity can only be accepted if present in two directions perpendicular to each other).

Beside these "direct" signs (changes of the tendons of the RC themselves), "indirect signs" were emphasized:
1. narrowing of the subacromial space;
2. fluid in two compartments;
3. cortical erosions on greater tuberosity [11, 25, 27].

The healthy, thick RC normally fills the SA space. An empty SA space is suspected for a (chronically) absent supraspinatus tendon. Gleno-

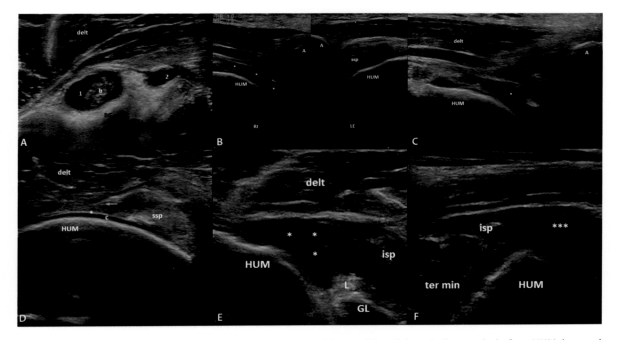

**Figure 5.18** Right shoulder, rotator cuff rupture in a 70-year-old man; fall with bicycle five weeks before. HUM, humeral head. A - Ventral horizontal view. Fluid in two compartments (1 intra-articular, 2 bursa). Bicipital groove (BG), biceps tendon (b), deltoid muscle (delt). B - Coronal view. Right (RI) and left (LE) shoulder. Absent supraspinatus tendon on the right side; the subacromial space is occupied by the fluid-filled bursa (*). Acromion (A), supraspinatus tendon (ssp). C - Coronal view. Detailed view. D - Lateral view. Naked humeral head; only a small stump of the supraspinatus tendon (ssp) is present; the cartilage (c) is uncovered, the interface sign (*) is an artifact indicative of fluid covering the cartilage; deltoid muscle (delt). E - Dorsal horizontal view. Infraspinatus tendon (isp) is also torn; a fluid-filled gap is visible. Glenoid (GL), labrum (L), deltoid muscle (delt). F - Dorsal vertical view. A small stump of the infraspinatus (isp) is visible, teres minor (ter min) is intact.

humeral joint and bursa are normally separated by the tendons of the intact RC. Posttraumatic fluid in the two compartments means that there must be a connection between them and thus a full thickness RC rupture (see figure 5.18 a).

With increasing quality of machines and probes, more details became visible and new criteria were proposed [11, 27, 28]. This made it possible to depict partial thickness tears and to evaluate the extent of the rupture (a rupture has 3 dimensions: the thickness-full or partial thickness; the width-expressed in cm; the length called retraction). The dimensions thickness and width of the tear should be evaluated and measured; the third dimension, the retraction, remains difficult to visualize (because covered by the acromion). In case of partial tear, the exact location of the lesion should be described: articular side, bursal side or midportion rupture. Classification of ruptures is difficult (what is a "massive tear"? width more than 3 cm? 5 cm? desinsertion of two tendons?).

New criteria that were put forward:

1. hypoechoic lesion with either articular or bursal extension (Figure 5.20);
2. fluid-filled defect;
3. compressibility.

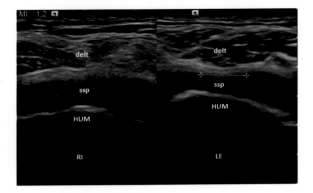

**Figure 5.19** Lateral view of right (RI) and left (LE) shoulder. Focal thinning of the supraspinatus (ssp) with image of "flat tire" over a width of 8 mm. Humeral head (HUM), deltoid muscle (delt).

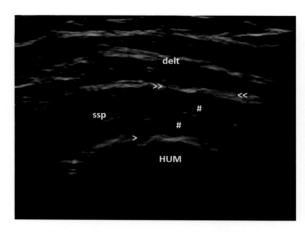

**Figure 5.20** Right shoulder, lateral view. Focal hypoechoic zone with articular and bursal contact (#) in the supraspinatus tendon (ssp); notice that the surface of the tendon is not perfectly convex, but a bit flattened (>><<) and that there are small irregularities on the cortex (>). Humerus (HUM), deltoid muscle (delt).

An additional indirect criterion was described: interface sign or "uncovered cartilage" sign: when a small bright line is noticed on top of the cartilage on the humeral head, this is suspicious of

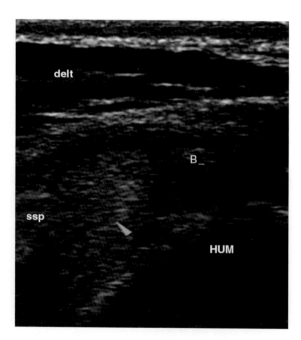

**Figure 5.21** Right shoulder, lateral view. Recent trauma. Hypoechoic zone in the anterior part of the supraspinatus tendon (ssp), filled with compressible (on dynamic examination) rather homogeneous fluid (arrowhead): full thickness tear, filled with blood. Humerus (HUM), deltoid muscle (delt).

fluid on top of it (so an articular side partial rupture or a full thickness rupture of the overlying supraspinatus tendon) [11, 27] (see figure 5.18 D).

Sensitivity and specificity increased, also in comparison with the new magnetic resonance imaging (MRI) techniques, that were developed during the same period. The main sources of error were put forward: improper equipment, insufficient knowledge of sonographic anatomy and incomplete examination technique [29]. The supraspinatus tendon is involved in most RC ruptures. However, isolated subscapularis and infraspinatus tears do occur, and massive supraspinatus ruptures may also involve the subscapularis and infraspinatus. This stresses the need for a complete antero-posterior examination of the shoulder. Additional dynamic testing is also indicated: most supraspinatus tears involve the distal lateral part of the tendon (which is routinely visualized in neutral position). The rare, more proximal tears become visible if the arm is moved into retroversion and internal (midportion) or external (anterior portion) rotation.

Other pitfalls are: acute/chronic lesions, degenerative cuff/cuff tear, post-surgery evaluation [30]. At the very acute stadium, it may be difficult to diagnose a rupture (the gap may be filled with blood, which is relatively echogenic) (Figure 5.21). At the other spectrum, a chronic rupture can be filled by a thickened bursa (Figure 5.22) - the compressibility sign might be helpful here and there is also another indirect sign, "signe du dédoublement de la ligne" [27] (Figure 5.23). The triangular insertion of the supraspinatus is absent and the area is filled by the expanding bursa with separation of lines. Notice that no separate criteria for traumatic/degenerative ruptures were designed. This is still not the case.

When evaluating RC (ruptures/neuropathy), it is possible to look at the muscle belly and check for atrophy and fatty degeneration (it becomes thin and echogenic) (although there are no international criteria and classification yet). Fatty degeneration is a poor prognostic factor for surgery of the RC.

In the beginning publications on US were mainly descriptive. As for MRI asymptomatic abnormalities are often found. An attempt was made to answer which RC ruptures become symptomatic (mainly those accompanied by a tendinopathy of the long biceps tendon or a hyperemic bursitis) [31]. There is also more pain if the anterior part of the supraspinatus is torn (the thickness of it pro-

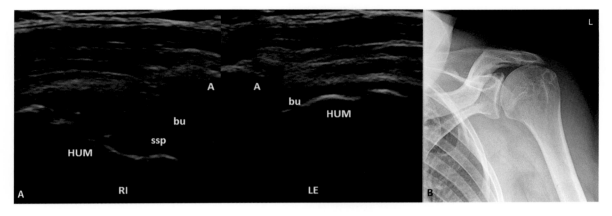

**Figure 5.22** A - Right (RI) and left (LE) shoulder, coronal view. Absent supraspinatus tendon with narrowed subacromial space on the left side; this space is filled by bursa. The right tendon is hypoechoic, with several calcifications. Humerus (HUM), acromion (A), supraspinatus tendon (ssp), subacromial bursa (bu). B - Corresponding radiograph of the left shoulder: ascending arthrosis.

tects the biceps) and more pain if the infraspinatus also is torn (this means also a worse prognosis, as well for conservative therapy as for surgery).

In conclusion, US is non-invasive, safe, inexpensive and has a good sensitivity/specificity compared with (arthro) computed tomography and a nearly equivalent accuracy compared with (arthro) MRI scanning and is consequently the ideal initial examination for diagnosing RC ruptures [32].

## Degenerative tendinopathy or tendinosis enthesopathy

Pathology of the RC tendons (mainly the supraspinatus tendon) can be caused by macrotrauma (see above traumatic RC avulsions and ruptures), or by repetitive microtraumata. These repetitive traumata can cause intrinsic impingement (degenerative changes inside the tendon), external or outlet impingement (at the bursal side) or internal impingement (at the articular side). Intrinsic impingement is the most frequent pathology of the RC, it is a "natural" phenomenon of aging. The term tendinopathy is used for clinical conditions arising from overuse; tendinosis is theoretically used after histological confirmation. Above the age of 60, more than 50% of supraspinatus tendons will become ruptured [33, 34]. This will become painful when there is a disturbed gliding-capacity (for example by a thickened, inflamed bursa) or a disturbed antero/posterior force couple (for example the biceps tendon "cutting" its way through the subscapularis). In case of macrotrau-

ma and rupture, retraction occurs soon; in case of microtraumata there will be less retraction.

External impingement can be caused by an anterior-superior conflict (supraspinatus tendon under acromion and coraco-acromial ligament, as described by Neer) or an anterior conflict (subscapularis against coracoid). In case of internal impingement, there is a posterior-superior conflict (supraspinatus/infraspinatus against posterior-superior glenoid, as described by Jobe father and son) often in overhead throwing [27].

Neer's three-stage classification of impingement syndrome was supposed to correlate with changes in echogenicity and shape of the tendons [33]:

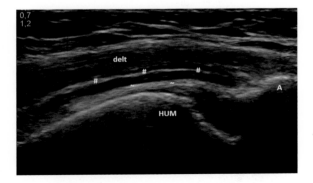

**Figure 5.23** Right shoulder, coronal view. *Dédoublement des lignes* (duplication of lines): the supraspinatus tendon is absent, the subacromial space is filled by bursa. This bursa extends over the tubercle (~~), while the supraspinatus tendon should insert on the tubercle. Acromion (A), humerus (HUM), deltoid muscle (delt), septum in the muscle (##).

- Stage I (reversible edema and hemorrhage in the bursa and RC): abnormal echogenicity, normal thickness or thickening;
- Stage II (fibrosis and thickening of subacromial soft tissue and sometimes a partial rupture of RC): abnormal echogenicity and thinning:
- Stage III reveals a complete rupture of the RC.

Van Holsbeeck, on the other hand, developed criteria taking into account the thickness of the bursa:
- Stage 1: bursa 1.5 to 2 mm;
- Stage 2: bursa over 2 mm;
- Stage 3: partial or full-thickness tear of RC [34].

Changes in shape (swelling, global thinning- not focal thinning) and changes in echogenicity (inhomogeneous aspect, multiple hypoechoic foci) can be sonographic degenerative signs. In chronic degenerative tendons, there can be multiple punctate calcifications in the tendon or rather in the insertion (see type D of the sonographic classification of calcifications) (or is the latter also fibrocartilagineous metaplasia?). Insertional calcifications are very often present in the subscapularis tendon in asymptomatic shoulders.

*Luxation of long biceps tendon*

The RC interval is composed of coracohumeral ligament (CHL) (which divides into a medial and lateral part, inserting on respectively lesser and greater tuberosity), superior glenohumeral ligament and capsular fibers, which all blend together along insertions medial and lateral to the bicipital groove, maintaining the long biceps tendon within this groove [35]. When there is a lesion of one or more of the components of this RC interval, a (sub)luxation of the biceps tendon will happen, almost always medially. The biceps groove will be empty (or eventually filled with blood, fluid or fibrotic tissue). Subluxation/luxation are ill defined (Figure 5.24). Almost always, a (sub)luxation of the biceps tendon is accompanied by a subscapularis rupture [35].

### 5.3.3 Ligaments

*The coracohumeral ligament and frozen shoulder*

The term "frozen shoulder" as a clinical presentation with decreased mobility was introduced by Codman in 1934, while Neviaser was the author who described "adhesive capsulitis" as an operative finding in 1945 [36, 37]. In 1969 Lundberg drew a distinction between primary (idiopathic) and secondary (post-traumatic) frozen shoulder [38]. The "adhesive capsulitis" described by Neviaser matches the primary frozen shoulder.

Zuckerman proposed a classification of frozen shoulder in 1994 [39, 40]. "Primary frozen shoulder" and "idiopathic adhesive capsulitis" are identical and not associated with underlying pathology. "Secondary frozen shoulder" is divided in three subcategories:
- systemical (due to underlying systemic connective tissue disease processes in diabetes, hypo/ hyperthyroidism...);
- extrinsic (known underlying disorder, but no shoulder pathology: cardiopulmonary disease, cerebrovascular accident, Parkinsons disease, cervical discopathy, humerus fracture...);
- intrinsic (underlying shoulder pathology: RC tendinitis, RC ruptures, biceps tendinitis, AC arthritis).

Hannafin and Chiaia described four stages in the course of adhesive capsulitis in 2000 [40, 41]:
- Stage 1 or preadhesive stage, with mild erythematous synovitis in the anterosuperior cap-

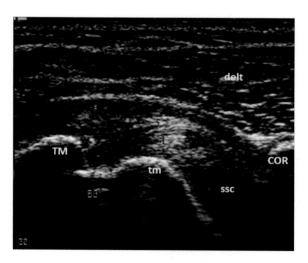

**Figure 5.24** Right shoulder, ventral horizontal view. (Sub) luxation of the biceps tendon (b) on top of lesser tubercle (tm). Bicipital groove (BG), greater tubercle (TM), coracoid (COR), subscapularis (ssc), deltoid muscle (delt), bursa (*).

sule (lasting 0-3 months, mild pain at the end of range of motion);
- Stage 2 or freezing stage (acute adhesive stage), with thickened and red synovitis (3-9 months, very painful during range of motion);
- Stage 3 or frozen stage, with less synovitis and more adhesions, no hypervascularisation (9-15 months, more stiffness and less pain);
- Stage 4 or thawing phase, with restrictive capsule (15-24 months, with a very stiff shoulder).

At the same time Watson et al. described four arthroscopic stadia:
- Stage 1, vascular synovitis;
- Stage 2, red synovium and early adhesions;
- Stage 3, pink synovium and extensive adhesions;
- Stage 4, mature capsular adhesions [42].

The etiology of adhesive capsulitis is unclear: synovitis or focal hypervascularity, synovial angiogenesis and thickening of the capsule.

Two regions are particularly affected: the RC interval and the axillary pouch [43]. The RC interval is a triangular anatomic area in the anterosuperior aspect of the shoulder, defined by the coracoid process at its base, by the anterior margin of the supraspinatus tendon superiorly and by the superior margin of the subscapularis tendon inferiorly [35]. The RC interval capsule is reinforced on top by the CHL and internally by the superior glenohumeral ligament and traversed by the intraarticular biceps tendon [35]. The axillary pouch is the inferior part of the glenohumeral joint, from humeral head to inferior glenoid labrum, between the anterior and posterior parts of the inferior glenuhumeral ligament.

Characteristic MRI findings of adhesive capsulitis have been documented: thickening of the RC interval, a thickened and edematous appearance of the axillary pouch. A biceps tendon sheath effusion is a further indicator. For glenohumeral MRI arthrography the same characteristic findings have been reported as well as restriction of the volume of contrast able to be injected [35, 43].

Ultrasound is not useful for the study of the axillary pouch, but it can of course be used for the study of the RC interval (use the coraco-acromial view). In a study presented at the Getroa-gel congress in 2005, the authors conclude that CHL depiction can be achieved in a reasonable proportion of shoulders. A thickened CHL is suggestive of

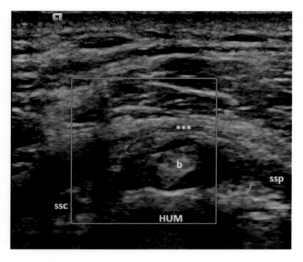

**Figure 5.25** Coraco-acromial view of the left shoulder. Frozen shoulder with hyperemia in coracohumeral ligament. Humerus (HUM), long biceps tendon (b), subscapularis (ssc), supraspinatus (ssp), bursa (***).

adhesive capsulitis [44] (Figure 5.25). Other specific findings of adhesive capsulitis on US examination include increased vascular flow and thickening of the RC interval structures and supraspinatus tendon bulging rather than smoothly gliding beneath the acromion during abduction. Here also, a biceps tendon sheath effusion has been described, without arguments for biceps tenosynovitis (the tendon sheath effusion presumably being joint fluid displaced into the sheath due to reduced capsular volume) [43-46]. It is important to recognize the difference between pure RC interval vascularity and bursal vascularity or a combination of the two. Pure bursal vascularity may simply represent subacromial-subdeltoid bursitis [46].

Still, in the consensus paper of ESSR, the indication for US in adhesive capsulitis is graded as "not indicated" by the experts [24].

### 5.3.4 Nerves

It is possible to visualize the suprascapular notch and mainly the spinoglenoid notch and check the suprascapular nerve. Labral cysts can cause a compression of the nerve, for example described in volley ball players (Figure 5.26). Accompanying muscle atrophy and fatty degeneration can be looked for.

In the ESSR the indications for US are graded as follows: in suprascapular nerve entrapment

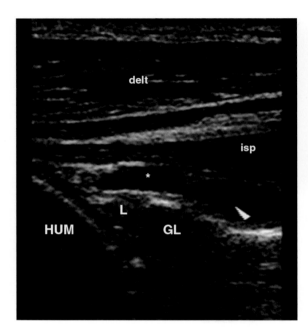

**Figure 5.26** Dorsal horizontal view of the right shoulder. Bilobular (* and arrowhead) labral cyst. Humerus (HUM), glenoid (GL), labrum (L), infraspinatus (isp), deltoid muscle (delt).

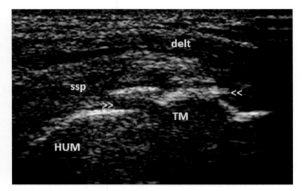

**Figure 5.27** Left shoulder, retroversion/adduction: irregular cortex of fractured tubercle. Humeral head (HUM), greater tubercle (TM), supraspinatus tendon (ssp), deltoid muscle (delt).

"equivalent to other imaging techniques - other techniques might provide significant information", in quadrilateral space syndrome and thoracic outlet syndrome only 'if other imaging techniques are not appropriate', and in Parsonage-Turner syndrome "not indicated" [24].

### 5.3.5 Masses and Foreign Bodies

Ultrasound is the first choice for an initial evaluation of a soft tissue swelling. The two important questions to answer are: is there a lesion yes/no? Is it a cyst or a soft tissue mass?

Around the shoulder there are some anatomical variants, causing "a swelling": the Langer arch (possibly interesting in the evaluation of thoracic outlet syndrome), sternalis muscle.

Foreign bodies (metal, glass, wood) are more frequently seen in the distal parts of the extremities. Ultrasound can be useful in the examination of plugs/osteosynthesis material/prostheses.

### 5.3.6 Bone

Ultrasound is above all a soft tissue exam, but when the cortex is abnormal it can also offer very interesting information about bony pathology [16].

In cortical lesions such as fractures of greater tubercle or the Hill-Sachs lesion after an anterior shoulder luxation, US soon offered the advantage of being able to look around the bone, thus avoiding eventual masking of erosions by superposition (such as in radiographs) (Figures 5.27 and 5.28). For the same reason, cortical destruction by tumours is sometimes better (sooner) visible on US. Changed relations between bones such as occurring in posterior shoulder luxation, can also be more obvious during ultrasound than on radiography. In bony pathology (for example stressfractures) the term "sono-palpation" was introduced (explicit pain when the probe is moved over the bony pathology, even without compressing).

In the ESSR consensus paper, the indications for US in bony pathology are as follows: AC trauma/instability, AC osteoarthritis, sternoclavicular disease and occult tuberosity fracture are graded "equivalent to other imaging techniques - other techniques might provide significant information". Loose bodies, on the contrary, are only graded "if other imaging techniques are not appropriate", whereas glenohumeral traumatic and dynamic instability are graded as "not indicated" [24].

## 5.4 ULTRASOUND IN PHYSICAL AND REHABILITATION MEDICINE CLINICAL SETTING

Patient history and clinical examination are of course keye-stones in the working-out of shoulder problems. The clinical examination should consist of inspection, passive and active mobility testing, iso-

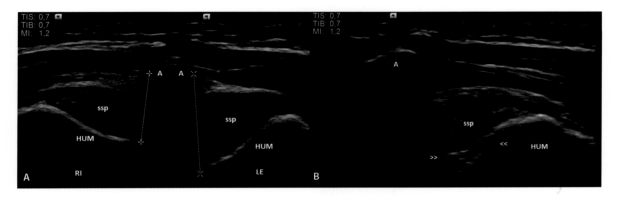

**Figure 5.28** A - Right (RI) and left (LE) shoulder, coronal view. Five years after luxation on the left side: wider subacromial space on the left side (RI 9.6 mm, LE 13.9 mm) (probably due to weakness of the deltoid and cuff). B - Hill-Sachs lesion (>> <<) more dorsally. Humerus (HUM), acromion (A), supraspinatus tendon (ssp).

metrical testing, specific testing. Clinical examination of the cervical spine and neurological exam should be included. Radiography and US will often be complementary. As mentioned above, sonographic abnormalities are frequently found in asymptomatic patients, mainly in the older population.

### 5.4.1 The Acute Painful Shoulder, Traumatic (Fractures, Dislocations, RC Ruptures)

For the diagnosis of fractures and dislocations, radiography is mandatory. Fractures of greater tubercle are sometimes more easily visible on US ("occult fractures"). As mentioned before, the indication for US in occult tuberosity fracture has been judged "equivalent to other imaging techniques" [24].

Ultrasound is mainly interesting if radiography is negative. As mentioned before, if fluid is present, this is indicative of accompanying pathology. Ultrasound is the first choice exam for diagnosis of ruptures of long biceps tendon and the different RC tendons. In the ESSR consensus paper the indications for US in full thickness cuff tears, biceps tendon rupture, and biceps tendon dislocation are graded "first choice level technique - other techniques rarely provide more information", and in partial thickness cuff tears "equivalent to other imaging techniques - other techniques might provide significant information"; on the contrary, in RC muscle atrophy is judged as "not indicated" [24].

On the contrary, RC muscle atrophy is only rated B 1 [24].

### 5.4.2 The Acute Painful Shoulder, Non Traumatic (Calcifying Tendinitis)

As mentioned in the paragraph on calcifying tendinitis, in acute shoulder pain a calcification of faint density with an impure shadow in the presence of hyperemic bursitis is definitely symptomatic [21]. An excellent correlation between color Doppler findings and symptoms was found [22].

### 5.4.3 The Chronic Painful Shoulder

In chronic pain, a dense calcification with a complete shadow which deforms the tendon and is sometimes accompanied by bursitis, is probably the cause of pain [21].

In the working out of RC tendinopathy ± rupture ± bursitis and eventual secondary ascending arthrosis, the combination of US and radiography will often lead to a diagnosis and give enough information to start conservative treatment or to decide to refer to an orthopedic surgeon. As mentioned, biceps tendinopathy should be looked for as the cause of pain in case of rupture of the supraspinatus and in case of subscapularis rupture and biceps luxation. In the ESSR consensus paper, the indication for US in bicipes rupture and dislocation is graded "first choice level technique", whereas that in biceps tendinopathy is "equivalent to other imaging techniques" [24].

In impingement, the combination of radiography (type of acromion?) and US (state of the different tendons of the RC? bursitis?) with dynamic testing (elevation/abduction) is also advised. Under the age of 40, work-up could even be complete only with US [32].

For AC pathology, radiography (arthrosis, sequelae of fracture, osteolysis) and US (fluid, synovitis, the age of 40, bone irregularities) are also complementary.

### 5.4.4 The Stiff Shoulder (Primary/ Secondary Frozen Shoulder, Omarthrosis)

Here again, the combination of US (see abnormalities in the RC interval, intra-articular fluid; evaluation of RC and bursa, of AC) and radiography will help to differentiate primary/secondary frozen shoulder and help to find the cause in the latter.

For omarthrosis, radiography demonstrates the bony abnormalities; US is needed to evaluate the state of the RC and thus help to decide whether a reversed prosthesis may be indicated (in case of rupture).

### 5.4.5 The Unstable Shoulder

In the ESSR consensus paper, the experts come to the conclusion that ultrasound is not indicated for glenohumeral joint instability [24].

### 5.4.6 The Hemiplegic Shoulder Pain

Shoulder pain following stroke can have many causes, such as RC disease, adhesive capsulitis, complex regional pain syndrome, shoulder joint subluxation, spasticity. Poor arm motor function and the presence of supraspinatus tendon pathology were found to be associated with hemiplegic shoulder pain in several studies [47, 48]. Effusion, tenosynovitis or tendinopathy of the biceps and supraspinatus tendinopathy were described during both acute and chronic stages [47].

Other authors found that patients with adhesive capsulitis, glenohumeral subluxation, or long head of biceps tendon effusion showed a higher prevalence of hemiplegic shoulder pain only one month after stroke [48]. Unaffected shoulders also show abnormalities, but affected shoulders received sonographic rating scores that reflected significantly more impairment than those of unaffected shoulders [49] (see also Chapter 14 - "Ultrasound Imaging in Rehabilitation Settings").

### 5.4.7 Wheelchair Users and Shoulder Pain

Increased age, duration of wheelchair use, and body mass are risk factors for shoulder pathology in wheelchair users. Collinger et al. [50] developed a numerical score for seven ultrasound signs (joint effusion, bursal thickening, bicipital and supraspinatus tendinopathy, greater tuberosity cortical surface, dynamic evaluation of supraspinatus and subscapularis tendon impingement). Older individuals tended to have a more degenerated biceps tendon appearance, while duration of wheelchair use was more affecting the supraspinatus tendon. Heavier individuals tended to have degeneration of both biceps and supraspinatus tendons. However, quantitative US features did not discriminate between people with and without shoulder pain [50, 51].

## 5.5 INTERVENTIONS

There is growing interest to use US for guiding interventions such as aspirations and infiltrations. It allows real-time imaging of target and needle and surrounding vulnerable structures such as vessels and nerves. Interventions under US guidance have been proven to be more accurate. Infection is the most dreaded complication. Further studies are required to prove better clinical results and less complications [52].

Needling means repeatedly puncturing for fragmentation of the calcification. Often lavage with irrigation and aspiration is added. There is no standardization of the technique: sometimes one needle is used, sometimes two, one acting as an inflow, the other as an outflow. For the lavage saline solution and/or an anaesthetic and/or corticosteroids are used. A corticosteroid can be injected after the lavage, eventually in the overlying bursa. Little attention is paid to the aspect and staging of the calcifications that are treated. Further research might help to distinguish subgroups of potential responders. The same applies to extracorporeal shock wave therapy [52].

# Ultrasound Evaluation of the Elbow

Kevin DE COCK, Wouter SABBE

## 6.1 INTRODUCTION

The elbow joint is a common site for musculo-skeletal pathologies. In addition to the several advantages (already mentioned in this book), its multiplanar capability and clear visualization of major vessels and nerves makes ultrasound (US) a paramount diagnostic or therapeutic guide for elbow involvement.

One of the most common applications of elbow US has always been lateral epicondyle tendinopathy. In former times, while only important swelling of the tendon could be detected; today, with high-end machines and high frequency probes it is possible to visualize even minor alterations in tendon structure and vascularisation. For some injuries, magnetic resonance imaging might be necessary as it gives more information about deep soft tissue structures, bones and parts of the joint cavities that cannot be fully evaluated with US [1]. Nevertheless it is more expensive, time consuming and less available. Further, magnetic resonance imaging cannot be performed in patients who are claustrophobic or who have implanted devices such as cardiac pacemakers. Therefore, in most cases of soft tissue pathology around the elbow, US should be the first choice. Of note, US is superior as regards its high resolution as well.

On the other hand, US is highly operator-dependent. As such, a good knowledge of anatomy, scanning techniques and the associated artifacts is mandatory.

## 6.2 EXAMINATION TECHNIQUE

The elbow joint is a rather superficial articulation and should be examined with a high frequency linear transducer (9-14 MHz). There are four regions to be explored: the anterior view, posterior view, lateral view and the medial view. Different anatomical structures can be visualized: cortex and joint surfaces, joint recesses, tendons, bursae, muscles and nerves.

Doppler US can be used for evaluating inflammation or vascularization pertaining to various structures or pathologies. Again, all findings should be documented in two perpendicular planes whereby comparison with the contralateral (asymptomatic) site is crucial/valuable.

For elbow imaging, the patient is usually seated in front of the examiner. Different aspects of the elbow can be scanned with varying positioning of the joint. Keeping a pillow -or the examination bed- in between might help for the comfort of the patient and the technique of the sonographer alike.

### 6.2.1 Anterior View

The best position for evaluating the anterior elbow would be the forearm in supination. The examiner first evaluates the bony structures and then the overlying soft tissues from deep to superficial. Either with transverse or longitudinal images, the humeroulnar (trochlea-coronoid process) and humeroradial (capitellum-radial head) joints and the proximal fossae (coronoid, radial) on the humerus would be the places to check for articular fluid (Figures 6.1 and 6.2). The fossae are usually filled with the anterior fat pad, seen as hyperechoic on US [2], and may sometimes contain a small (normal) amount of fluid. The joint surfaces will be seen as regular, continuous hyperechoic lines (bones) which are covered with the hypo-/an-echoic smooth, regular layers of hyaline cartilage and the overlying hyperechoic anterior joint capsule [2].

Axially, pronator teres muscle with the under-

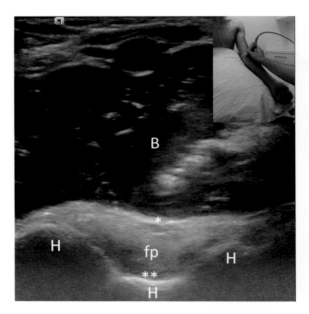

**Figure 6.1** Left elbow, anterior transverse view above the elbow joint space: the anterior recess (**) with the fat pad (fp) is seen between the humerus (H) and the joint capsule (*). This is the place to look for intra-articular fluid in the anterior view. The brachialis muscle (B) is seen above the joint capsule (*).

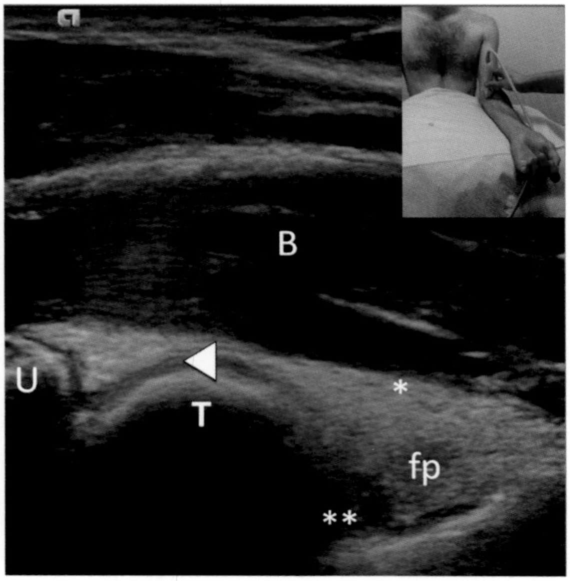

**Figure 6.2** Left elbow, anterior longitudinal view: the anterior recess (**) with the fat pad (fp) is seen proximal to the trochlea (T). This is the place to look for intra-articular fluid in the anterior view. The brachialis muscle (B) is seen superficial to the joint capsule (*). The cartilage or the trochlea appears hypoechoic (arrowhead). U, ulna.

lying median nerve, median artery, brachialis muscle and the distal biceps tendon, and brachio-

radialis muscle and the underlying radial nerve can be nicely visualized (Figures 6.3 and 6.4).

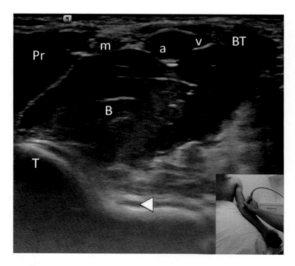

**Figure 6.3** Left elbow, anterior transverse view at elbow joint space: the trochlea (T) is covered with cartilage (arrowhead). Superficial to the trochlea, the pronator muscle (Pr), brachialis muscle (B), median nerve (m), median artery (a), median vein (v) and biceps tendon (BT) can be seen.

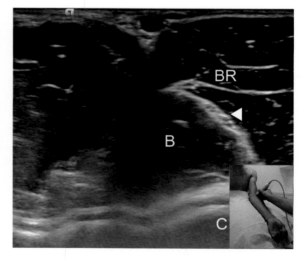

**Figure 6.4** Left elbow, anterolateral transverse view at elbow joint space: the capitellum (C) is covered with cartilage. Superficial to the capitellum, the brachialis muscle (B), brachioradialis muscle (BR) and in between the radial nerve (arrowhead) are seen.

The biceps brachii muscle generally (>78%) consists of two heads: the short one originating from the coracoid process, and the long one originating from the supraglenoid tubercle. Both heads descend and keep a quasi-complete separation of the two muscle bellies along their entire course ending in two separate distal tendons. The distal tendon of the short head attaches at the radial tuberosity (slightly anteriorly), whereas the tendon of the long head attaches more proximally. These two parts of the distal biceps tendon (DBT) cannot always be distinguished with US. Besides, there is also the lacertus fibrosis which typically arises from the proximal DBT (mostly from the short head) and fans out medially in the fascia of the forearm. It may prevent a ruptured biceps tendon from retracting proximally [3, 4]. Evaluation for the DBT is technically challenging because of its oblique course. The arm of the patient is best placed in full extension and forced supination whereby the radial tuberosity becomes more anterior and superficial. On longitudinal view, the tendon will be seen superficial to the brachialisis (proximally) and supinator muscles (distally), eventually inserting on the radial tuberosity. Nonetheless, anisotropy for its distal portion is almost inevitable (Figure 6.5).

Accordingly, different additional techniques have also been described [4-6]. Most popular ones are the lateral and medial approaches. With a supinated forearm flexed in 90 degrees, the probe is placed parallel with the distal humerus. The distal tendon is visualized deep to the extensor (lateral) or flexor (medial) muscles and its insertion onto the radial tuberosity is clearly visible as well. A great advantage of this approach is the ability to perform a dynamic evaluation of the biceps in pronation and supination (impossible with an anterior approach). This provides important information regarding continuity of the tendon parts in case of a suspected tear. Posterior visualization (with extended and supinated elbow) of the distal insertion is more difficult and less frequently used [4, 5].

The vascularisation of the DBT can be divided into three zones. A proximal zone 1 is supplied by the brachialis artery. The distal zone 3 is supplied by the posterior recurrent artery. In between there is zone 2, approximately 2 cm proximal to the insertion, representing a relatively hypovascular zone. During pronation, the proximal radioulnar space is reduced to its half. Thus, mechanical im-

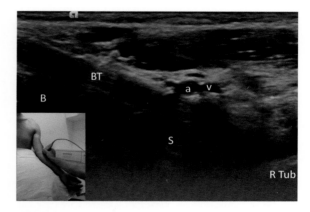

**Figure 6.5** Left elbow, anterior longitudinal view: the biceps tendon (BT) lies superficial to the brachialis muscle (B) and the supinator muscle (S) and inserts on the radial tuberosity (R Tub); a, brachialis artery; v, brachialis vein.

pingement of the tendon together with the relatively hypovascularity may contribute to tendinosis and (partial) tendon tears [7].

The bicipitoradial bursa is a serous bursa consisting of a synovial membrane enveloping a film of liquid. It surrounds the distal biceps tendon as it approaches the radial tuberosity and lies between the DBT (anterior) and the anterior aspect of the radial tuberosity (posterior). In the absence of a synovial tendon sheath, its function lies in decreasing friction between the tendon and the radial tuberosity during pronation and supination. It is a fairly large bursa, with dimensions ranging from 2.4 to 3.9 cm, sometimes divided by different septae. The bursa does not communicate with the joint cavity, but it may communicate with the interosseous bursa of the elbow. The bicipitoradial bursa is normally flattened and difficult to visualize with US [3, 4, 8].

### 6.2.2 Posterior View

The elbow is in 90° flexion and neutral pro-supination with the shoulder in internal rotation. The patient putting his/her hand on the thigh/knee (pointing the elbow towards the examiner) can even be more comfortable. Evaluation usually starts with the longitudinal plane, evaluating the bony edges of the olecranon and the olecranon fossa, a concavity at the posterior surface of the humerus filled with the posterior fat pad [2]. A small amount of fluid may normally be seen in the posterior recess between the fat pad and the humerus. More

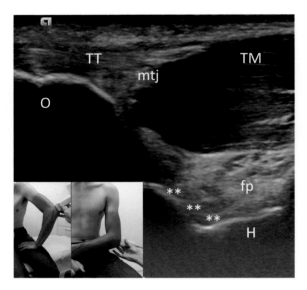

**Figure 6.6** Left elbow, posterior longitudinal view: the posterior recess (**) with the fat pad (fp) is seen proximal to the olecranon (O) and superficial to the humerus (H). This is the place to look for intra-articular fluid in the posterior view. More superficial, the triceps muscle (TM), the musculo-tendinous junction (mtj), and the triceps tendon (TT) with its insertion on the olecranon (O) are seen.

superficially, the triceps muscle, its musculotendineus junction, and its insertion on the olecranon are seen. The olecranon bursa can only be seen as a very thin hypoechoic line overlying the olecranon and the triceps tendon (Figure 6.6).

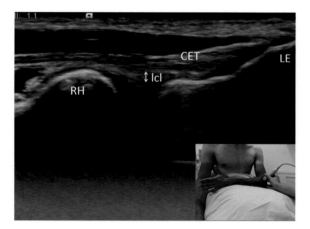

**Figure 6.7** Left elbow, lateral longitudinal view: the common extensor tendon (CET) arises from the lateral epicondyle (LE). The lateral collateral ligament (lcl) lies deep to the CET and is difficult to distinguish from the CET, since they have a similar echo texture. RH, radial head.

The ulnar nerve can best be evaluated in a transverse plane. At the level of the elbow, the nerve lies in the ulnar nerve groove (proximally), than enters the cubital tunnel under the retinaculum of Osborne and continues its course under the fascia between the two heads of the flexor carpi ulnaris muscle. The nerve is a round or oval hypoechoic honeycomb-like structure situated next to the medial epicondyle. It is not unusual to see a bifid or multifascicular ulnar nerve at this level. Longitudinally, the ulnar nerve has a tortuous course around the elbow. Additionally, dynamic evaluation with flexion-extension of the elbow can be performed to check if the ulnar nerve subluxates, partially or completely (snapping ulnar nerve).

### 6.2.3 Lateral View

The elbow is in 90° flexion, a neutral pro-supination and the upper arm is in partial internal rotation, preferably resting on the pillow/bed. When the probe is positioned in a longitudinal plane, the lateral epicondyle and the radial head and the overlying common extensor tendon (CET), seen as a hyperechoic "beak", are visualized (Figure 6.7). The CET contains fibers from extensor carpi radialis brevis and a minor part of the extensor carpi radialis longus, extensor digitorum, extensor digiti minimi and extensor carpi ulnaris tendons [5]. Although, it is impossible to distinguish these tendons on US, the extensor carpi radialis brevis makes up most of the deep layer and the extensor digitorum most of the superficial layer [6]. The major part of the extensor carpi radialis longus and the brachioradialisis muscles emerge more proximally on the humerus. The lateral collateral ligament, extending from the lateral epicondyle down to the radial head, lies between the bone and the CET. Normally, because they both have a similar fibrillar echotexture, it is not easy to differentiate it from the CET. When the probe is positioned in a transverse plane at the anterolateral site of the elbow, the brachioradialisis muscle and the underlying radial nerve (a round or oval hypoechoic structure) can be visualized (Figure 6.8A). More distally, the radial nerve splits into superficial and the deep branch (Figure 6.8B). The latter one pierces the supinator muscle (between the two heads) where it may possibly be entrapped (posterior interosseous nerve syndrome) (Figures 6.8C-6.8E).

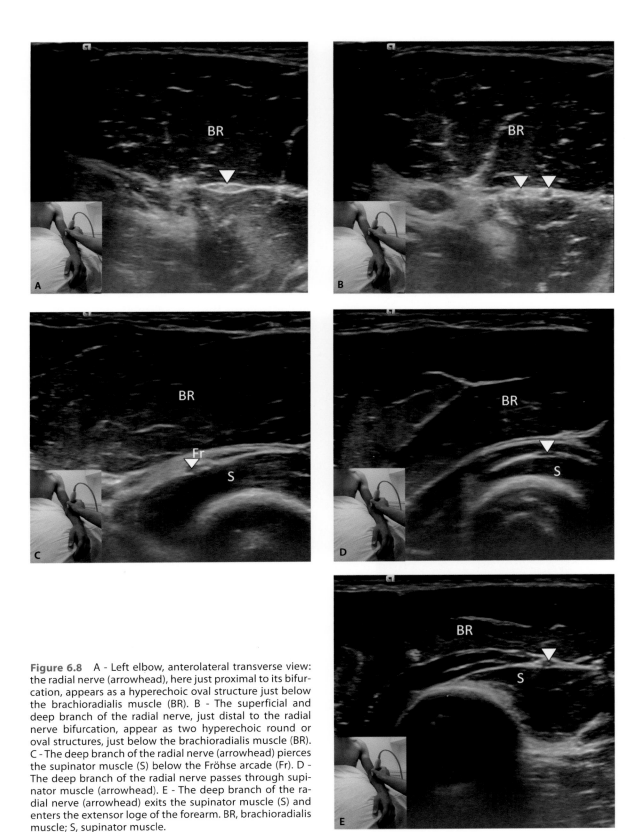

**Figure 6.8** A - Left elbow, anterolateral transverse view: the radial nerve (arrowhead), here just proximal to its bifurcation, appears as a hyperechoic oval structure just below the brachioradialis muscle (BR). B - The superficial and deep branch of the radial nerve, just distal to the radial nerve bifurcation, appear as two hyperechoic round or oval structures, just below the brachioradialis muscle (BR). C - The deep branch of the radial nerve (arrowhead) pierces the supinator muscle (S) below the Fröhse arcade (Fr). D - The deep branch of the radial nerve passes through supinator muscle (arrowhead). E - The deep branch of the radial nerve (arrowhead) exits the supinator muscle (S) and enters the extensor loge of the forearm. BR, brachioradialis muscle; S, supinator muscle.

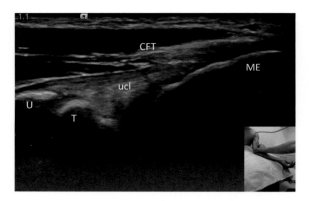

**Figure 6.9** Left elbow, medial longitudinal view: the common flexor tendon (CFT) arises from the medial epicondyle (ME). The ulnar collateral ligament (ucl) lies deep to the CFT and is difficult to distinguish from the CFT, since they have a similar echo texture. T, trochlea; U, ulna.

### 6.2.4 **Medial View**

The elbow is in extension, forearm in supination and the arm in external rotation, again suggested to rest on a pillow or the examination table.

On longitudinal plane, the bony edges of the medial epicondyle and the proximal ulna are visualized. Superficial to these bony landmarks the common flexor tendon (CFT) is seen as a hyperechoic "beak" or triangle, normally broader and

shorter than the CET. It contains fibers from the tendons of pronator teres, flexor carpi radialis, flexor digitorum superficialis, palmaris longus, flexor carpi ulnaris (humeral head) muscles. The ulnar collateral ligament (UCL) lies between the CFT and the joint (Figure 6.9).

## 6.3 ELBOW PATHOLOGIES

### 6.3.1 **Effusion, Synovitis and Arthritis**

For the evaluation of intra-articular (IA) fluid, both the anterior and posterior joint recesses are examined in two planes. The fluid is usually detected in the anterior or posterior fossae as hypo- or anechoic accumulation elevating the fat pads and distending the joint capsule (Figures 6.10 and 6.11) [5]. A typical pitfall would be to mix articular cartilage and fluid. Differentiation can be done with pressure application whereby the cartilage would remain the same but fluid is expected to be displaced [5]. Otherwise, it should always be kept in mind that probe compression needs to be avoided while searching for fluid.

Ultrasound is more sensitive for diagnosing joint fluid with the elbow flexed: 1-3 ml joint fluid can be better identified, due to gravity on the posterior side [9]. Ultrasound with the elbow in extension is of little value in detecting small effusions. Yet, the anterior fat pad is drawn closer to the coronoid fossa, preventing fluid from collecting anteriorly [10]. Dynamic evaluation, with

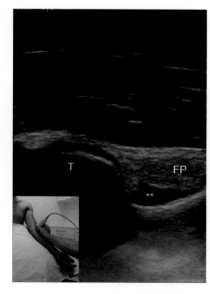

**Figure 6.10** Left elbow, anterior longitudinal view above joint space: intra-articular fluid appears in the anterior recess (**) as an anechoic collection pushing the fat pad (FP) away. T, trochlea.

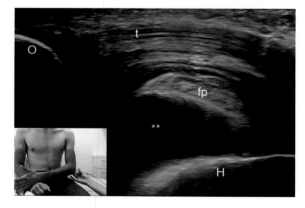

**Figure 6.11** Left elbow, posterior longitudinal view: a big amount of intra-articular fluid appears in the posterior recess (**) as an anechoic collection pushing the fat pad (fp) away. H, humerus; O, olecranon; t, triceps tendon.

pro-supination in the anterior view and flexion-extension in the posterior view, is valuable to visualize small amounts of IA fluid and also to assist in the detection of loose bodies in the elbow joint [9].

The normal synovial membrane is thin and difficult to see when no pathology is present [2, 5]. Thickening of the synovial membrane (pannus) will be seen as hypoechoic vegetations located inside the synovial cavity. The pannus can protrude in the synovial fluid or can fill completely the articular space [2]. Such synovial swelling will occur in rheumatic disorders, and haemophilic arthropathy, but can also been seen in degenerative osteoarthritis. Graded compression helps to differentiate between IA fluid (fully compressible) and synovial swelling (partially compressible). In inflammatory conditions, hyperaemia can also be detected with the use of color or power Doppler US, helping to monitor disease activity and response to treatment [2, 5]. Although the etiology regarding the IA fluid cannot be ascertained only with the use of US imaging, the presence of particular findings may be contributory, i.e. hyperechoic fluid (bloody effusion, fibrin clots), complex fluid containing hyperechoic spots (air) and debris (infection) [2]. On the other hand, US definitely aids for aspirations and further laboratory analyses.

Given its capability for dynamic assessment, US can effectively be used also for detection of intra-articular loose bodies [11, 12]. In the presence of IA fluid, they can actually be identified more easily. Absence of loose bodies on US evaluation however does not exclude their presence. When clinically suspected and negative US, an MRI examination is advised [12]. Loose bodies are most often found in the anterior recess, with the surrounding IA fluid enhancing their visualization [6]. Lastly, hyaline cartilage alterations that ensue in various disorders (degenerative, rheumatic or hemophilic) can be followed with US imaging as well [2].

## 6.3.2 Lateral and Medial Epicondyle Tendinopathy

Lateral epicondyle tendinopathy, commonly referred to as "tennis elbow", is an overuse tendinopathy of the CET. It is the most common cause of disability concerning the elbow, with an incidence of 1 to 3% in the general population. The use of US for diagnosing lateral epicondyle tendi-

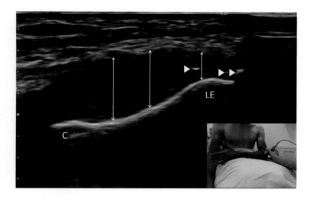

**Figure 6.12** Left elbow, lateral longitudinal view: a lateral epicondyle tendinopathy is seen with swelling at origin and swelling distal to origin (arrows), calcifications at origin and a bone spur (arrowheads), loss of the normal fibrillar pattern and diffuse hypoechoic zones. C, capitellum; LE, lateral epicondyle.

nopathy is widely accepted, with a sensitivity of 65-95% and specificity of 67-100% [10].

Similarly, medial epicondyle tendinopathy -commonly referred to as "golfer's elbow"- is an overuse tendinopathy of the CFT.

The US features of epicondyle tendinopathy include loss of the normal fibrillar pattern of the tendons, swelling, focal/diffuse hypo- or anechoic zones, calcification at the origin of the tendons or 1 to 3 cm distally, hyperaemia on power Doppler imaging, and cortical irregularities or spurs at the origin of the tendons [5]. Tears or clefts are often identified in tendons with diffuse changes of tendinopathy, and in chronic tendinopathy tendon thinning may also occur (Figures 6.12-6.15).

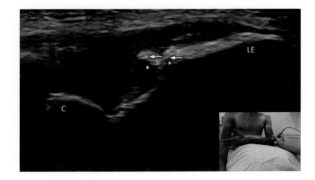

**Figure 6.13** Left elbow, lateral longitudinal view: a lateral epicondyle tendinopathy is seen, with calcifications (arrow) and acoustic shadow (*), swelling distal to origin, loss of the normal fibrillar pattern and diffuse hypoechoic zones. C, capitellum; LE, lateral epicondyle.

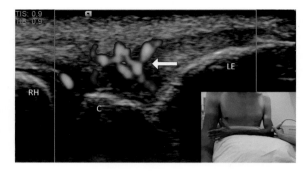

**Figure 6.14** Left elbow, lateral longitudinal power Doppler view: a lateral epicondyle tendinopathy is seen, with important hyperaemia distal to the tendon origin (arrow). C, capitellum; LE, lateral epicondyle; RH, radial head.

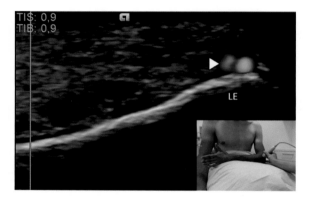

**Figure 6.15** Left elbow, lateral longitudinal power Doppler view: a lateral epicondyle tendinopathy is seen, with hyperaemia at the tendon origin (arrowhead). LE, lateral epicondyle.

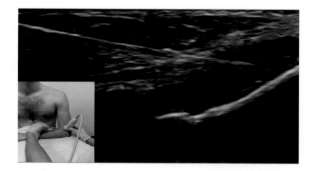

**Figure 6.16** Left elbow, lateral longitudinal view: US guided infiltration at the common extensor tendon. The procedure is performed with a sterile probe cover and sterile gloves.

The CET and CFT have a hyperechoic triangular configuration. On the other hand, appropriate probe positioning is needed to avoid anisotropy.

Proper left-right comparison is important to detect subtle differences and sonopalpation is definitely noteworthy [9]. The thickness of the CET can be measured at different points: the deepest point of the capitellum, the level of the radiocapitellar joint, and the level of the radial head. Care should be taken not to compress the tendon and to avoid inadvertent inclusion of the lateral collateral ligament [13]. Other authors suggest to measure the cross sectional area and the thickness of the CET in a transverse plane. Cut-off values of 32 $mm^2$ (sensitivity 86.3%, specificity 82.5%) and 4.2 mm (sensitivity 78.4%, specificity 95.2%) measured midway between the lateral epicondyle and the capitellum -respectively- were used for the diagnosis [13].

In daily practice, the thickness is often subjectively estimated: measured at the site of swelling and compared with the contralateral side. Mild sonographic alterations in the CET or CFT and bone spurs should be considered with caution when assessing epicondylar pain (especially in patients older than 55 years and those with a history of epicondylalgia), and should be correlated to the clinical examination [14].

Indisputably, US can be used to guide any infiltration for these patients (Figure 6.16).

### 6.3.3 Ulnar Collateral Ligament Lesions

Evaluation of the UCL is usually confined to the anterior band which is the most superficial and visible portion, located between the antero-inferior medial epicondyle and the coronoid process [9]. It is the primary stabilizer against valgus stress in extension. The normal ligament appears as an echogenic fibrillar cord-like structure. The posterior band forms the floor of the cubital tunnel and therefore has a direct relationship with the ulnar nerve, but a less stabilizing function. The transverse ligament lies between the ulnar insertions of the anterior and posterior bands, and its function is yet unclear [15].

Tears of the UCL are often due to trauma or sports injuries that cause abnormal valgus stress. While an acute partial thickness tear is seen as diffuse thickening and decreased echogenicity of the ligament with focal hypoechoic zones and surrounding hypoechoic edema, a full thickness tear (less common) will be seen as a fluid filled gap or a complete lack of visualization of the ligament [1, 10]. In case the ligament is only elongat-

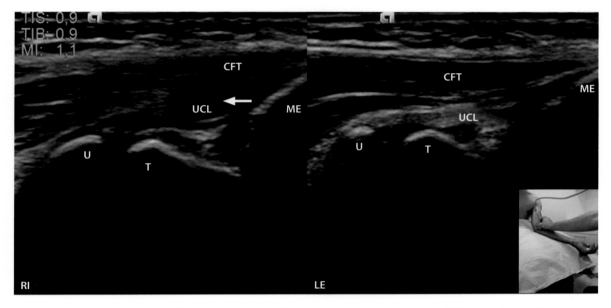

**Figure 6.17**  Right (RI) and left (LE) elbow. At the right elbow, he ulnar collateral ligament (UCL) is swollen and hypoechoic (arrow) when compared with the left elbow. CFT, common flexor tendon; ME, medial epicondyle; T, trochlea; U, ulna.

ed, but the bone at its origin or insertion is avulsed, the fragment can be seen as a hyperechoic particle with acoustic shadowing. Since the deep layers of the anterior bundle are mostly affected, dynamic evaluation can also demonstrate an asymmetric widening of the humeroulnar joint [16]. When the anterior bundle of the UCL is compromised, the radial head is the second stabilizer to abnormal valgus stress. As such, this can lead to intra-articular damage and degenerative osteophyte formation. These osteophytes can be seen on US as a sign of chronic instability. Consequently, when evaluating lesions of the UCL, the investigation of the lateral aspect should not be overlooked. Furthermore, 40% of these patients with chronic instability will develop ulnar nerve traction injuries [16]. Lastly, chronic repetitive injuries might cause degeneration of the UCL demonstrating diffuse (Figure 6.17) or focal swelling, hypoechoic zones, loss of normal lamellar structure, cortical alterations at its origin and insertion and intraligamentous calcifications [1, 10].

### 6.3.4 Lateral Collateral Ligament Lesions

The lateral collateral ligament (LCL) is a complex formed by the radial collateral ligament, fan-shaped, originating from the lateral epicondyle and blending distally with the annular ligament; the annular ligament, surrounding the radial head; and the lateral ulnar collateral ligament, starting from the lateral epicondyle to the supinator crest of the ulna.

The US assessment of the LCL pathology can show similar findings with the UCL. Due to its oblique course, however, it is technically challenging to see it with US. Actually, it becomes better visible when injured, and Teixeira et al. [17] even described the possibility of visualisation of all the components of the LCL. Nevertheless, US might not be fully adequate for the detection of LCL pathology [11].

### 6.3.5 Biceps Tendon Pathologies

*Distal biceps tendon tears*

Distal biceps tendon (DBT) tears are less common than proximal ones (less than 3% of all biceps tendon tears). They typically arise during an eccentric load of the muscle in middle-aged men. Fully retracted tears are often clinically diagnosed, whereas US plays an important role in evaluating partial or non-retracted tears. Distinction between complete and partial tears is impor-

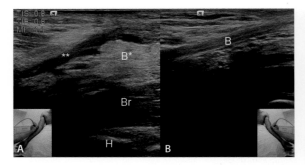

**Figure 6.18** Elbow, anterior longitudinal view. A - At the right elbow, the distal biceps tendon is ruptured (**) and retracted (B*). B - At the left elbow, the normal comparative image is seen. B, biceps tendon; Br, brachioradialis muscle; H, humerus.

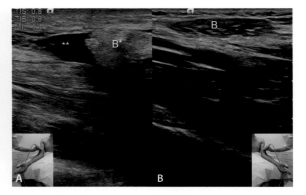

**Figure 6.19** Elbow, anterior transverse view. A - At the right elbow, the distal biceps tendon is ruptured and retracted (B*). The retracted tendon is surrounded by a fluid collection (**). B - At the left elbow, the normal comparative image is seen. B, biceps tendon.

tant, as complete tears are treated surgically and partial tears may be managed conservatively. Due to an intact lacertus fibrosus or excessive edema and hemorrhage, a complete tendon rupture can clinically be overlooked [1, 7, 18].

A tear in the DBT is visualized best in the longitudinal axis. It can appear as an anechoic fluid-filled gap distal to the joint, typically accompanied with an acoustic shadow (Figures 6.18 and 6.19). These findings usually indicate a complete rupture of the DBT. Complete long tendon head ruptures often lead to retraction, in contrast with short tendon head ruptures. A hypoechoic discontinuity of the tendon fibers with contour waviness and thickening/thinning of the tendon, sometimes accompanied with peritendinous fluid (without acoustic shadowing) can indicate a partial tear. Partial tears are even more uncommon and are more linked with fluid in the bicipitoradial bursa as compared to complete ruptures. US has been reported to differentiate between complete and partial tears with 95% sensitivity, 71% specificity and 91% accuracy [1, 7, 18]. While a concomitant tear of lacertus fibrosus can lead to further retraction of a complete rupture, the degree of tendon retraction should not be considered as a direct reflection of intact or absent lacertus fibrosus [1, 7, 18].

### Distal biceps tendinosis

While tears demonstrate contour irregularity and hypo- or anechoic disruption of tendon fibers, tendinosis appears as hypoechoic thickening of the tendon (Figure 6.19). This distinction might sometimes be difficult and arbitrary, since all patients with tendinosis have micro-tearing and degeneration. The presence of hyperaemia or calcification can partially be help [1, 18]. As quoted before, repetitive pro- and supination activities (leading to a mechanical impingement because of the narrowing of the radioulnar space) together with the relatively hypovascular zone of the tendon may contribute to tendinosis and further degeneration of the tendon [1, 7]. Tenosynovitis of the DBT does not exist since it lacks a synovial sheath.

### Bicipitoradial bursitis

This bursa functions to compensate for the impingement of the middle part of the distal biceps tendon. It is normally flattened and hardly visible on US; however, with increased fluid ac-

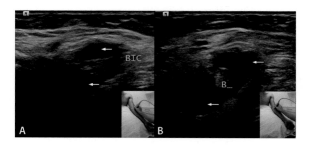

**Figure 6.20** A - Left elbow, anterior longitudinal view: the biceps tendon (BIC) is swollen and surrounded by fluid: bicipitoradial bursitis (arrows). B - Left elbow, anterior transverse view. The biceps tendon (B) is swollen and surrounded by fluid: bicipitoradial bursitis (arrows).

cumulation it can readily/effectively be detected with US imaging (Figure 6.20). Partial/complete tears of the tendon, repetitive mechanical microtrauma and overuse and rheumatic or infectious diseases are usually the underlying causes for bursitis [8, 18]. Clinically, bursitis may present as a mass in the cubital fossa or with sensory/motor symptoms related to compression of the radial nerve, which can also be seen with US [8].

### 6.3.6 Triceps Tendon Pathologies

The three parts of the triceps muscle come together into a single distal tendon, inserting onto the olecranon process of the ulna [5, 19]. On US, the continuity of the tendon can be easily imaged throughout, on longitudinal view [5, 19]. Rupture of the distal triceps tendon is a rare injury. It is generally suspected when a patient presents with pain and swelling on the posterior elbow after forced flexion with contracted triceps muscle. The most common form of disruption is avulsion from its insertion on the olecranon. The sonographic findings of a triceps tendon tear include absence of the distal triceps tendon, anechoic fluid-filled gap within the tendon and peritendinous fluid. The degree of retraction of a torn triceps tendon may be assessed on longitudinal US images and especially in patients with a torn but non-retracted triceps tendon, dynamic imaging (elbow flexion and extension) may be quite helpful [1, 5, 19]. Tendinosis of the distal triceps tendon is uncommon. Classical US images would comprise thickening of the tendon and hypoechoic areas sometimes with neovascularization or calcification as well [1, 19].

### 6.3.7 Olecranon Bursitis

The olecranon bursa, also consisting of a synovial membrane enveloping a film of liquid, lies superficial to the olecranon process and the distal part of the triceps tendon. It is the most commonly involved bursa of the elbow. The quantity of fluid in the bursa increases with age and the dominant side contains usually more fluid than the non-dominant side. In a young healthy person, US examination shows no swelling or fluid collection [5, 20].

Olecranon bursitis occurs after repetitive trauma of the elbow (Figure 6.21) or, less frequently, in patients with inflammatory diseases or infection (Figures 6.22 and 6.23). As elsewhere, the sono-

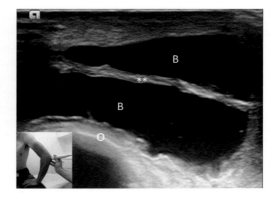

**Figure 6.21** Left elbow, posterior transverse view. Traumatic olecranon bursa (B) is filled with fluid and divided in two compartments by a septum (**). O, olecranon.

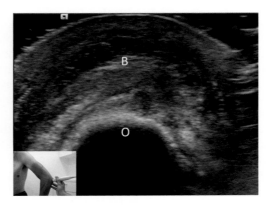

**Figure 6.22** Left elbow, posterior transverse view. Septic bursitis (B) is seen as a filled bursa with synovial thickening (hyperechoic regions) and fluid (hypoechoic regions). O, olecranon.

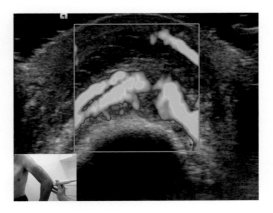

**Figure 6.23** Left elbow, posterior transverse view. Septic bursitis (B) is seen as a filled bursa with synovial thickening (hyperechoic regions) and fluid (hypoechoic regions). The power Doppler view shows an important amount of hyperemia.

graphic appearance of the fluid content may indirectly reflect the underlying cause, e.g. hyperechogenic in hemorrhagic and septic conditions or containing hyperechoic deposits in gout or pseudogout. Synovial hypertrophy and hyperemic flow on power Doppler imaging can be other findings in favor of inflammatory/rheumatic diseases. Again, (US-guided) aspiration and further analyses of the fluid may help for definite diagnosis.

### 6.3.8 Ulnar Nerve Problems

They will be discussed in Chapter 12 - "Ultrasound Imaging for Peripheral Nerve Problems".

### 6.3.9 Radial and Median Neuropathies at the Elbow

When compared with other common peripheral nerve entrapments of the upper limbs, radial and median neuropathies at the elbow are far less common. Nevertheless, besides the electrodiagnostic evaluation, US imaging can definitely yield useful information.

The radial nerve lies in the spiral groove of the humerus, where it can easily be detected with US, adjacent to the bone (the forearm of the patient is placed in pronation, the upper arm is adducted with a 45° of internal rotation). After starting the scanning at the middle of the posterolateral upper

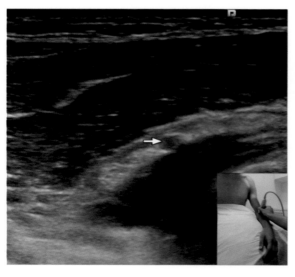

**Figure 6.24** Left elbow, anterolateral transverse view. The radial nerve (arrow) is swollen at supinator entrance (posterior interosseus nerve syndrome).

arm, the nerve can be followed (axially) as it penetrates the lateral intermuscular septum about 10 cm proximal to the elbow, entering the anterior compartment of the upper arm. The radial nerve then (3-5 cm proximal to the supinator muscle) bifurcates into superficial radial and a deep branch (see figure 6.8A, B). The latter runs distally deep to the brachioradialisis muscle before penetrating the supinator muscle. Anatomically, there are five potential sites of compression for the posterior interosseus nerve: fibrous bands anterior to the radiocapitellar joint between the brachialisis and brachioradialisis muscles; the recurrent radial vessels at the level of the radial neck ("leash of Henry"); the proximal edge of the extensor carpi radialis brevis muscle; the proximal edge of the supinator (arcade of Fröhse) see figure 6.8C); and the distal edge of the supinator muscle (see figure 6.8E) [21]. The arcade of Fröhse, which appears as a thin hyperechoic structure at the proximal edge of the supinator muscle [22], is described to be the most common site of primary compression. Of note, US can readily discriminate between such primary and secondary compressions (e.g. due to lipomas, ganglia, heterotopic ossification, callus, synovial overgrowth). In case of entrapment, the radial nerve will be seen as more hypoechoic with loss of normal fascicular structure and swollen proximal to the site of compression (Figure 6.24). A cut-off value of 0.15 cm for the anteroposterior diameter of the nerve just proximal to the arcade of Fröhse can be used as a diagnostic criterion [22].

The median nerve at the upper arm lies at the medial side between the biceps and brachialisis muscles, and dives below the ligament of Struthers in the distal 1/3 of the upper arm (a possible site of compression). At the level of the elbow, the median nerve lies medial to the biceps tendon and the brachialis artery, superficial to the brachialisis muscle. The nerve then passes between the two heads of the pronator muscle, a second site of possible compression. Exact diagnostic cut-off values do not exist for these sites, however the above described US changes are valid as elsewhere in peripheral nerve entrapment syndromes. Distal to the pronator muscle, the median nerve lies between the deep and superficial flexor digitorum muscles. Approximately 5 to 8 cm distal to the lateral epicondyle, the anterior interosseus nerve leaves off the main trunk [23]. Comparison with the asymptomatic side would again be reasonable to assess a likely entrapment.

# REFERENCES

1) Kijowski R, De Smet AA. The role of ultrasound in the evaluation of sports medicine injuries of the upper extremity. Clin Sports Med. 2006; 25: 569-90, viii.

2) Bianchi S, Martinoli C, Bianchi-Zamorani M, Valle M. Ultrasound of the joints. Eur Radiol. 2002; 12: 56-61.

3) Cho CH, Song KS, Choi IJ, Kim DK, Lee JH, Kim HT, et al. Insertional anatomy and clinical relevance of the distal biceps tendon. Knee Surg Sports Traumatol Arthrosc. 2011; 19: 1930-5.

4) Brigido MK, De Maeseneer M, Morag Y. Distal biceps brachii. Semin Musculoskelet Radiol. 2013; 17: 20-7.

5) Martinoli C, Bianchi S, Zamorani MP, Zunzunegui JL, Derchi LE. Ultrasound of the elbow. Eur J Ultrasound. 2001; 14: 21-7.

6) Radunovic G, Vlad V, Micu MC, Nestorova R, Petranova T, Porta F, et al. Ultrasound assessment of the elbow. Med Ultrason. 2012; 14: 141-6.

7) Lobo Lda G, Fessell DP, Miller BS, Kelly A, Lee JY, Brandon C, et al. The role of sonography in differentiating full versus partial distal biceps tendon tears: correlation with surgical findings. AJR Am J Roentgenol. 2013; 200: 158-62.

8) Draghi F, Gregoli B, Sileo C. Sonography of the bicipitoradial bursa: A short pictorial essay. J Ultrasound. 2012; 15: 39-41.

9) Finlay K, Ferri M, Friedman L. Ultrasound of the elbow. Skelet Radiol. 2004; 33: 63-79.

10) Tran N, Chow K. Ultrasonography of the elbow. Semin Musculoskelet Radiol. 2007; 11: 105-16.

11) Klauser AS, Tagliafico A, Allen GM, Boutry N, Campbell R, Court-Payen M, et al. Clinical indications for musculoskeletal ultrasound: a Delphi-based consensus paper of the European Society of Musculoskeletal Radiology. Eur Radiol. 2012; 22: 1140-8.

12) Allen G, Wilson D. Ultrasound of the upper limb: when to use it in athletes. Semin Musculoskelet Radiol. 2012; 16: 280-5.

13) Ustuner E, Toprak U, Baskan B, Oztuna D. Sonographic examination of the common extensor tendon of the forearm at three different locations in the normal asymptomatic population. Surg Radiol Anat. 2013; 35: 547-52.

14) Jaen-Diaz JI, Cerezo-Lopez E, Lopez-de Castro F, Mata-Castrillo M, Barcelo-Galindez JP, De la Fuente J, et al. Sonographic findings for the common extensor tendon of the elbow in the general population. J Ultrasound Med. 2010; 29: 1717-24.

15) Schaeffeler C, Waldt S, Woertler K. Traumatic instability of the elbow - anatomy, pathomechanisms and presentation on imaging. Eur Radiol. 2013; 23: 2582-93.

16) Lee KS, Rosas HG, Craig JG. Musculoskeletal ultrasound: elbow imaging and procedures. Semin Musculoskelet Radiol. 2010; 14: 449-60.

17) Teixeira PA, Omoumi P, Trudell DJ, Ward SR, Lecocq S, Blum A, et al. Ultrasound assessment of the lateral collateral ligamentous complex of the elbow: imaging aspects in cadavers and normal volunteers. Eur Radiol. 2011; 21: 1492-8.

18) Konin GP, Nazarian LN, Walz DM. US of the elbow: indications, technique, normal anatomy, and pathologic conditions. Radiographics. 2013; 33: E125-47.

19) Tagliafico A, Gandolfo N, Michaud J, Perez MM, Palmieri F, Martinoli C. Ultrasound demonstration of distal triceps tendon tears. Eur J Radiol. 2012; 81: 1207-10.

20) Blankstein A, Ganel A, Givon U, Mirovski Y, Chechick A. Ultrasonographic findings in patients with olecranon bursitis. Ultraschall Med. 2006; 27: 568-71.

21) Dang AC, Rodner CM. Unusual compression neuropathies of the forearm, part I: radial nerve. J Hand Surg. 2009; 34: 1906-14.

22) Djurdjevic T, Loizides A, Loscher W, Gruber H, Plaikner M, Peer S. High resolution ultrasound in posterior interosseous nerve syndrome. Muscle Nerve. 2014; 49: 35-9.

23) Dang AC, Rodner CM. Unusual compression neuropathies of the forearm, part II: median nerve. J Hand Surg. 2009; 34: 1915-20.

# Ultrasound Evaluation of the Wrist and Hand

Alper Murat ULAŞLI

**7**

## 7.1 INTRODUCTION

The role of ultrasound (US) imaging in the assessment of disorders affecting the wrist/hand has increased in the last decade in parallel with advances in technology. Yet, high frequency transducers, improvement in resolution, and color/power Doppler imaging allow comprehensive evaluation of soft tissue disorders. US can provide dynamic and real time examination of the affected tissue; as such, it appears to be a unique imaging modality in the evaluation of the wrist/hand whereby a wide range of disorders may be encountered in clinical practice. Adequate knowledge about specific examination techniques, normal appearance of the target tissues and specific artifacts is essential for prompt examination. Accordingly, this chapter comprises the normal anatomy and the examination technique, and US imaging of the pathological conditions.

## 7.2 EXAMINATION TECHNIQUE

During the US examination, patients are seated in a comfortable position with the hands supported or resting on a pillow. Shoulders are kept in neutral position with the elbows flexed and the forearms in supination/pronation depending on the side of the wrist/hand to be imaged.

Ultrasound imaging of the wrist/hand is performed with high-frequency linear array probes (preferably >10 MHz) and a standard gel interface. In particular conditions -especially when examining small and round structures or fingers with deformities- higher amounts of gel may be needed. Further, gel pads may also be used or imaging can be performed while the hand is kept inside water.

Bilateral examination, which allows a right-left comparison, is recommended [1]. Dynamic examination of the tendons, ligaments, and joints with active and passive mobilization may be quite helpful in the diagnosis [2]. Color/power Doppler imaging may provide valuable information about the vascularization of the structures/pathologies [1, 2]. Of note, during the examination, the sonographer should avoid much compression with the probe since small amount of fluid in B-mode and low resistance blood flow during Doppler imaging may be reluctantly overlooked.

A healthy bone cortex may be identified by its relatively smooth, sharp, and continuous hyperechoic layer on US examination [3]. Tendons are depicted as round or oval hyperechoic fibrillar structures in transverse scans, while they have a cord-like appearance in longitudinal scans [4]. Ligaments have a fibrillar echotexture and, like tendons, they appear hyperechoic [5]. Nerves display a fascicular pattern; hypoechoic between hyperechoic tendons, superficially, or hyperechoic between hypoechoic muscles deeply. Hyaline cartilage is seen as an anechoic layer over the articular surfaces, while fibrocartilage (e.g. triangular cartilage) appears as hypo- or hyperechoic due to its fibrillary echotexture.

### 7.2.1 Dorsal Wrist

The routine US examination of the wrist starts with the dorsum of the hand. The longitudinal scan of the wrist shows the radiocarpal (radio-scaphoid, radio-lunate), intercarpal, carpa-metacarpal (CMC), and metacarpophalangeal (MCP) joints, as well as the sagittal view of the extensor tendons (Figure 7.1A). The longitudinal scan starts from the radial side and the transducer is slowly moved towards the ulnar side without losing contact with the skin surface. To view the triangular cartilage, the US probe is placed immedi-

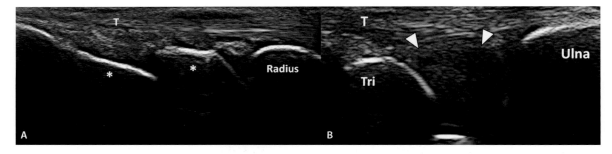

**Figure 7.1** Longitudinal views of the normal dorsal wrist. A - The US probe is placed in line with radius and second metacarpal joint. The radio-lunate joint, the dorsum of the carpal bones (white asterisks), and extensor tendon (T) are depicted. B - The US probe is placed in line with the ulna, immediately distal to the ulnar styloid. The sagittal views of triangular cartilage (white arrowheads), extensor carpi ulnaris tendon (T), ulna and triquetrum (Tri).

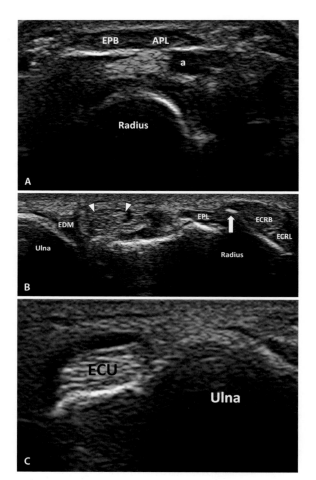

**Figure 7.2** Transverse views of the normal dorsal wrist. A - Abductor pollicis longus tendon (APL), extensor pollicis brevis tendon (EPB) and radial artery (a). B - From right to left; Extensor carpi radialis longus (ECRL) and brevis (ECRB) tendons, Lister's tubercle (white arrow), extensor pollicis longus tendon (EPL), extensor digitorum communis tendons (white arrowheads), and extensor digiti minimi tendon (EDM). C - Extensor carpi ulnaris (ECU) tendon on the ulnar side.

ately distal to the ulnar styloid, longitudinally and in line with the ulna [6] (Figure 7.1B).

In the transverse scan, the Lister's tubercle of the radius may easily be used as a landmark to get better oriented to the six extensor compartments. Starting from the radial side, they harbor the following tendons: 1st, abductor pollicis longus (APL) and extensor pollicis brevis (EPB); 2nd, extensor carpi radialis longus and brevis (ECRL and ECRB); 3rd, extensor pollicis longus (EPL); 4th, extensor digitorum communis (EDC); 5th, extensor digiti minimi (EDM) and 6th, extensor carpi ulnaris (ECU). Lister's tubercle separates the 2nd and 3rd compartments (Figure 7.2). To avoid anisotropy during the examination, correct inclination of the probe is recommended. The distal radioulnar joint and the scapholunate ligament are the other structures that may be evaluated during the transverse scan. The latter appears as a compact triangular echogenic fibrillar structure between the lunate and scaphoid bones, immediately distal to the Lister's tubercle [6].

## 7.2.2 Volar Wrist

In order to better recognize each and every flexor tendon, the examination needs to start with the transverse scan. Aside from the tendons of flexor carpi radialis (FCR), flexor digitorum superficialis (FDS) (N=4), flexor digitorum profundus (FDP) (N=4), flexor pollicis longus (FPL), palmaris longus tendon, flexor carpi ulnaris, flexor retinaculum (FR), median/ulnar nerves, radial/ulnar arteries and the carpal bones can readily be visualized (Figure 7.3A).

The FR lies transversely between the scaphoid

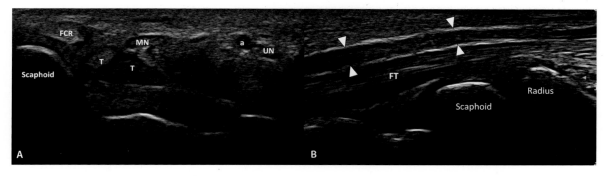

**Figure 7.3**   Transverse and longitudinal views of normal volar wrist. A - Transverse view of median nerve (MN), flexor tendons (T), flexor carpi radialis tendon (FCR), ulnar artery (a) and ulnar nerve (UN) at scaphoid level. B - Longitudinal view of the volar wrist. Median nerve (white arrowheads) lies over flexor tendons (FT).

tubercle and pisiform proximally, and between the trapezium and hook of hamate distally. It is a thin, convex band forming the roof of the carpal tunnel through which the tendons of FDS, FDP and FPL and the median nerve traverse. Laterally, the FR splits into 2 laminae. On the ulnar side, the ulnar artery and nerve lie between the 2 laminate of the FR [6]. Because of its convex shape, the FR may be visualized as hypoechoic or hyperechoic throughout its alignment in the wrist. The FCR lies over the FR on the radial side near the scaphoid.

The median nerve lies over the flexor tendons and immediately below the FR in the carpal tunnel. Proximal to the tunnel, it lies between the superficial and deep flexor muscles, with a hyperechoic appearance. As the probe is moved from proximal to distal, the nerve becomes superficial and hypoechoic. In transverse images, the median nerve displays a round/ovoid shape also depending on the wrist position and varying among subjects [7]. Longitudinally, it does not have a straight alignment troughout the wrist. Proximal to the tunnel, it is localized more radially; whereas after entering the tunnel, it has a more central alignment. As such, fine probe positioning may be necessary to nicely observe an anechoic tubular structure with a few intrinsic hyperechoic lines (Figure 7.3B). During dynamic imaging with finger flexion/extension, the median nerve normally accompanies the movement of the gliding flexor tendons but to a lesser extent.

The ulnar nerve is usually found ulnar/medial to the ulnar artery in the distal forearm (Figure 7.3A). Accordingly, the pulsatility of the ulnar artery or the use of Doppler imaging may help distinguish the nerve readily on transverse scans.

### 7.2.3  **Palm and Fingers**

Since there are plenty of structures that can be scanned in the hand, the US examination needs to be performed in light of the history and physical examination. One of the commonly evaluated structures would be FPL tendon. After passing through the carpal tunnel, it lies between the superficial and deep bellies of the flexor pollicis brevis muscle. Characteristically, it may be visualized as hyperechoic round structure ("full moon") with proper placement of the US probe in the thenar region (transverse scan) (Figure 7.4A). For sure, longitudinal assessment is pos-

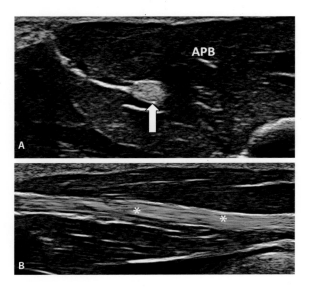

**Figure 7.4**   Flexor pollicis longus (FPL) tendon at the thenar area. A - Transverse view of the tendon (white arrow), and abductor pollicis brevis muscle (APB). B - Longitudinal view of the FPL tendon (white asterisks).

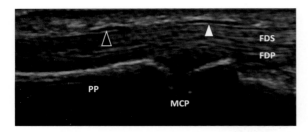

**Figure 7.5** Longitudinal view of flexor tendons (FDS, FDP), A1 (white arrowhead), and A2 (black arrowhead) pulleys. PP, proximal phalanx; MCP, metacarpophalangeal joint.

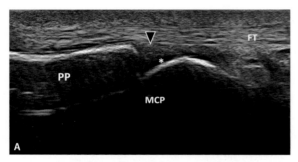

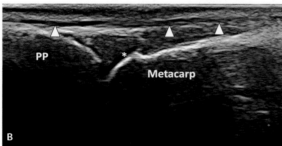

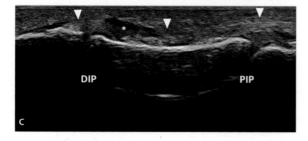

**Figure 7.6** Palmar and dorsal longitudinal views of the finger joints and tendons. A - Palmar longitudinal view of the metacarpophalangeal joint, flexor tendons (FT), and volar fat pad (black arrowhead). PP, proximal phalanx; MCP, metacarpophalangeal joint. B - Dorsal longitudinal view of the metacarpophalangeal joint, and extensor tendon (white arrowheads). C - Palmar longitudinal view of the proximal and distal interphalangeal joints (PIP and DIP), flexor tendons (white arrowheads) and its' insertion to the distal phalanx. Note the anechoic area due to anisotropy artefact (white asterisk).

sible/necessary as well (Figure 7.4B).

In the palm, the tendons of the FDS are located over the FDP tendons. They then split into 2 parts (chiasm) at the level of proximal phalanges and insert on both sides of the middle phalanges [6]. These tendons can substantially be evaluated from proximal to distal and also dynamically. Small, passive and selective movements of the phalanges can be applied in this regard. Additionally, depending on the technical capabilities of the US machine, the pulleys of these flexor tendons can be imaged as well [8-10] (Figure 7.5). Likewise, the extensor tendons (quite thinner than the flexors) on the dorsal side of the fingers can also be examined statically and/or dynamically.

Another structure to be scanned would be the ulnar collateral ligament of the thumb, running from the ulnar side of the metacarpal head to the lateral tubercle of the proximal phalanx of the thumb. It can be visualized by longitudinally placing the US probe on the ulnar side of the thumb [6].

Ultrasound may provide valuable information as regards the radiocarpal, intercarpal, metacarpophalangeal (MCP), proximal interphalangeal (PIP) and distal interphalangeal (DIP) joints (Figure 7.6). The examination of these joints starts with longitudinal scans of both the volar and dorsal surfaces. The bone cortex, articular cartilage, intra-articular fat pad and the joint capsule can be conveniently imaged from multiplanar views (especially important for patients with rheumatic diseases) [11]. The intrinsic hand muscles and the related neurovascular structures can also be examined where needed and if technically available.

## 7.3 WRIST AND HAND PATHOLOGIES

The use of musculoskeletal US is well accepted in a variety of clinical conditions involving the muscles, tendons, ligaments, nerves, and joints in the wrist/hand. Likewise, herein, we describe several common pathologies that are encountered in daily clinical practice.

### 7.3.1 De Quervain's Disease

De Quervain's disease -a stenosing tenosynovitis of the 1st extensor compartment of the wrist- has been linked to overuse [12, 13]. Although the

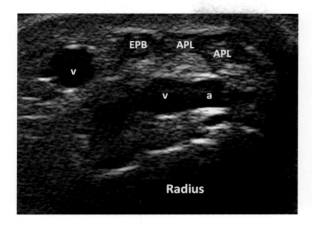

**Figure 7.7** Anatomical variation in the first dorsal extensor compartment of the wrist. Note the two tendineous slips of abductor pollicis longus (APL), extensor pollicis brevis tendon (EPB) and radial artery (a), and veins (v).

exact pathogenesis of the disease has not been fully determined, previous anatomical studies have suggested that variations in the compartment may play role (Figure 7.7). In a cadaveric study of sixty-six specimens [14], the APL was found to have a single tendinous slip in nine specimens, two slips in fourty-six specimens, three slips in nine specimens, and four slips in two specimens. Moreover, the 1st extensor compartment was found to be subdivided, partially or completely, by a septum forming two distinct tunnels in 20-60% of the specimens studied. The thickening of the synovial sheath leads to irritation of the APL and EPB tendons, causing pain and swelling over the radial side of the wrist, exacerbated by repetitive movements of the thumb and wrist i.e. gripping or forceful pinching of the objects [15]. The differential diagnosis includes intersection syndrome, osteoarthritis or Wartenberg's syndrome and becomes easy with the use of US. US examination may yield thickening of the tendon sheath with a hypoechoic appearance, increased anechoic or hypoechoic fluid surrounding the tendons, swelling of the tendons, and synovial hyperemia with Doppler imaging. In chronic cases, the tendons may have a heterogeneous echotexture with eventual tear/ruptures. Additionally, aforementioned anatomic variations can also be observed as potential trigerring mechanisms [16]. In this sense, US may also be helpful for guiding precisely different local injections -with better treatment outcome when compared with blind injections [17].

## 7.3.2 Intersection Syndrome

This is a relatively uncommon overuse syndrome which is associated with repeated radial deviation of the wrist. The clinical scenario is that of pain, tenderness, swelling and crepitus in the intersected region [18]. The syndrome is described as two types; proximal and distal. In proximal intersection -a region located 4-8 cm proximal to the Lister's tubercle- the musculotendinous junctions of the first extensor compartment (APL and EPB) cross over the tendons of the second extensor compartment (ECRL and ECRB). In distal intersection, the third extensor compartment tendon (EPL) crosses over the tendons of the second extensor compartment distal to the Lister's tubercle (Figure 7.8). During wrist movements, friction can ensue between the relevant groups of tendons at either point, more commonly at the proximal intersection [19]. Accordingly, in suspected patients, each tendon of the first three extensor compartments need to be evaluated from the musculotendinous junction to the insertion with both transverse and longitudinal scans, with special attention given to the intersecting areas. The US examination may reveal local soft tissue edema and other above quoted tendonitis/tenosynovitis findings.

Similarly, other wrist extensor/flexor tendons may also undergo inflammatory or overuse injuries whereby the US imaging findings again en-

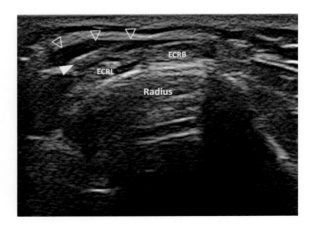

**Figure 7.8** Normal transverse view of the distal intersection. Distal to the Lister's tubercle, the extensor pollicis longus tenton -the third extensor compartment- (white arrowheads show the musculous component) crosses over the extensor carpi radialis brevis (ECRB) and longus (ECRL) tentons -the second extensor compartment.

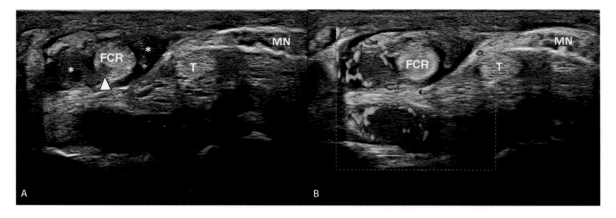

**Figure 7.9** Transverse view of flexor carpi radialis (FCR) tenosynovitis in a patient with Rheumatoid arthritis. A - The heterogenous echogenicity of the FCR tendon and the hypoechoic synovial proliferation (white asterisks) surrounding the tendon. Note the hypoechoic synovial tissue invading the FCR tendon (white arrowhead). T: Flexor tendon, MN: Median nerve. B - Doppler imaging of the volar wrist, showing marked hyperemia around the tendon (the Doppler signals imaged below the FCR represents as mirror image artifact).

compass hypo- or anechoic fluid around the injured tendon (target sign) and/or hypoechoic synovial thickening with or without Doppler signals representing hyperemia [2, 20, 21] (Figure 7.9). Tears, ruptures and subluxations can be seen depending on the underlying disease [22, 23].

### 7.3.3 Trigger Finger, Pulley Syndrome

Trigger finger or stenosing tenosynovitis of the flexor digitorum tendons is generally due to overuse; however certain diseases affecting the soft tissues (diabetes mellitus, hepatic failure, etc.) might well be accompanying. On US, retinaculum or pulley hypertrophy as well as restricted tendon movements in the osseofibrous tunnels can typically be observed (Figure 7.10) [24]. Tendinosis (loss of homogenous fibrillary pattern), intra- or peritendinous nodules, peritendinous effusion and hypervascularisation on power Doppler imaging or even problems of the nearby joints may also be present. Currently there is no valid grading system for evaluating trigger finger severity; however Guerini et al. [25] reported an average thickness of 0.5 mm in normal pulleys and increased thickness with an average of 1.8 mm in pulleys with hypertrophy on US. Lastly, owing to the capability of detailed imaging with US, interventions targeted to these small pulleys or particular areas of the related soft tissues are

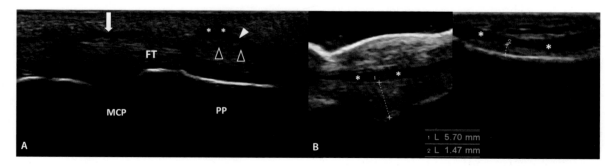

**Figure 7.10** Pulley syndrome. A - Longitudinal view of the thickened A1 pulley (white arrow), and the fibrous nodules on the flexor tendons (black arrowheads) accompanying hypoechoic fluid (white arrowhead) and synovial proliferation (white asterisks) (PP, Proximal phalanx; MCP, metacarpophalangeal joint; FT, flexor tendons). B - Longitudinal views of a normal (right) and ruptured (left) pulley. The indirect way to demonstrate a pulley rupture is measuring the distance between the bone cortex and the flexor tendon (between + +) and comparing with the normal side. Ultrasound examination in a water bath clearly depicts, on the left side, separation of the tendon (white asterisks) and bone.

Musculoskeletal Ultrasound in Physical and Rehabilitation Medicine

### 7.3.4 Tendon Ruptures

Given the possibility of dynamic evaluation with US, tendon injuries seem to be one of the most appropriate pathologies that need to be examined with it. In case of partial or complete ruptures, passive or active movement of the tendons will indisputably help for prompt diagnosis and follow up [27]. US can also show the gap in the tendon substance, the empty or fluid filled sheath, the distal or retracted proximal ends [28]. Particular attention must be paid concerning anisotropy; yet while it may challenge the examination, once it is recognized (like many other artifacts), it may facilitate the assessment as well. Relevant US findings are generally classified as tendon echotexture derangement (hypoechoic loss of fibrillar echotexture), partial tear (focal discontinuity) or complete tear (complete loss of the tendon) [29, 30]. Of additional note, US imaging can also help guide a likely surgery (in advance) or follow postoperatively for complications i.e. re-rupture or adhesions.

### 7.3.5 Space-occupying Lesions

*Ganglia* are the most common cystic lesions of the hand and wrist occurring in patients of all ages [4, 20, 31]. These round or lobulated masses, usually containing thick viscous fluid and epithelial lining, often develop from mucinous degeneration of the periarticular soft tissues secondary to repetitive trauma [32-34]. Dorsal ganglia are more common and patients usually describe either pain or cosmetic disturbance, and less movement limitations. In addition to these symptoms, ganglia on the volar side may present with neuropathic symptoms if they are in/close to the carpal or Guyon's canal [35].

At the dorsum of the wrist, ganglia usually arise at the attachment of the joint capsule to the dorsal aspect of scapholunate ligament, taking origin from the scapholunate joint (Figure 7.11). The volar ganglia originate from the triscaphoid joint (between the scaphoid, trapezium, and trapezoid) and are located on the radial side of the wrist [28]. On US examination, these cystic lesions appear as round or oval shaped masses with well-defined external margins and sometimes with internal septa. They contain anechoic fluid and are weakly or non-compressible.

*Giant cell tumor* of the tendon sheath is another mass commonly detected in the hand and wrist. It is also known as "localized pigmented villonodular synovitis". This slow-growing lobulated mass is locally aggressive and can even cause bone erosions [36]. Close to the finger flexor tendons, on US, it usually appears as an hypoechoic mass with well-defined margins and high Doppler signals interiorly [37].

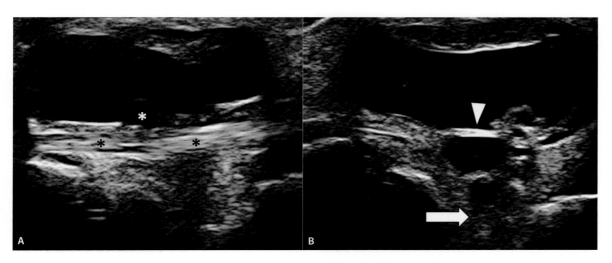

**Figure 7.11**   The oval shaped, lobulated ganglion cyst (GC) over the dorsum of the wrist containing anechoic fluid. A - Longitudinal view of the GC, synovial septae (white asterisk) and the extensor tendon (black asterisks). Note the enhancement artifact of the tendon under anechoic fluid. B - Transverse view of the GC, the septa (white arrowhead) and the probable origin of the cyst (white arrow).

## 7.3.6 Carpal Tunnel Syndrome

Carpal tunnel syndrome (CTS) is the most frequent peripheral entrapment neuropathy, with a higher prevalence in females [38]. The underlying pathophysiology has not been clearly identified; however, congestion of the epineural and endoneural veins, nerve edema and impaired blood supply are reported to play role [39]. Other than morphological confirmation as regards the nerve entrapment, US examination can also depict possible causes of CTS e.g. anatomical variations (bifid median nerve, persistent median artery, etc.), flexor tenosynovitis, displaced bone, ganglia or other space occupying lesions in the tunnel [10, 40-42].

As usual, transverse and longitudinal images are both necessary for the sonographic diagnosis

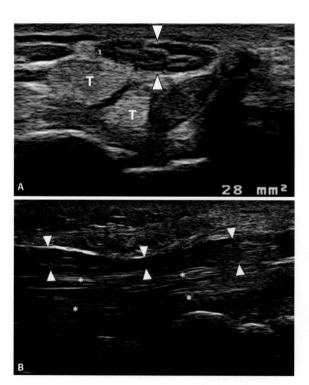

**Figure 7.12** Transverse and longitudinal views and the corresponding cross-sectional area (CSA) of the median nerve (dashed circle) in a patient with severe carpal tunnel syndrome (CTS). A - Median nerve (white arrowheads) CSA measured at the carpal tunnel (T, tendon). B - The longitudinal view of the median nerve (white arrowheads). Note the characteristic "dumble sign" as the median nerve is thicker at the tunnel inlet and outlet and it is thinner because it is compressed between flexor retinaculum and flexor tendons in the mid-tunnel.

(Figure 7.12). The nerve is examined in short axis planes with sweeping of the probe from the distal forearm to the palm. Typically, the nerve is observed to be thinner at the site of entrapment and enlarged (and less echogenic) just proximal to it. Quantification is usually carried out via measuring the cross-sectional area (CSA) -using the continuous trace of the nerve boundary excluding the surrounding echogenic rim- at the tunnel inlet, mid-tunnel and tunnel outlet (Figure 7.12A). Herewith, the first measurement -which pertains to the swollen site- is most commonly taken into consideration for sonographic cut-off values, ranging between 9-15 mm$^2$ in different studies [38, 39, 43-45]. These CSA values have shown to be significantly correlated with the electrophysiogical studies [40, 46] and their discrepancies were attributed to different measurement techniques and/or demographics [40, 47, 48]. The addition of measurements at the outlet or swelling ratio (in comparison with the proximal portion of the nerve in the forearm) may increase the sensitivity/specificity of US examination in the diagnosis [40, 49].

Entrapment may cause nerve ischemia and affect the microvasculature within the neural fascicles [50] and due to inflammation and ischemia, the intraneuronal microvasculature of the median nerve may dilate [51]. It has been shown that the presence of intraneuronal vascularity with Doppler imaging revealed good concordance with electrodiagnostic testing in the diagnosis of CTS [52]. Further, power Doppler signal grading has also been suggested in the diagnosis [53] (Table 7.1).

Due to non-inflammatory fibrosis and thickening of the connective tissue in the carpal tunnel, dynamic scanning may reveal limited motion of the compressed median nerve beneath the flexor retinaculum [54]. The displacement measurements (endpoint displacement and path displacement) of the nerve and the flexor tendons has revealed moderate to good results for CTS diagnosis [55]. Hand blood flow (the flow volume, peak systolic velocity, end-diastolic velocity) was also reported to be different in CTS patients (as compared to normal hands) both at rest and during provocative maneuvers [56].

Lastly, sonoelastography is another method recently studied in CTS diagnosis. The idea is mainly to detect the scar tissue (fibroblast invasion) which develops due to increased intracarpal tunnel pressure, affected circulation and long-term edema of the median nerve [57, 58].

Musculoskeletal Ultrasound in Physical and Rehabilitation Medicine

**Table 7.1** Power Doppler grading of median nerve in carpal tunnel syndrome

| | |
|---|---|
| Grade 0 | No power Doppler signal |
| Grade 1 | 1 single vessel within the MN |
| Grade 2 | 2-3 single, or 2 confluent vessels |
| Grade 3 | >3 single, or >2 confluent vessels in the transverse images |

MN: Median nerve. A power Doppler score of grade 2 or higher obtained from the level of the largest MN cross-sectional area observed between the area proximal to the carpal tunnel inlet and the tunnel outlet yielded low sensitivity (47.4%) and high specificity (92%).

### 7.3.7 Guyon's Tunnel Syndrome

The ulnar tunnel originates at the proximal edge of the carpal ligament and extends distally to the fibrous arch of the hypothenar muscles at the level of the hook of hamate. The medial wall is formed by the pisiform bone, FCU tendon, and abductor digiti minimi (ADM); the lateral wall is formed by the hook of hamate and transverse carpal ligament; the flexor retinaculum, pisohamate ligament and pisometacarpal ligament form the floor and palmar carpal ligament and hypothenar fibroadipose tissue form the roof [28, 59-61]. The ulnar artery (UA) may be used as a landmark for finding the ulnar nerve at the wrist as they cross the ulnar tunnel together. The UN lies medially and slightly deep to the UA. Three types of UN compression syndromes, at 3 anatomical zones, have been described [59]. Zone 1 compression may occur proximal to or within Guyon's tunnel before bifurcation of the UN into the superficial and deep branches. Zone 2 compression may occur where the deep motor branch exits Guyon's tunnel and affects the motor branch of the UN. This is the most frequent compression type in Guyon's tunnel. Zone 3 compression affects the superficial sensory branch of the UN.

Ulnar nerve compression syndrome may be caused by anomalous muscles (particularly the accessory ADM), GCs and tumors, fractures or dislocations, direct compression from trauma, and thrombosis of the UA. The frequency of the UN compression syndrome at the wrist level is higher in patients with CTS [62, 63].

Transverse US images of the UN during its course at the wrist and Guyon's tunnel can be observed. The UN and/or its branches may be enlarged and thickened. US can show space-occupying lesions compressing the UN. GCs originating from the hamate-triquetrum or the piso-triquetrum joints are the most frequent cause of UN compression in Guyon's tunnel. Anechoic masses with well-defined margins may be easily differentiated with US; however, the origin of the cyst is difficult to identify [64]. UA thrombosis can be depicted with color Doppler imaging. The anomalous accessory ADM can be depicted anterior to the ulnar neurovascular bundle. Comparing the thickness of this muscle with the contralateral side or normal subjects may give valuable information in patients with clinical UN entrapment symptoms and signs [65].

### 7.3.8 Wartenberg Syndrome

Wartenberg syndrome (WS) is a neuropathy affecting the superficial branch of the radial nerve (SBRN) presenting with abnormal sensation and pain in the distribution of the SBRN, namely over the dorsal lateral surface of the wrist and hand [66]. It can mimic dQD as both diseases have similar presentations. WS is usually secondary to trauma of the SBRN distal to its perforation through the superficial fascia of the forearm. Other causes including watchband or handcuff compression, braces, fractures, or iatrogenic events such as vein cannulation may also cause SBRN neuropathy [66-68]. The US examination can depict the SBRN segment between ECRL tendons, and the SBRN passage through the forearm fascia, and SBRN at the wrist segment lateral to the first extensor compartment tendons. Furthermore, it may reveal swelling of the nerve, which can be seen as increased at the level of the injury compared to a more proximal site of the nerve or the SBRN on the contralateral wrist. The treatment of WS includes corticosteroid injections at the injury site. Finally, US examination may be useful in the treatment of WS as US-guided perineural injections to the SBRN were found to be feasible [66].

### 7.3.9 Foreign Bodies

Foreign bodies (FB) are seen frequently after soft tissue penetration traumas, and detection is often difficult, especially when the material is radiolucent [69]. The FB may lead pain, soft tissue infection and abscess [70]. Radiodense materials like earth and metal may be detected with plain radiography. However, the radiolucent materials like vegetable, wood, and glass and their relationship with surrounding tissues such as nerves, tendons and vessels can be effectively shown with US [71]. Moreover, US may guide the surgeon for removal of FB. Metallic FB may seem hyperechoic with acoustic shadowing and a comet-tail artefact may accompany (Figure 7.13). Wood, glass and vegetables do not reflect sound waves as much as metals. The reactive inflammation or granuloma formation surrounding the FB may be seen as a hypoechoic halo in subacute and chronic lesions. This can be used as an indirect method to detect radiolucent FB. Even for radiodense objects, US provides better localization within the soft tissues. Radiodense FB may show posterior reverberation artefact which may help sonographers to detect

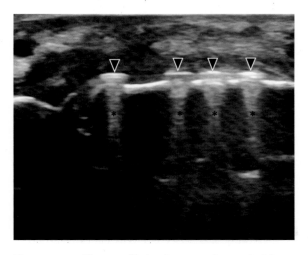

**Figure 7.13** The metallic implants on the cortical bone (black arrowheads) and the comet-tail artefacts (black asterisks).

small FB [70]. Musculoskeletal US may aid during the initial management or followup of patients with soft tissue injuries with potential FB.

### 7.3.10 Ulnar Collateral Ligament Injury of the Thumb

Ulnar collateral ligament (UCL) injury of the thumb, frequently referred to as gamekeeper's thumb, is one of the common injuries of the hand. UCL injuries occur due to forced hyperextension or abduction of the MCP joint, and may result with strain, or partial or full-thickness tear. A displaced full-thickness tear has been referred to as a Stener lesion [72]. The UCL arises from the distal metacarpal bone and attaches on the medial tubercle of the proximal phalanx of the thumb. The UCL is normally typically 4-8 mm in width and 12-14 mm in length [73-75]. The normal UCL has a linear fibrillary pattern with hyperechoic appearance with US. It is covered by the adductor pollicis aponeurosis, with a thin linear hyperechoic appearance [76]. Both tissues may seem hypoechoic or anechoic if the US probe is not placed perpendicular to the ligaments. The UCL tears are mostly seen at its insertion site into the proximal phalanx of the thumb [77]. Pain, swelling, ecchymosis, and instability on MCP joint, may be noted during examination of the thumb. An avulsion fracture may occur and plain radiographs can show a bone fragment.

Ulnar collateral ligament tears can be effectively demonstrated with US, including Stener lesions [72]. The differentiation of displaced from non-displaced tears is important as it can change the type of the management. The displaced ligament mostly has a heterogeneous echogenicity due to a combination of echogenic ligament, hypoechoic ligament from anisotropy, and possible refraction shadowing at the torn ligament stump [77]. A hyperechoic avulsion bone fragment and acoustic shadowing artifact may also be seen. Additional Doppler imaging may show hyperemia in certain cases. Performing manual valgus stress to the MCP joint of the thumb may help better visualization of UCL.

### 7.3.11 Arthritis of the Wrist and Hand

Various inflammatory diseases may affect the joints in wrist and hand. The wrist is the most affected joint in rheumatoid arthritis, and has been selected as the target joint in clinical trials evaluating the disease activity scoring systems [1].

The US evaluation of an arthritic joint will be discussed in detail in another section. Here, we will discuss arthritis of the wrist and hand in brief. The US evaluation starts with the longitudinal imaging of the dorsal aspect of the wrist, as the probe is placed between distal radius and second or third MCP joint. The probe is slowly swifted from radial side to ulnar side without applying any compression towards underlying soft tissue. On the ulnar side, the insertion of the ECU and triangular cartilage are areas of interest during examination. The examination continues with transverse imaging of the extensor compartments on the dorsal aspect of the wrist. On the volar aspect, carpal tunnel including flexor tendons and MN, and Guyon's tunnel including ulnar nerve and ulnar artery, and carpal bones are areas of interest.

Both the dorsal and volar aspects of the joints are evaluated during US evaluation to detect joint effusion and synovial hypertrophy. The multiplanar scanning technique is recommended for proper joints [1] as a radial distribution of the synovial hypertrophy at the level of PIP joint was suggested [78]. However, palmar evaluation of the finger joints alone was found to be highly sensitive [78, 79]. On longitudinal scan of the finger joints (MCP, PIP and DIP), the probe is moved medially and laterally as much as possible, to circumferentially image each joint.

Joint synovial fluid is defined as an abnormal hypoechoic or anechoic intra-articular material that is displaceable and compressible and does not exhibit a Doppler signal. Synovial hypertrophy is not displaceable but weakly compressible, and seems hypoechoic with US [80].

Several methods have been reported for the quantification of synovitis. The method commonly used is a semiquantitative scale graded between 0-3, as follows: grade 0, absence of synovitis; grade 1, mild synovial hypertrophy; grade 2, moderate synovial hypertrophy; and grade 3, marked synovial hypertrophy [81]. In addition to this grading system, Szkudlarek et al. proposed a

different classification with good interobserver agreement (kappa coefficient 0.63). They defined grade 2 as synovial hypertrophy bulging over the line between the top of the bones forming the joint without extension along bone diaphyses, and divided grade 3 into extension to one of the two diaphyses (grade 3) and extension to both diaphyses (grade 4) [82].

Power or color Doppler US evaluation helps in synovitis activity assessment with differentiation between the inflamed synovium and inactive pannus or fibrous tissue. Various studies have confirmed that power Doppler is useful for the detection of inflammation, estimation of disease severity, and determination of response to treatment [1, 83-85]. The color Doppler in new generation US equipment is highly sensitive in detecting synovial inflammation, and may provide the quantification of the inflammation using color fraction [86]. Power Doppler quantification is usually graded on a 0-3 semiquantitative scale, as follows: grade 0, absence of signal with no intra-articular flow; grade 1, mild with up to 3 single vessel signals or 2 single vessels plus 1 confluent signal; grade 2, moderate with a signal occupying <50% of the synovium; grade 3, marked with a vessel signal in >50% of the synovial area [83]. In healthy subjects, power Doppler signals may be seen especially in the carpometacarpal joint area, which may be mistakenly considered as a pathological sign of inflammation. Depending on the stage and the severity of the disease, ultrasonographic findings of the arthritic joints may vary from mild effusion in early arthritis to marked effusion, synovial hypertrophy, cortical bone erosions and deformities. US is also helpful in guidance of intra-articular injections and synovial biopsy.

## 7.4 CONCLUSION

The wide availability of US equipment and the increasing interest of clinicians on musculoskeletal imaging has placed the US as the first line imaging modality. The wrist and hand are involved in various overuse, inflammatory, and traumatic conditions.

# REFERENCES

1) Vlad V, Micu M, Porta F, Radunovic G, Nestorova R, Petranova T, et al. Ultrasound of the hand and wrist in rheumatology. Med Ultrason. 2012; 14: 42-8.

2) Wong DCM, Wansaicheong GKL, Tsou IYY. Ultrasonography of the hand and wrist. Singapore Med J. 2009; 50: 219-26.

3) Filippucci E, Iagnocco A, Meenagh G, Riente L, Delle Sedie A, Bombardieri S, et al. Ultrasound imaging for the rheumatologist. Clin Exp Rheumatol. 2006; 24: 1-5.

4) Jacobson JA, van Holsbeeck MT. Musculoskeletal ultrasonography. Orthop Clin North Am. 1998; 29: 135-67.

5) Erickson SJ. High-resolution imaging of the musculoskeletal system. Radiology. 1997; 205: 593-618.

6) Lee JC, Healy JC. Normal sonographic anatomy of the wrist and hand. Radiographics. 2005; 25: 1577-90.

7) Kuo MH, Leong CP, Cheng YF, Chang HW. Static wrist position associated with least median nerve compression: sonographic evaluation. Am J Phys Med Rehabil. 2001; 80: 256-60.

8) Bianchi S, Martinoli C, de Gautard R, Giagnot C. Ultrasound of the digital flexor system: Normal and pathological findings. J Ultrasound. 2007; 10: 85-92.

9) Hauger O, Chung CB, Lektrakul N, Botte MJ, Trudell D, Boutin RD, et al. Pulley system in the fingers: normal anatomy and simulated lesions in cadavers at MR imaging, CT, and US with and without contrast material distention of the tendon sheath. Radiology. 2000; 217: 201-12.

10) Martinoli C, Bianchi S, Nebiolo M, Derchi LE, Garcia JF. Sonographic evaluation of digital annular pulley tears. Skeletal Radiol. 2000; 29: 387-91.

11) Filippucci E, Iagnocco A, Meenagh G, Riente L, Delle Sedie A, Bombardieri S, et al. Ultrasound imaging for the rheumatologist II. Ultrasonography of the hand and wrist. Clin Exp Rheumatol. 2006; 24: 118-22.

12) Lalonde DH, Kozin S. Tendon disorders of the hand. Plast Reconstr Surg. 2011; 128: 1-14.

13) Kay NR. De Quervain's disease. Changing pathology or changing perception? J Hand Surg Br. 2000; 25: 65-9.

14) Wolfe SW, Hotchkiss RN, Pederson WC, Kozin SH. Green's Operative Hand Surgery. 6th ed. Vol. 2. Philadelphia, PA: Elsevier, 2010: 2067-88.

15) Hazani R, Engineer NJ, Cooney D, Wilhelmi BJ. Anatomic landmarks for the first dorsal compartment. ePlasty. 2008; 8: 489-93.

16) Nagaoka M, Matsuzaki H, Suzuki T. Ultrasonographic examination of de Quervain's disease. J Orthop Sci. 2000; 5: 96-9.

17) Hajder E, de Jonge MC, van der Horst CM, Obdeijna MC. The role of ultrasound-guided triamcinolone injection in the treatment of De Quervain's disease: Treatment and a diagnostic tool? Chir Main. 2013; 32: 403-7.

18) Pantukosit S, Petchkrua W, Stiens SA. Intersection syndrome in Buriram Hospital: a 4-year prospective study. Am J Phys Med Rehabil. 2001; 80: 656-61.

19) Draghi F, Bortolotto C. Intersection syndrome: ultrasound imaging. Skeletal Radiol. 2014; 43: 283-7.

20) Chiou HJ, Chou YH, Chang CY. Ultrasonography of the wrist. Can Assoc Radiol J. 2001; 52: 302-11.

21) Lin J, Jacobson JA, Fessell DP, Weadock WJ, Hayes CW. An illustrated tutorial of musculoskeletal sonography: part 2, upper extremity. AJR Am J Roentgenol. 2000; 175: 1071-9.

22) Chang CY, Huang AJ, Bredella MA, Kattapuram SV, Torriani M. Association between distal ulnar morphology and extensor carpi ulnaris tendon pathology. Skeletal Radiol. 2014; 43: 793-800.

23) Parellada AJ, Morrison WB, Reiter SB. Flexor carpi radialis tendinopathy: spectrum of imaging findings and association with triscaphe arthritis. Skeletal Radiol. 2006; 35: 572-8.

24) Vuillemin V, Guerini H, Bard H, Morvan G. Stenosing tenosynovitis. J Ultrasound. 2012; 15: 20-8.

25) Guerini H, Pessis E, Theumann N, Le Quintrec JS, Campagna R, Chevrot A, et al. Sonographic appearance of trigger fingers. J Ultrasound Med. 2008; 27: 1407-13.

26) Bodor M, Flossman T. Ultrasound-guided first annular pulley injection for trigger finger. J Ultrasound Med. 2009; 28: 737-43.

27) Kürklü M, Bilgiç S, Kömürcü M, Özçakar L. Sonographic evidence for the absence of abductor pollicis longus, extensor poliicis longus, and brevis. Orthopedics. 2010; 33(4).

28) Tagliafico A, Rubino M, Autuori A, Bianchi S, Martinoli C. Wrist and hand ultrasound. Semin Musculoskelet Radiol. 2007; 11: 95-104.

29) Schmidt WA. Value of sonography in diagnosis of rheumatoid arthritis. Lancet. 2001; 357: 1056-7.

30) Grassi W, Filippucci E, Farina A, Cervini C. Sonographic imaging of tendons. Arthritis Rheum. 2000; 43: 969-76.

31) McAlinden PS, Teh J. Imaging of the wrist. Imaging. 2003; 5: 180-92.

32) Capelastegui A, Astigarraga E, Fernandez-Canton G, Saralequi I, Larena JA, Merino A. Masses and pseudomasses of the hand and wrist: MR findings in 134 cases. Skeletal Radiol. 1999; 28: 498-507.

33) Miller TT, Potter HG, McCormack RR Jr. Benign soft tissue masses of the wrist and hand: MRI ap-

pearances. Skeletal Radiol. 1994; 23: 327-32.

34) Peh WC, Truong NP, Totty WG, Gilula LA. Pictorial review: magnetic resonance imaging of benign soft tissue masses of the hand and wrist. Clin Radiol. 1995; 50: 519-25.

35) Nguyen V, Choi J, Davis KW. Imaging of wrist masses. Curr Probl Diagn Radiol. 2004; 33: 147-60.

36) De Schepper AM, Hogendoorn PC, Bloem JL. Giant cell tumors of the tendon sheath may present radiologically as intrinsic osseous lesions. Eur Radiol. 2007; 17: 499-502.

37) Jacob D, Cohen M, Bianchi S. Ultrasound imaging of nontraumatic lesions of wrist and hand tendons. Eur Radiol. 2007; 17: 2237-47.

38) de Krom MC, Knipschild PG, Kesster AD, Thijs CT, Boekkooi PF, Spaans F. Carpal tunnel syndrome: prevalence in general population. J Clin Epidemiol. 1992; 45: 373-6.

39) Beekman R, Visser LH. Sonography in the diagnosis of carpal tunnel syndrome: a critical review of the literature. Muscle Nerve. 2003; 27: 26-33.

40) Ulaşli AM, Duymuş M, Nacir B, Erdem HR, Koşar U. Reasons for using swelling ratio in sonographic diagnosis of carpal tunnel syndrome and a reliable method for its calculation. Muscle Nerve. 2013; 47: 396-402.

41) Propeck T, Quinn TJ, Jacobson JA, Paulino AF, Habra G, Darian VB. Sonography and MR imaging of bifid median nerve with anatomic and histologic correlation. AJR Am J Roentgenol. 2000; 175: 1721-5.

42) Kuvat SV, Ozcakar L, Yazar M. A foregoing thenar muscular branch of the median nerve. Indian J Plast Surg. 2010; 43: 106-7.

43) Buchberger W, Judmaier W, Birbamer G, Lener M, Schmidauer C. Carpal tunnel syndrome: diagnosis with high-resolution sonography. AJR Am J Roentgenol. 1992; 159: 793-8.

44) Visser LH, Smidt MH, Lee ML. High-resolution sonography versus EMG in the diagnosis of carpal tunnel syndrome. J Neurol Neurosurg Psychiatry. 2008; 79: 63–7.

45) Duncan I, Sullivan P, Lomas F. Sonography in the diagnosis of carpal tunnel syndrome. AJR Am J Roentgenol. 1999; 173: 681-4.

46) Bayrak IK, Bayrak AO, Tilki HE, Nural MS, Sunter T. Ultrasonography in carpal tunnel syndrome: comparison with electrophysiological stage and motor unit number estimate. Muscle Nerve. 2007; 35: 344-8.

47) Mondelli M, Filippou G, Gallo A, Frediani B. Diagnostic utility of ultrasonography versus nerve conduction studies in mild carpal tunnel syndrome Arthritis Rheum. 2008: 59; 357-6.

48) Hobson-Webb LD, Massay JM, Juel VC, Sanders DB. The ultrasonographic wrist-to forearm median nerve area ratio in carpal tunnel syndrome. Clin Neurophysiol. 2008; 119: 1353-7.

49) Paliwal PR, Therimadasamy AK, Chan YC, Wilder-Smith EP. Does measuring the median nerve at the carpal tunnel outlet improve ulrasound CTS diagnosis? J Neurol Sci. 2014; 339: 47-51.

50) Boland RA, Adams RD. Vascular factors in carpal tunnel syndrome. J Hand Ther. 2002; 15: 22-30.

51) Kobayashi S, Meir A, Baba H, Uchida K, Hayakawa K. Imaging of intraneural edema by using gadolinium-enhanced MR imaging: experimental compression injury. AJNR Am J Neuroradiol. 2005; 26: 973-80.

52) Ghasemi-Esfe AR, Khalilzadeh O, Vaziri-Bozorg SM, Jajroudi M, Shakiba M, Mazloumi M, et al. Color and power doppler US for diagnosing carpal tunnel syndrome and determining its severity: A quantative image processing method. Radiology. 2011; 261: 499-506.

53) Dejaco C, Stradner M, Zauner D, Seel W, Simmet NE, Klammer A, et al. Ultrasound for diagnosis of carpal tunnel syndrome: comparison of different methods to determine median nerve volume and value of power Doppler sonography. Ann Rheum Dis. 2013; 72: 1934-9.

54) Ettema AM, Amadio PC, Zhao C, Wold LE, An KN. A histological and immunohistochemical study of the subsynovial connective tissue in idiopathic carpal tunnel syndrome. J Bone Joint Surg Am. 2004; 86: 1458-66.

55) Filus A, Korstanje JWH, Selles RW, Hovius SER, Slijper HP. Dynamic sonographic measurements at the carpal tunnel inlet: reliability and reference values in healthy wrists. Muscle Nerve. 2013; 48: 525-31.

56) Ozcan HN, Kara M, Ozcan F, Bostanoğlu S, Karademir MA, Erkin G, et al. Dynamic doppler evaluation of the radial and ulnar arteries in patients with carpal tunnel syndrome. AJR Am J Roentgenol. 2011; 197: 817-20.

57) Uchiyama S, Itsubo T, Yasutomi T, Nakagawa H, Kamimura M, Kato H. Quantitative MRI of the wrist and nerve conduction studies in patients with idiopathic carpal tunnel syndrome. J Neurol Neurosurg Psychiatry. 2005; 76: 1103-8.

58) Orman G, Ozben S, Huseyinoğlu N, Duymuş M, Orman KG. Ultrasound elastographic evaluation in the diagnosis of carpal tunnel syndrome: Initial findings. Ultrasound in Med and Biol. 2013; 39: 1184-9.

59) Gross MS, Gelberman RH. The anatomy of the distal ulnar tunnel. Clin Orthop Relat Res. 1985; 196: 238-47.

60) Pierre-Jerome C, Moncayo V, Terk MR. The Guyon's canal in perspective: 3-T MRI assessment of the normal anatomy, the anatomical variations

and the Guyon's canal syndrome. Surg Radiol Anat. 2011; 33: 897-903.

61) Zeiss J, Jakab E, Khimji T, Imbriglia J. The ulnar tunnel at the wrist (Guyon's canal): normal MR anatomy and variants. AJR Am J Roentgenol. 1992; 158: 1081-5.

62) Gozke E, Dortcan N, Kocer A, Cetinkaya M, Akyuz G, Us O. Ulnar nerve entrapment at wrist associated with carpal tunnel syndrome. Neurophysiol Clin. 2003; 33: 219-22.

63) Seror P. Electrophysiological pattern of 53 cases of ulnar nerve lesion at the wrist. Neurophysiol Clin. 2013; 43: 95-103.

64) Tagliafico A, Cadoni A, Fisci E, Gennaro S, Molfetta L, Perez MM, et al. Nerves of the hand beyond the carpal tunnel. Semin Musculoskeletal Radiol. 2012; 16: 129-36.

65) Harvie P, Patel N, Ostlere SJ. Prevalence and epidemiological variation of anomalous muscles at Guyon's canal. J Hand Surg [Br]. 2004; 29: 26-9.

66) Dang AC, Rodner CM. Unusual compression neuropathies of the forearm, part I: radial nerve. J Hand Surg. 2009; 34: 1906-14.

67) Dellon AL, Mackinnon SE. Radial sensory nerve entrapment in the forearm. J Hand Surg. 1986; 11: 199-205.

68) Dellon AL, Mackinnon SE. Susceptibility of the superficial sensory branch of the radial nerve to form painful neuromas. J Hand Surg. 1984; 9: 42-5.

69) Erol O, Ozcakar L, Çetin A. Sonography streamlines the diagnosis in hand injuries with small foreign bodies. J Emerg Med. 2010; 39: 502-3.

70) Bianchi S, Martinoli C, Abdelwahab IF. High-frequency ultrasound examination of the wrist and hand. Skeletal Radiol. 1999; 28: 121-9.

71) Karabay N. US findings in traumatic wrist and hand injuries. Diagn Interv Radiol. 2013; 19: 320-5.

72) Shinohara T, Horii E, Majima M, Nakao E, Suzuki M, Nakamura R, et al. Sonographic diagnosis of acute injuries of the ulnar collateral ligament of the metacarpophalangeal joint of the thumb. J Clin Ultrasound. 2007; 35: 73-7.

73) Ebrahim FS, De Maeseneer M, Jager T, Marcelis S, Jamadar DA, Jacobson JA. US diagnosis of UCL tears of the thumb and Stener lesions: technique, pattern-based approach, and differential diagnosis. Radiographics. 2006; 26: 1007-20.

74) Canella Moraes Carmo C, Cruz GP, Trudell D, Hughes T, Chung C, Resnick D. Anatomical features of metacarpal heads that simulate bone erosions: cadaveric study using computed tomography scanning and sectional radiography. J Comput Assist Tomogr. 2009; 33: 573-8.

75) Kataoka T, Moritomo H, Miyake J, Murase T, Yoshikawa H, Sugamoto K. Changes in shape and length of the collateral and accessory collateral liga-ments of the metacarpophalangeal joint during flexion. J Bone Joint Surg Am. 2011; 93: 1318-25.

76) Stener B. Displacement of the ruptured ulnar collateral ligament of the metacarpo-phalangeal joint of the thumb: a clinical and anatomical study. J Bone Joint Surg Br. 1962; 44: 869-79.

77) Melville D, Jacobson JA, Haase S, Brandon C, Brigido MK, Fessel D. Ultrasound of displaced ulnar collateral ligament tears of the thumb: the Stener lesion revisited. Skeletal Radiol. 2013; 42: 667-73.

78) Backhaus M, Ohrndorf S, Kellner H, Strunk J, Backhaus TM, Hartung W, et al. Evaluation of a novel 7-joint ultrasound score in daily rheumatologic practice: a pilot project. Arthritis Rheum. 2009; 61: 1194-201.

79) Ostergaard M, Szkudlarek M. Ultrasonography: a valid method for assessing rheumatoid arthritis? Arthritis Rheum. 2005; 52: 681-6.

80) Wakefield RJ, Balint PV, Szudlarek M, Filipucci E, Backhaus M, D'Agostino MA, et al. Musculoskeletal ultrasound including definitions for ultrasonographic pathology. J Rheumatol. 2005; 32: 2485-7.

81) Weidekamm C, Koller M, Weber M, Kainberger F. Diagnostic value of high resolution B mode and Doppler sonography for imaging of hand and finger joints in rheumatoid arthritis. Arthritis Rheum. 2003; 48: 325-33.

82) Szudlarek M, Court-Payen M, Jacobsen S, Klarlund M, Thomsen HS, Ostergaard M. Interobserver agreement in ultrasonography of the finger and toe joints in rheumatoid arthritis. Arthritis Rheum. 2003; 48: 955-62.

83) Dougados M, Jousse-Jolin S, Mistretta F, D'Agostino MA, Backhaus M, Bentin J, et al. Evaluation of several ultrasonography scoring systems for synovitis and comparison to clinical examination: results from a prospective multicenter study of rheumatoid arthritis. Ann Rheum Dis. 2010; 69: 828-33.

84) Filippucci E, Farina A, Carotti M, Salaffi F, Grassi W. Gray scale and power Doppler sonographic changes induced by intra-articular steroid injection treatment. Ann Rheum Dis. 2004; 63: 740-3.

85) Terslev L, Torp-Pedersen E, Qvistgaard E, Kristoffersen H, Rogind H, Danneskiold-Sampsoe B, et al. Effects of treatment with etanercept (Enbrel, TNRF:Fc) on rheumatoid arthritis evaluated by Doppler ultrasonography. Ann Rheum Dis. 2003; 62: 178-81.

86) Ellegaard K, Torp-Pedersen S, Terslev L, Danneskiold-Samsoe B, Henriksen M, Bliddal H. Ultrasound Colour Doppler measurements in a single joint as measure of disease activity in patients with rheumatoid arthritis-assessment of current validity. Rheumatology (Oxford). 2009; 48: 254-7.

# Ultrasound Evaluation of the Hip

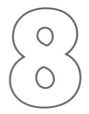

Adelheid STEYAERT

## 8.1 INTRODUCTION

In 1979, Kramps and Lenschow mentioned the opportunity of visualising the hip with ultrasound (US). However, for a long time this investigation has had a relatively limited role in the assessment of hip pathologies, due to the deep location of the joint [1]. Developmental dysplasia of the hip was the first focus in the 20th century [2, 3]: for this topic we refer to the chapter "Ultrasound Imaging in Pediatric Conditions", in this book. Thereafter, technological improvements made US of the adult hip more applicable, accurate and popular since the turn of the century [4, 5]. Effusion of the hip joint is the most important indication for this technical investigation.

## 8.2 EXAMINATION TECHNIQUE

The hip joint is a deep articulation and can be examined using transducers with wide frequency range. Superficial structures are well visualized with linear multi-frequency (9-15 MHz) transducers. The joint recess of the hip is better visualized with lower-frequency transducers (5-7.5 MHz). In obese patients, sometimes 3.5-5 MHz would be necessary.

There are four major sites (quadrants) to be explored for the US examination of the hip: anterior (groin), lateral (trochanter), medial (adductor) and posterior (buttock). Various structures including the pertinent tendons, muscles, nerves, bursae, cartilage, joint etc. can be visualized. Doppler US imaging can be interesting in case of inflammatory pathologies. All findings should be documented in two perpendicular planes, and comparison with the contralateral hip is absolutely warranted [6].

### 8.2.1 Anterior Quadrant

For the examination of the anterior side, the patient should be in a supine position with the legs in extension and a mild external rotation. It is important to recheck the position of the legs during the examination; yet a false positive left-right difference for joint effusion may result with different joint positioning, e.g. a minimal unilateral internal rotation (Figure 8.1). The probe should be kept in a sagittal oblique way, parallel to the long axis of the femoral neck (Figure 8.2). From proximal to distal, the cortex of the acetabulum, femoral head and neck can be seen as hyperechoic structures. The femoral head is covered by a thin hypoechoic layer, which represents the hyaline articular cartilage [7-9]. In between the acetabulum and the femoral head, the hyperechoic triangular structure corresponds to the labrum (fibrocartilage), whereby only its anterior superior portion can be effectively visualized [7, 8] (Figure 8.3).

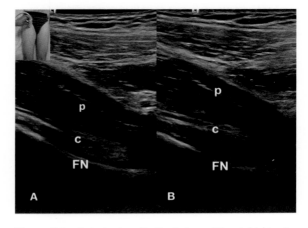

**Figure 8.1** Anterior longitudinal view of the right hip. A - In slight exorotation. B - In slight endorotation. FN, femoral neck; c, capsule, p, psoas muscle.

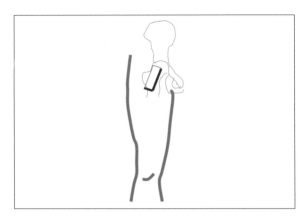

Figure 8.2    Position of the transducer for the anterior longitudinal view in an oblique way parallel to the long axis of the femoral neck.

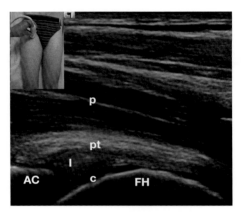

Figure 8.3    Anterior longitudinal proximal view of the right hip. AC, acetabulum; c, cartilage; FH, femoral head; l, labrum; p, psoas muscle; pt, psoas tendon.

From the acetabular rim the capsule runs as a hyperechoic structure inserting onto the femoral neck. On the inner side of the capsule lies the synovium and on the outer side the iliofemoral and pubofemoral ligaments. Normally the capsule appears concave or flat, however about 9% of a-symptomatic hips exhibit anterior capsular bulging in the absence of effusion [5].

Although it might vary, the distance between the cortex of the femur (neck) and the upper line of the capsule is normally 7-9 mm. Anterior to the capsule the iliopsoas muscle can be seen. Its tendon -a homogeneously hyperechoic fibrillar structure- runs posteriorly and medially in the muscle

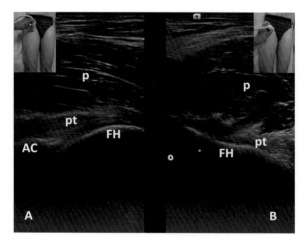

Figure 8.4    Anterior view of the right hip over the femoral head. A - Longitudinal. B - Transverse. FH, femoral head; p, psoas muscle; pt, psoas tendon; AC, acetabulum.

belly, anteromedial to and parallel with the joint capsule (Figure 8.4).

Medially to the iliopsoas muscle, the femoral nerve can be visualized as a honeycomb structure consisting of several small hypoechoic spaces each surrounded by a hyperechoic thin rim. More medially, femoral artery and vein are seen whereby the use of Doppler -venous collapse on probe compression or distension during Valsalva maneuver- can be used to distinguish the femoral vein [7, 8].

While the mean cross-sectional area of the femoral nerve in the infrainguinal area measures approximately 22,7 mm², 3-4 cm distal to the inguinal ligament, it suddenly gets smaller as it divides into multiple branches in the groin [10].

Medial to these neurovascular structures, the pectineus muscle takes its origin from pubis. Subcutaneously the inguinal lymph nodes can be seen as oval hypoechoic structures, with hyperechoic centers (usually with less than 1 cm in diameter).

On the lateral side, the cortex of the anterior inferior iliac spine is visualized, possibly preceded by palpation. With the probe in the sagittal plane the cortex can be seen as a hyperechoic curved line where the direct tendon of the rectus femoris starts (Figure 8.5). The indirect tendon originates from the superolateral margin of the acetabulum. The indirect tendon travels with the central aponeurosis whereas the direct tendon travels with the superficial fascia. On transverse view, the oblique indirect tendon causes an artifact as a posterior acoustic shadowing to the overlying hyperechoic direct tendon [11].

More laterally and superiorly lies the anterior

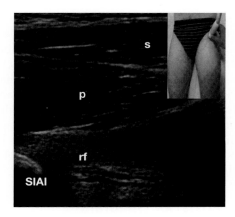

Figure 8.5 Anterior longitudinal view of the left hip starting at the spina iliaca anterior inferior (SIAI); p, psoas muscle; s, sartorius muscle; rf, direct tendon of rectus femoris muscle.

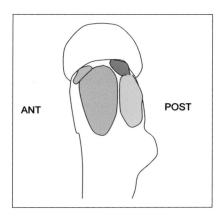

Figure 8.6 Four facets of lateral hip. Blue, anterior; pink, lateral; green, posterosuperior; yellow, posterior.

superior iliac spine with the origin of the sartorius and tensor fascia lata muscles. To distinguish them, the probe can be put in the axial plane and the pennate structure of the different muscles can be followed from proximal to distal. The sartorius muscle has a triangular shape and crosses the upper leg from proximal lateral to distal medial. The muscles pennate structure is seen as contiguous hypoechoic muscular bundles/fascicles, separated from one another by hyperechoic lines/perimysium. Typically, the tensor fascia lata is hypoechoic at proximal level, but it becomes more echogenic at distal level. The latter is the result of increased fat content among the myofibrils. Just proximal to the greater trochanter, the distal musculotendineous junction is encountered with the muscle inserting obliquely into the iliotibial tract over a distance of approximately 7 cm [8, 12, 13].

At the level of the inguinal ligament, about 2 cm medial to the anterior superior iliac spine, the lateral femoral cutaneus nerve can be viewed on axial view as a small, flat, oval hyper- to hypo-echoic structure in the subcutaneous tissue (or sometimes within/deep to the inguinal ligament). Than it dives vertically to run superficial to the sartorius muscle and, in approximately 60% of cases, splits into an anterior and a posterior division [14].

## 8.2.2 Lateral Quadrant

Imaging of the lateral side mainly comprises the greater trochanter and the insertions of gluteus medius and minimus tendons. The greater trochanter has four facets: anterior, lateral, super-

ola-teral (or superoposterior), and posterior (Figure 8.6). The gluteus minimus tendon has two components: the dominant portion attaching onto the anterior facet of the greater trochanter, and a smaller portion inserting onto the hip joint capsule. The gluteus medius tendon has a broad attachment on the lateral facet but has also a narrower attachment on the superolateral facet [15-17]. The gluteus maximus runs over the gluteus medius and inserts onto the tensor fascia lata.

For examining the trochanter region, the patient is suggested to lie either in supine or in contralateral decubitus position. The easiest way to start the examination of the trochanter is to view the lateral facet in the longitudinal way parallel to the femoral diaphysis (Figure 8.7). The cortex of the trochanter (that can also be palpated for better

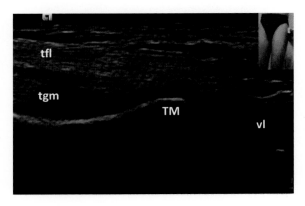

Figure 8.7 Lateral longitudinal view of the left trochanter. TM, greater trochanter (trochanter major); tgm, gluteus medius tendon; vl, vastus lateralis muscle; tfl, tensor fascia lata.

localization) is seen on US examination as a hyperechoic structure which can vary in shape (rounded or more hooked). The gluteus medius tendon can be seen proximally as a hyperechoic fibrillar triangle. To avoid anisotropic effects, the probe can be tilted a little bit, parallel to the insertion of the tendon. Distally the vastus lateralis takes its origin from the lateral facet and can be seen as a pennate structure. Superficial to the gluteus medius tendon and vastus lateralis origin, the iliotibial tract runs as a hyperechoic linear, fibrillar structure. Sometimes the muscle belly of the tensor fascia lata reaches the greater trochanter.

When the probe is moved in an anterosuperior way on the greater trochanter, the gluteus minimus tendon insertion is visualized as a hyperechoic fibrillar structure. The transition from the gluteus minimus tendon to the gluteus medius tendon is not well delineated.

The posterior facet is covered by the muscular structure of the gluteus maximus muscle. On the axial view, the trochanter can be seen as a relatively rounded hyperechoic line, on top of which hyperechoic fibrillar tendon structures of the gluteus medius and minimus (rotator cuff of the hip) reside.

### 8.2.3  Medial Quadrant

On the medial side, the gracilis and the adductor muscles can be scanned. The patient should lie in supine position with some hip and knee flexion, and hip external rotation. The probe should be held in a longitudinal position, parallel to the adductor tendons' origin on the pubic bone. While the pubis is seen as a hyperechoic structure, the origin/proximal portions of the adductor muscles can be seen as three hypoechoic triangular structures: from superficial to deep, as adductor longus, adductor brevis and adductor magnus (Figure 8.8). When the probe is moved a little more medially and vertically, the origin of the gracilis muscle can also be visualized.

### 8.2.4  Posterior Quadrant

On the posterior side, the origin of the hamstring muscles on the ischial tuberosity can be viewed. During the examination, the patient should lie in prone position, with the feet hanging over the edge of the examination table [18]. The ischial tuberosity can again be palpated and the probe should be held in longitudinal position. While the tuberosity is visualized as a hyperechoic structure, the origin of the hamstrings are seen as hyperechoic fibrillar beak-like structures, posterior to it (Figure 8.9). The semimembranosus muscle originates anterolaterally to the conjoined tendon of the biceps femoris and the semitendinosus muscles.

Lateral to the hamstrings' origin, halfway between the ischial tuberosity and the greater trochanter, the sciatic nerve can be observed as a

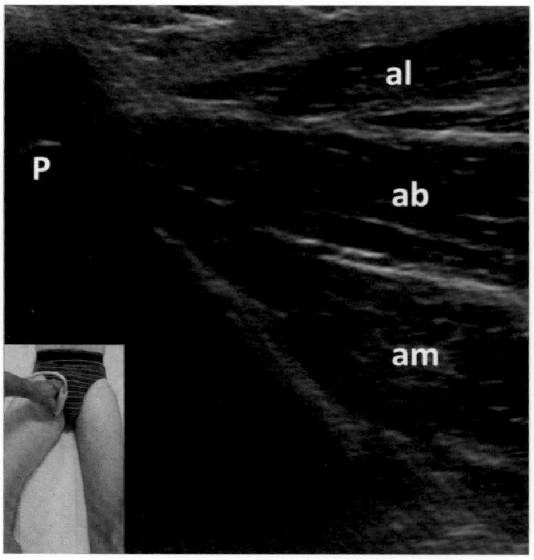

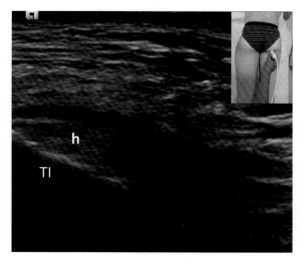

**Figure 8.8**  Medial longitudinal view of the right hip. P, pubis; al, adductor longus muscle; ab, adductor brevis muscle; am, adductor magnus muscle.

**Figure 8.9**  Posterior longitudinal view of the right ischial tuberosity (TI). h, hamstrings origin.

honeycomb structure deep to the gluteus maximus and piriformis muscles (sometimes superficial to it). More distally, it can be detected deep to the biceps muscle [18]. The normal diameter of the nerve is 5 to 9 mm [19].

## 8.3 HIP PATHOLOGIES

Due to its size and deep position, the diagnosis of intra-articular fluid cannot be made clinically. Since US is inexpensive, readily available and safe, it is the first choice for detection of hip effusion. Other indication could be the suspicion of bursitis at the trochanter region, psoas, and ischial tuberosity. However tendon (insertion) problems are more often the source of pain than bursae. There can be tendon swelling, calcifications or rupture (partial or full). Nevertheless, US findings of a tendon will often be normal even with complaints. Another tendon problem is snapping, internal or external. The internal snapping hip can be due to psoas snapping or to an intra-articular problem. The latter should be suspected if there is clinically locking of the hip. External snapping hip takes place at the lateral side due to snapping of the gluteus maximus muscle or tensor fascia lata over the greater trochanter.

Although all above indications are frequently a reason for referral, US is generally not indicated for intra-articular snapping hip, osteoarthritis and labral tears, while much more indicated for fluid detection and extra-articular snapping hip [20].

### 8.3.1 Effusion

A variety of clinical settings is accompanied by effusion: osteoarthritis, osteonecrosis, (transient) synovitis, septic arthritis, occult fracture, hip arthroplasty [21].

Using an accurate probe, as little as 1 ml of intra-articular fluid can be reliably seen [22].

However the differentiation of the kind of effusion (serous, bloody, infectious) cannot be made. The effusion is mostly hypoechoic, although the nature of the fluid content can influence the echogenicity. Hyperemia on power Doppler imaging should suggest synovitis. Arthrocentesis under US guidance can exclude septic arthritis [21, 23].

For the evaluation of effusion, the distance

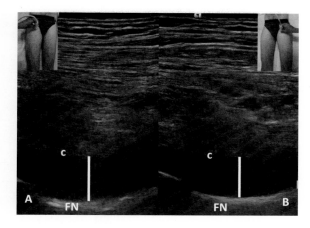

**Figure 8.10** Bilateral intra-articular effusion of the hip. Distance capsule (c) - femoral neck (FN): A - Right hip 10.9 mm. B - Left hip 9.8 mm.

from the top level of the capsule to the cortex of the neck should be measured. According to different studies, the absolute cut-off level is taken as 7-10 mm (Figure 8.10). However looking for a left-right difference of more than 1-2 mm is preferential above a unilateral measurement [5, 24-26]. Effusion is often depicted with US by convexity of the joint capsule; but a convex capsule can also be seen in normal individuals. On the other hand, a concave capsule effectively excludes joint effusion. In case of suspicion for septic arthritis, a blood control should be made and it is mandatory to perform an aspiration for evaluation of the fluid.

In osteoarthritis, US can yield an assessment which is correlated with the pain of the patient. A semiquantitative analysis can be made by scoring four parameters: osteophytes, femoral head, synovial profile, and joint effusion [27].

Ultrasound (US) is also an effective screening tool for post-traumatic hip pain with negative radiographic findings, in the absence of magnetic resonance imaging (MRI) availability. In those cases attention should be paid not only to joint effusion but also to fracture lines, bursal effusion and peritrochanteric edema (hypoechoic fluid collection or heterogeneous soft tissue swelling) [28].

### 8.3.2 Psoas Bursitis

The bursa of the psoas muscle is a virtual space which can be filled in case of pathology. The bursa

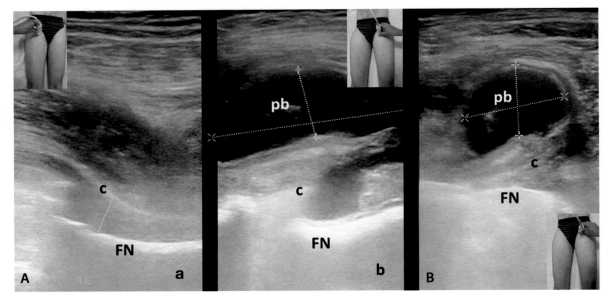

**Figure 8.11** Psoas bursitis. A - Ventral longitudinal view. a, right normal hip; b, left hip with psoas bursa (pb) in connection with hip joint capsule (c). B - Transverse view of the left hip with psoas bursa (pb). FN, femoral neck.

is situated medial to the psoas tendon or between the iliopsoas tendon and the hip joint, communicating with the joint cavity - through a foramen located between the iliofemoral and pubofemoral ligaments - in 10-15% of the cases [11, 29] (Figure 8.11A, B). If filled, it is seen as an anechoic/hypoechoic mass along the medial aspect of the hip joint. It is important to recognize that subtle bursitis can be overlooked easily, if too much pressure is applied on the transducer!

### 8.3.3 Labral Tear

Ultrasound can only visualize the anterior acetabular labrum and has a low sensitivity, specificity and accuracy for labral tears. Therefore, MR arthrography is recommended. If there are contraindications for MRI, US can be performed. Tears of the acetabular labrum are seen as irregular or linear hypoechoic fissures or clefts through the anterior labrum. Associated periarticular fluid collections (ganglion cysts) can also be readily evaluated with US. An intra-articular injection can help to confirm by filling the hypoechoic tear, yielding a sonoarthrographic effect. Another helpful indirect sign is the thickening of the labrum with a cross sectional area of 34.7 mm² or more. This should alert the examiner for the presence of a labral tear [30, 31].

### 8.3.4 Trochanter Pathology

Great trochanteric pain syndrome is a very common problem, sometimes referred as "trochanteritis" or bursitis. However, we know that the pain is often related to a gluteus medius tendinopathy. Different problems of the gluteus medius tendon can be seen. Calcifications can be visualized as hyperechoic structures with different size, mostly in the insertion and sometimes in the body of the tendon. A dense calcification can give a shadow with cortex interruption underneath the calcification. They should be reproduced on the longitudinal view as well as on the axial view. A tendinopathy can also be seen as a thickened hypoechoic tendon. But even with complaints of gluteus medius tendinopathy, US can be normal. Ruptures of the gluteus medius and/or minimus tendons are often associated with bursitis. A partial tear will give a discontinuity of the tendon with intervening anechoic or hypoechoic fluid. A full rupture of the glutei is visualized as a "bald" facet (Figure 8.12).

There are three bursae at the trochanteric region which can be filled in pathologic conditions. The trochanteric bursa lies between the tensor fascia lata and gluteus medius insertions. In the supine position, the fluid will move posteriorly between the cortex (posterior facet) and the glu-

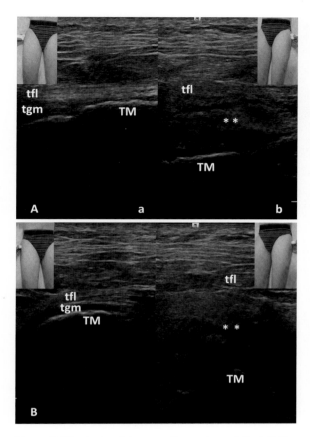

Figure 8.12 Acute gluteus medius rupture of the left hip. A - Longitudinal view of the greater trochanter (TM). a, right normal hip; b, left hip with absence of gluteus medius tendon and soft tissue swelling (*). B - Transverse view of the greater trochanter; tgm, gluteus medius tendon; tfl, tensor fascia lata.

teus maximus. The bursa is not always sharply bounded and part of the gluteus maximus should not be mistaken as the bursa. The examinator should be aware not to press too hard on the probe to visualize the fluid. Otherwise, a filled bursa should be compressible (Figure 8.13). A second one, the submedius bursa, can be found between the cortex of the trochanter (lateral facet) and the tendon of the gluteus medius. This one will not migrate posteriorly and is less frequently filled than the trochanteric bursa. The subminimus bursa can be seen as a hypoechoic halo between the gluteus minimus tendon and the anterior facet. This one is seldomly encountered.

The lateral aspect of the hip is also the peculiar site of the Morel-Lavallée lesion, a posttraumatic seroma that extends along the trochanteric region and the proximal thigh. This fluid collection derives from an injury of the vascular plexus that pierces the fascia lata and expands between the deep layer of the subcutaneous tissue and the fascia. Excessive pressure with the probe should be avoided when examining a Morel-Lavallée lesion to avoid squeezing the bloody effusion away from the field-of-view of the probe. In chronic lesions, the heterogeneous appearance of the hematoma may resemble a soft-tissue tumor [32-35].

### 8.3.5 Pathology of the Adductors

The adductor longus tendon is most commonly involved. In case of a tendinopathy, a hypoechoic

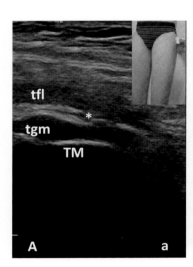
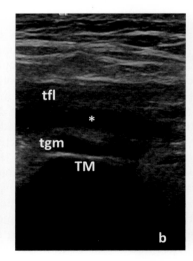
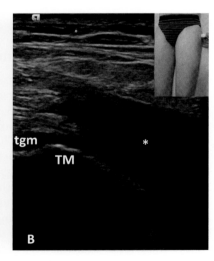

Figure 8.13 Bursitis trochanterica (*) of the left hip. A - Longitudinal view lateral facet. a, with compression; b, without compression. B - Transverse view lateral-posterior facet. TM, greater trochanter; tgm, gluteus medius tendon; tfl, tensor fascia lata.

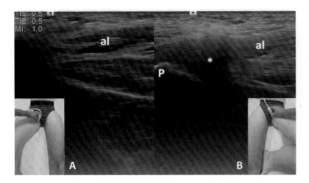

**Figure 8.14** Avulsion of the left adductor longus muscle. Longitudinal medial view of the adductors. A - Normal right hip. B - Retraction of the left adductor longus muscle over 2 cm (*). P, pubis; al, adductor longus muscle.

or inhomogeneous and thickened tendon can sometimes be seen with blurring of the sharp edges. Cortex irregularity can be seen in chronic tendinopathy. However, as with gluteus medius tendinopathy, a normal US does not exclude a tendinopathy. In low-grade injuries and chronic adductor tendinopathy, US has demonstrated low sensitivity in comparison to contrast enhanced MRI [36].

Calcifications can be seen as hyperechoic structures within the tendon. A rupture can be seen as an avulsion with cortex interruption at the pubis or with an intact pubis but hypoechoic fluid filled zone next to the pubis into the adductor longus. The adductor longus can also be retracted in case of a total rupture. And in major traumas the rupture may also involve the superficial fibers of the adductor brevis (Figure 8.14).

## 8.3.6 Snapping Hip Syndrome

Snapping hip syndrome consists of hip pain and audible or perceived snapping of the hip in young adults during movements [15, 16]. A difference should be made between an intra-articular and extra-articular snapping hip. The intra-articular snapping can ensue due to loose bodies, labral tears, osteochondral fractures and synovial chondromatosis. MRI is preferable for this pathology [37, 38]. Extra-articular snapping can occur both on the anterior and lateral side. On the anterior side, a snapping can be produced by the psoas tendon or iliofemoral ligament over the iliopectineal eminence or the lesser trochanter (internal snapping hip). Other proposed mechanisms involve accessory iliopsoas tendinous slips, stenosing tenosynovitis of the iliopsoas insertion and dynamic interaction between the iliopsoas tendon and its muscle [37, 39]. This snapping can be elicited by extending the leg to a neutral position starting out of a flexed, abducted and externally rotated hip. Normally, the tendon should make a smooth move from lateral to medial. In anterior snapping, a sudden movement from the psoas tendon can be seen whether or not associated with an audible click. This diagnosis can often be made clinically. With US, it is sometimes technically difficult to fix the transducer and to ask the patient to move slowly. A videorecording can be useful to review the images more closely [40]. Snapping at the lateral side is due to snapping of the gluteus maximus or the tensor fascia lata over the trochanter (external snapping hip). This can best be elicited by bringing the hip in flexion from an adducted extended position, often in a standing position and with the probe axial to the trochanter.

## 8.3.7 Tendinopathy at the Anterior Superior/Inferior Iliac Spine

Rectus femoris tendinopathy at the anterior inferior iliac spine can be seen as a hypoechoic and/or thickened tendon. Proximal tears of the rectus femoris occur less frequently than tears in the midsubstance of the muscle belly involving the central aponeurosis or the level of the deep distal aponeurosis. Complete proximal tears are rare and may mimic a soft-tissue mass as a result of retraction. In chronic injuries, tendon calcifications and hematoma ossification may be observed [3].

Tendinopathy of the sartorius muscle is rare, whereas tendinopathy of the tensor fascia lata can be seen as a hypoechoic and thickened tendon. The mean size of the tensor fascia lata on transverse view is 2.1 mm (1.5-3.1 mm). A thickening of more than 30% compared to the asymptomatic side can be considered significant. In chronic tendinopathies, cortical irregularity at the iliac crest can be seen [13] (Figure 8.15).

Apophyseal injuries of the iliac spine can also occur in young sporters. When evaluating those injuries, four criteria should be used: a hypoechoic zone in the region of the apophysis extending to the surrounding soft tissue (representing edema or hemorrhage), widening of the normally hypoechoic physis between the apophysis and the pelvis, tilting and dislocation of the apophysis and

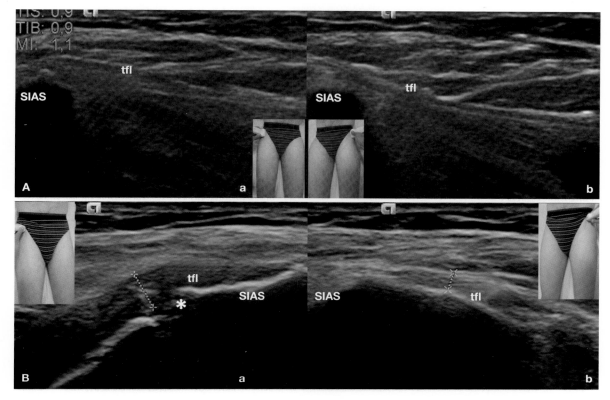

**Figure 8.15** Tendinopathy of the origin of the tensor fasciae latae muscle (tfl) of the right hip. A - Longitudinal anterior view at the spina iliaca anterior superior (SIAS). a, thickening of the origin; b, normal left hip. B - Transverse anterior view at the SIAS. a, thickening and hypoechogenic origin of tfl and cortex irregularity (*); b, normal left hip.

(on Doppler US) hyperemia within the affected region of the apophyseal injury [41].

## 8.3.8 Ischiogluteal Bursitis and Hamstring Tendinopathy

The ischiogluteal bursa is rarely filled in healthy persons. This pathology is also known as "weaver's bottom". If it is a filled, hypoechoic effusion located between the ischial tuberosity and the gluteus maximus. In patients with polymyalgia rheumatica it is more often observed [6, 18].

A tendinopathy of the hamstring origin can be seen as a hypoechoic swollen tendon. Calcifications can also be detected as irregular hyperechoic foci near the ischial tuberosity. In case of rupture, there can be cortex irregularity of the ischial tuberosity and/or a hypoechoic fluid filled zone at the hamstrings origin. The long head of the biceps femoris and the semitendinosus are more frequently affected than the semimembranosus [42].

## 8.3.9 Heterotopic Ossification

The appearance of a heterotopic ossification depends on the duration of the lesion, its rate of formation and the degree of mineralization.

Early in the process, when a radiograph is normal, US shows a nonspecific hypoechoic area that is hypervascular on Doppler imaging. Within 4 to 6 weeks, regions with differing echo properties will appear. A thin, hypoechoic zone is seen at the periphery, a broader reflective zone in the middle, and a small amorphous hypoechoic zone in the center. As the lesion matures, it mineralizes and becomes progressively more visible radiographically.

Calcified lesions have typical US features consisting of a strongly echogenic curvilinear rim and a posterior acoustic shadow.

The combination of radiographic and US findings is sufficient for diagnosis and follow-up [43, 44].

# REFERENCES

1) Kramps HA, Lenschow E. Investigations on hips and extremities by ultrasonics (author's translation). Z Orthop Ihre Grenzgeb. 1979; 117: 355-64.

2) Roberts CS, Beck DJ Jr, Heinsen J, Seligson D. Review article: diagnostic ultrasonography: applications in orthopedaedic surgery. Clin Orthop Relat Res. 2002; 401: 248-64.

3) Martinoli C, Garello I, Marchetti A, Palmieri F, Altafini L, Valle M, et al. Hip ultrasound. Eur J Radiology 2012; 81: 3824-31.

4) Moshe G. Ultrasound of the hip. Eur J Ultrasound. 2001; 14: 35-43.

5) Cho KH, Park BH, Yeon KM. Ultrasound of the adult hip. Semin Ultrasound CT MR. 2000; 21: 214-30.

6) Nestorova R, Vlad V, Petranova T, Porta F, Radunovic G, Micu MC, et al. Ultrasonography of the hip. Med Ultrason. 2012; 14: 217-24.

7) Naredo E, editor. Joint ultrasonography. Sonoanatomy and examination technique. Barcelona: Euromedice, 2007: 134-45.

8) O'Neill J, editor. Musculoskeletal ultrasound, anatomy and technique. New York: Springer, 2008: 167-78.

9) Valley VT, Stanhmer SA. Targeted musculoarticular sonography in the detection of joint effusions. Acad Emerg Med. 2001; 8: 361-7.

10) Gruber H, Peer S, Kovacs P et al. The ultrasonographic appearance of the femoral nerve and cases of iatrogenic impairment. J Ultrasound Med. 2003; 22: 163-72.

11) Molini L, Precerutti M, Gervasio A, Draghi F, Bianchi S. Hip: anatomy and US technique. J Ultrasound. 2011; 14: 99-108.

12) McNally EG. Practical musculoskeletal ultrasound. Philadelphia: Elsevier, 2005: 23-8; 136-41.

13) Bass CJ, Connell DA. Sonographic findings of tensor fascia lata tendinopathy: another cause of anterior groin pain; Skeletal Radiol. 2002; 31: 143-8.

14) Martinoli C, Miguel-Perez M, Padua L, Gandolfo N, Zicca A, Tagliafico A. Imaging of neuropathies about the hip. Eur J Radiol. 2013; 82: 17-26.

15) Blankenbaker DG, De Smet AA, Keen JS. Sonography of the iliopsoas tendon and injection of the iliopsoas bursa for diagnosis and management of the painful snapping hip. Skeletal Radiol. 2006; 35: 565-71.

16) Blankenbaker DG, Tuite MJ. The painful hip: new concepts. Skeletal Radiol. 2006; 35: 352-70.

17) Pfirrmann CW, Chung CB, Theumann NH, Trudell DJ, Resnick D. Greater trochanter of the hip: attachment of the abductor mechanism and a complex of three bursae – MR imaging an MR bursography in cadavers and MR imaging in symptomatic volunteers. Radiology. 2001; 221: 469-77.

18) Bianchi S, Martinoli C. Hip. In: Bianchi S, Martinoli C, editors. Ultrasound of the musculoskeletal system. Berlin: Springer, 2007: 551-610.

19) Graif M, Seton A, Nerubai J, Horoszowski H, Itzchak Y. Sciatic nerve: sonographic evaluation and anatomic-pathologic considerations. Radiology. 1991; 181: 405-8.

20) Klauser AS, Tagliafico A, Allen GM, Boutry N, Campbell R, Court-Payen M, et al. Clinical indications for musculoskeletal ultrasound: a Delphi-based consensus paper of the European society of musculoskeletal radiology. Eur Radiol. 2012; 22: 1140-8.

21) Bancroft LW, Merinbaum DJ, Zaleski CG, Peterson JJ, Kransdorf MJ, Berquist TH. Hip ultrasound. Sem Musculoskelet Rad. 2007; 11: 126-36.

22) Valley VT, Stanhmer SA. Targeted musculoarticular sonography in the detection of joint effusions. Acad Emerg Med. 2001; 8: 361-7.

23) Martino F, Silvestri E, Grassi W, Garlaschi G, editors. Musculoskeletal sonography - . Technique, Anatomy, Semeiotics and Pathological Findings in Rheumatic Diseases. Milan: Springer, 2006: 52-61; p. 97-107.

24) Iagnocco A, Filippucci E, Meenagh G, Delle Sedie A, Riente L, Bombardieri S, et al. Ultrasound imaging for the rheumatologist III. Ultrasonography of the hip. Clin Exp Rheumatol. 2006; 24: 229-32.

25) Schmidt WA, Schmidt H, Schicke B, Gromnica-Ihle E. Standard reference values for musculoskeletal ultrasonography. Ann Rheum Dis. 2004; 63: 988-94.

26) Koski JM, Isomaki H. Ultrasonography may reveal synovitis in a clinically silent hip joint. Clin Rheumatol. 1990; 9: 539-41.

27) Qvistgaard E, Torp-Pedersen S, Christensen R, Bliddal H. Reproducibility and inter-reader agreement of a scoring system for ultrasound evaluation of hip osteoarthritis. Ann Rheum Dis. 2006; 65: 1613-9.

28) Safran O, Goldman V, Applbaum Y, Milgrom C, Bloom R, Peyser A, et al. Sonography as a screening test for occult hip fractures. J Ultrasound Med. 2009; 28: 1447-52.

29) Bianchi S, Martinoli C, Keller A, Bianchi-Zamorani MP. Giant iliopsoas bursitis: sonographic findings with magnetic resonance correlations. J Clin Ultrasound. 2002; 30: 437-41.

30) Sofka CM, Adler R, Danon M. Sonography of the acetabular labrum. J Ultrasound Med. 2006; 25: 1321-6.

31) Kantarci F, Ozpeynirci Y, Unlu M, Gulsen F, Ozbayrak M, Botanlioglu H, et al. Cross-sectional area of the labrum: role in diagnosis of anterior ace-

tabular labral tears. Eur Radiol. 2012; 22: 1350-6.

32) Mukherjee K, Perrin SM, Hughes PM. Morel-Lavallée lesion in an adolescent with ultrasound and MRI correlation. Skelet Radiol. 2007; 36: 43-5.

33) Puig J, Pelaez I, Banos J, Balliu E, Casas M, Maroto A, et al. Long-standing Morel-Lavallée lesion in the proximal thigh: ultrasound and MR findings with surgical and histopathological correlation. Australas Radiol. 2006; 50: 594-7.

34) Kalaci A, Karazincir S, Yanat AN. Long-standing Morel-Lavallée lesion of the thigh simulating a neoplasm. Clin Imaging. 2007; 31: 287-91.

35) Choskhi FH, Jose J, Clifford PD. Morel-Lavallée lesion. Am J Orthop. 2010; 39: 252-3.

36) Robinson P, Barron DA, Parsons W, Grainger AJ, Schilders EM, O'Connor PJ. Adductor-related groin pain in athletes: correlation of MR imaging with clinical findings. Skeletal Radiol. 2004; 33: 451-7.

37) Schaberg JE, Harper MC, Allen WC. The snapping hip syndrome. Am J Sports Med. 1984; 12: 361-5.

38) Wahl CJ, Warren RF, Adler RS, Hannafin JA, Hansen B. Internal coxa saltans (snapping hip) as a result of overtraining. Am J Sports Med. 2004; 32: 1302-9.

39) Deslandes M, Guillin R, Cardinal E. The snapping iliopsoas tendon: new mechanisms using dynamic sonography. Am J Roentgenol. 2008; 190: 576-81.

40) Bureau N. Sonographic evaluation of snapping hip syndrome. J Ultrasound Med. 2003; 32: 895-900.

41) Pisacano RM, Miller TT. Comparing sonography with MR imaging of apophyseal injuries of the pelvis in four boys. Am J Roentgenol. 2003; 181: 223-30.

42) Slavotinek JP, Verrall GM, Fon GT. Hamstrings injury in athletes: using MR imaging measurements to compare extent of muscle injury with amount of time lost from competition. Am J Roentgenol. 2002; 179: 1621-8.

43) Fornage BD. Soft tissue masses. In: Fornage BD, editor. Musculoskeletal ultrasound. New York: Churchill Livingstone, 1995: 21-42.

44) Thomas EA, Cassar-Pullicino VN, Mc Call IW. The role of ultrasound in the early diagnosis and management of heterotopic bone formation. Clin Radiol. 1991; 43: 190-6.

# Ultrasound Evaluation of the Knee

İbrahim BATMAZ, Fevziye ÜNSAL MALAS, Levent ÖZÇAKAR

## 9.1 INTRODUCTION

Ultrasound (US) is increasingly being considered as a valuable diagnostic modality for the evaluation of the knee joint [1]. It has been used to evaluate tendons, vessels, nerves, joints and para-articular structures of the knee [2]. However, there are still limitations as regards the evaluation of menisci, cartilage and bone [1]. While magnetic resonance imaging is preferred for relevant pathologies of those structures, US has significant advantages i.e. easily accessible, convenient, user/patient friendly, cost-effective, does not contain radiation, provides dynamic imaging of the knee joint [2, 3].

## 9.2 EXAMINATION TECHNIQUE AND PATIENT POSITION

A high-resolution linear-array transducer with a frequency band range of 7–10 MHz is most commonly used for the evaluation of the knee. However, there are some specific situations when a lower frequency probe (approximately 5 MHz) may be more suitable, e.g. during the visualization of deeply located cysts in the popliteal region or during the assessment of the posterior cruciate ligament [4].

The routine US examination of the knee begins with the anterior compartment, which is followed by the evaluation of the medial, lateral and posterior compartments. The anterior compartment of the knee is typically examined with the patient in supine position. A pillow beneath the popliteal fossa helps to passively stretch the extensor mechanism providing better visualization with less anisotropy-related artifacts [5]. For the medial compartment of the knee, the patient remains supine, with the knee slightly flexed. The hip should be mildly flexed and externally rotated. For US examination of the lateral compartment of the knee joint, the leg may be internally rotated, with the patient either remaining supine, or in a lateral decubitus position [6]. The posterior compartment is examined while the patient lies in prone position with the knee extended. However, imaging the posterior structures with slight flexion can reduce tension on the posterior tendons. Additionally, knee flexion increases the internal pressure of the posterior veins, so that they can obtain their full distension [7]. A variety of structures, such as para-articular ligaments, tendons and related muscles can be(tter be) examined at rest, with stress maneuvers, or during active movements as well.

### 9.2.1 Anterior Compartment

The suprapatellar, juxtapatellar and infrapatellar regions are imaged in succession. Initially, the transducer is swept in a longitudinal plane, from medial to lateral or lateral to medial in the suprapatellar region. The quadriceps tendon, the suprapatellar synovial recess, the suprapatellar fat pad, the prefemoral fat, the distal femoral metaphysis and the trochlea can be visualized in this region.

The normal quadriceps tendon is a hyperechoic, well-defined fibrillar structure extending from the quadriceps muscle inserting to the patella. It is bordered anteriorly by the subcutaneous fat and posteriorly by the suprapatellar fat and bursa. The suprapatellar bursa, also called as the suprapatellar recess, lies deep in the distal part of the quadriceps tendon between the hyperechoic suprapatellar and prefemoral fat pads. With US, the normal suprapatellar bursa is seen as a thin-walled, well-defined anechoic line deep to the quadriceps tendon (Figure 9.1). The same

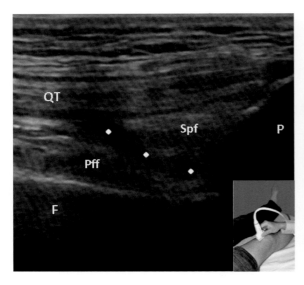

**Figure 9.1** Suprapatellar region. Long axis image over the quadriceps tendon (QT). The synovial recess (rhombi) is bordered anteriorly by the suprapatellar fat (Spf) and posteriorly by the prefemoral fat (Pff) pads. P, patella; F, femur.

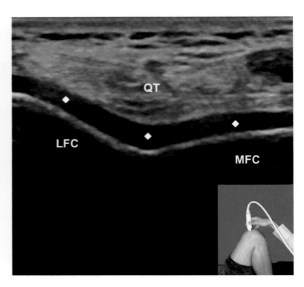

**Figure 9.2** Normal trochlear cartilage. US demonstrates the trochlear cartilage (rhombi) as a homogeneous anechoic band overlying the bright hyperechoic line of the subchondral bone plate. QT, quadriceps tendon; LFC, lateral femoral condyle; MFC, medial femoral condyle.

structures can (needs to) be scanned in the axial view as well.

The knee joint can be further flexed (as much as possible) for scanning the femoral trochlea and the overlying cartilage on transverse plane. Deep to the quadriceps tendon the cartilage is seen as a well-defined, smooth hypo-/an-echoic line covering the highly reflective subchondral bone (Figure 9.2).

Depending on the local measurement, its mean thickness can range between 1.8 and 2.5 mm [8].

The infrapatellar region includes the patellar tendon, the prepatellar and infrapatellar bursae and the Hoffa's fat pad. The patellar tendon is similar in appearance to the quadriceps tendon; a well-defined, hyperechoic, fibrillar structure. The tendon lies between the hyperechoic subcutane-

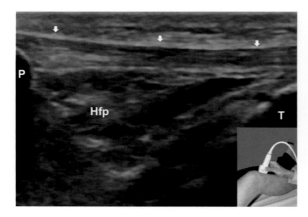

**Figure 9.3** Longitudinal US image over the patellar tendon (arrows). Hoffa's fat pad (Hfp) is seen deep to the patellar tendon with heterogeneous, hypoechoic appearance. P, patella; T, tibia.

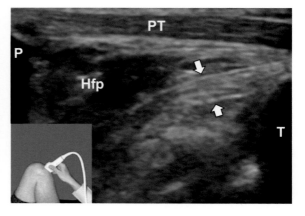

**Figure 9.4** Longitudinal US image over the patellar tendon (PT) depicts the anterior cruciate ligament (arrows) in its long axis, deep to the Hoffa's fat pad (Hfp). P, patella; T, tibia.

Musculoskeletal Ultrasound in Physical and Rehabilitation Medicine

ous fat and Hoffa's fat pad, which is normally seen as a collection of hypoechoic fat lobules separated by thin, hyperechoic fibrous septae (Figure 9.3). Two bursae (superficial and deep infrapatellar) are present at the insertion of the patellar tendon to the tibia. While a small amount of fluid posterior to the distal patellar tendon insertion (deep infrapatellar bursa) is usually observed; the small superficial infrapatellar bursa is typically not visualized on US [1]. The prepatellar bursa is located in the subcutaneous tissue, which overlies the lower pole of the patella and the proximal patellar tendon. In normal conditions, the bursa is again not seen with US because of its thin walls and absence of internal fluid [7].

Imaging the anterior cruciate ligament (ACL) with US can be difficult due to its deep location and oblique orientation. However, positioning the probe (infrapatellar midline) 30 degrees (counter clockwise for the right and clockwise for the left knee) during maximum flexion can help visualize the ligament in long axis. Due to anisotropy, the echogenicity of the ligament may vary and usually its distal part can be seen better/easier (Figure 9.4) [2].

## 9.2.2 Medial Knee Compartment

Major components of the medial knee are medial collateral ligament (MCL), medial meniscus and pes anserine tendons. On US, the MCL appears as an elongated band 1-3 mm thick that is formed by two definite hyperechoic layers, reflecting the superficial part and the deep meniscofemoral and meniscotibial parts of the ligament, and a hypoechoic layer of connective tissue separating these layers [9] (Figure 9.5).

Imaging the medial meniscus on US can be difficult, due to artifacts and limited visualization. However, its outer portion is nicely observed as a triangular-shaped hyperechoic structure positioned at the joint space deep to the MCL (Figure 9.5).

The tendons of sartorius, gracilis and semitendinosus muscles insert on the anteromedial aspect of the tibial metaphysis. The concavity on the anteromedial surface of the proximal tibia is thus covered by thin, hyperechoic fibers from these three tendons. They lay together and cannot be differentiated by US (Figure 9.6). The pes anserine bursa is located between and beneath the tendon insertions on the tibia; sonographically visible only when distended [2].

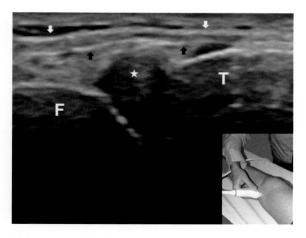

**Figure 9.5** Coronal US image over the medial collateral ligament. The superficial layer appears as a thick, straight fibrillar (white arrows) band and the deep layer is formed by the meniscofemoral and the meniscotibial (black arrows) ligaments which are seen as hyperechoic bands connecting the meniscus (star). F, femur; T, tibia.

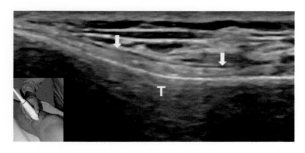

**Figure 9.6** Long-axis US image over the pes anserinus complex demonstrates a hyperechoic band (white arrows) inserting into the anterolateral aspect of the proximal tibial metaphysis (T).

## 9.2.3 Lateral Knee Compartment

Major components of the lateral knee are the distal aspect of the iliotibial band (ITB), lateral meniscus, the lateral collateral ligament (LCL) and the biceps tendon. These structures can be properly identified by the sonographic anatomy and specific bony landmarks [10]. On the most anterior localization, the ITB extends from the fascia lata distally and anteriorly to Gerdy's tubercle, which can be found on the anterolateral aspect of the tibia. The distal segment of the iliotibial band is best imaged on long-axis scans, appearing as a thin, hyperechoic sheath extending broadly over the anterolateral aspect of the knee (Figure 9.7)

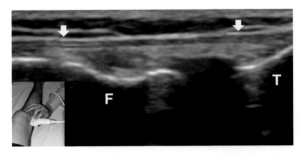

**Figure 9.7** Coronal oblique US image over the iliotibial band shows a hyperechoic band (arrows) inserting to the Gerdy's tubercle on the tibia (T). F, femur.

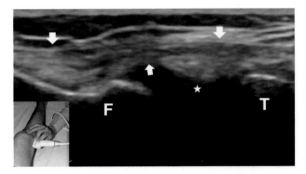

**Figure 9.8** Coronal oblique US image demonstrates the lateral collateral ligament (arrows) and the lateral meniscus (star). F, femur; T, tibia.

lateral. The major components of the posterior knee to be visualized are the gastrocnemius muscle, the semimembranosus tendon, the semimembranosus-gastrocnemius bursa, and the posterior cruciate ligament (PCL).

On US, the semimembranosus-gastrocnemius bursa is a thin-walled, hypoechoic structure located between the medial head of the gastrocnemius muscle and the semimembranosus tendon with little or no fluid. When this bursa becomes pathologically distended, it is named as the Baker's cyst. Herein, in order not to overdiagnose a cystic lesion, sonographers should be cautious as regards the anisotropy artifact pertaining to the semimembranosus or gastrocnemius tendons and the bursa. The bursa will always be relatively hypoechoic, irrespective of the inclination angle of the sound beam, while the tendons are hyperechoic when the US beam is perpendicular to their surfaces (Figure 9.9).

On longitudinal US images, the PCL can be seen as a deep thick hypoechoic band extending into the joint from the posterior lip of the tibia. The transducer should be placed in a sagittal oblique orientation, with the proximal end of the transducer oriented medially. The femoral insertion (proximal part) of the PCL can hardly be evaluated with US (Figure 9.10) [3, 11].

When the probe is moved a little posteriorly, again in long axis, the LCL (extracapsular, 5-7 cm long) can be seen as a hypoechoic, compact structure bridging the lateral femoral condyle and the anterior aspect of the fibular head (Figure 9.8). LCL is 3-4 mm thick and lies in a more anterior plane than does the biceps tendon (seen a little more posteriorly with the same positioning). When imaged with 20-30 degrees of knee flexion, the LCL assumes a vertical oblique orientation, which is quite different from that of the iliotibial band [10].

While scanning from anterior to posterior, deep to the aforementioned three structures, the lateral meniscus can be imaged with an overall appearance similar to that of the medial meniscus i.e. hyperechoic and triangular in shape (Figure 9.8).

### 9.2.4 Posterior Knee Compartment

The patient lies prone while a systematic posterior joint evaluation is performed from medial to

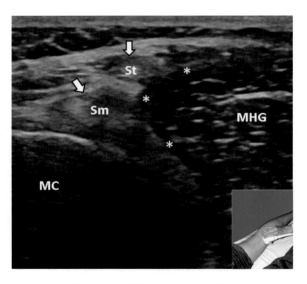

**Figure 9.9** Transverse US image showing the bursa (asterisks) between the medial head of the gastrocnemius muscle (MHG) and the semitendinosus (St) and semimembranosus tendons (Sm) (arrows). MC, medial condyle.

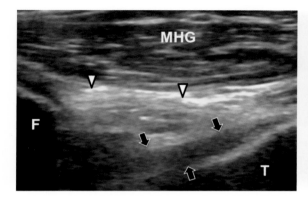

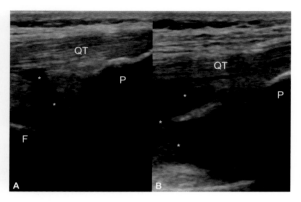

**Figure 9.10**  A sagittal oblique US image shows the posterior cruciate ligament as a thick hypoechoic cord-like structure (arrows). Posterior to the ligament, a triangular fat pad (arrowheads) and the medial head of the gastrocnemius (MHG) can be seen. F, femur; T, tibia.

**Figure 9.11**  A - Small amount of fluid in the suprapatellar bursa under the quadriceps tendon (QT) (asterisk). B - Larger amount of fluid in the suprapatellar bursa (asterisk) consistent with hematoma. F, femur; P, patella.

## 9.3  KNEE PATHOLOGIES

### 9.3.1  Anterior Knee

*Joint effusion and synovial hypertrophy*

Examination starts with evaluation of the suprapatellar area. The knee joint may either be positioned in mild flexion (to detach the layers of the bursa and make it easier) to find fluid in the midline; or in full extension for better localization of the fluid in the medial and lateral pouches of the suprapatellar bursa. As such, prompt evaluation should comprise appropriate medial to lateral fan-like movements of the probe without much compression, to avoid displacement/disappearance of the fluid. In this regard, while fluid more than 3 ml can be detected in the knee joint with US [7], it should always be kept in mind that the position of the knee joint and the contraction of the quadriceps muscle are contributory [4, 12].

When effusion is suspected, transducer compression can be applied to differentiate fluid from synovial hypertrophy. While compressible and displaceable abnormal hypo-/an-echoic intrarticular material which does not exhibit Doppler signal is accepted as effusion, it is more like to be synovial hypertrophy if poorly compressible and exhibiting Doppler signal [13]. A joint effusion can be anechoic suggesting a more acute problem or hypoechoic if it contains some debris. The debris or internal echoes may arise from small loose bodies, inflammation, hemorrhage, or fat globules

(Figure 9.11). Although it may sometimes not possible to conclude on the exact underlying cause, US is definitely an initial imaging tool to guide further investigation in such cases [14].

*Quadriceps tendon*

The quadriceps tendon extends from the four quadriceps muscles and attaches to the upper pole of the patella. The normal quadriceps tendon is hyperechoic and consists of a bundle of fibrillary structures. Quadriceps tendinitis results from focal inflammation or overuse injuries. The tendon loses its fibrillary appearance, becomes hypoechoic and thickened; and in chronic conditions calcifications may also be seen within the tendon [3] (Figure 9.12).

Quadriceps muscle or tendon tears are commonly seen in young athletes [2, 9]. Forced muscle contraction and direct trauma are major causes. Although ruptures are often traumatic; they can

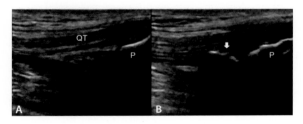

**Figure 9.12**  Comparative imaging of the quadriceps tendon (QT). A - Normal side. B - Quadriceps tendinitis. The fibrillary structure of the tendon is lost with hypoechoic appearance and calcification (arrow).

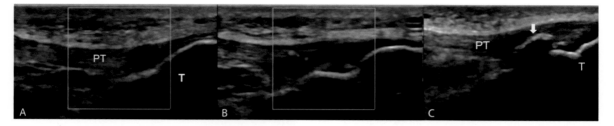

**Figure 9.13** Longitudinal imaging over the patellar tendon (PT) during 30° of knee flexion. When compared to the normal side (A, upper left), PT is enlarged and hypoechoic with power Doppler activity on the side of tendinitis (B, upper right). Arrow show calcified areas over the tuberosity of tibia (T) in Osgood Schlatter disease (C, below).

also be idiopathic or due to systemic diseases e.g. systemic lupus erythematosus, gout, rheumatoid arthritis, hyperpararthyroidism, diabetes, chronic renal failure. Partial ruptures present as anechoic or hypoechoic areas with distorted fibrillary

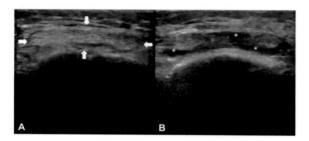

**Figure 9.14** Axial view of the patellar tendon. While arrows show the borders of the patellar tendon on the normal side (A), asterisks show the ruptured areas on the symptomatic side of the patient (B).

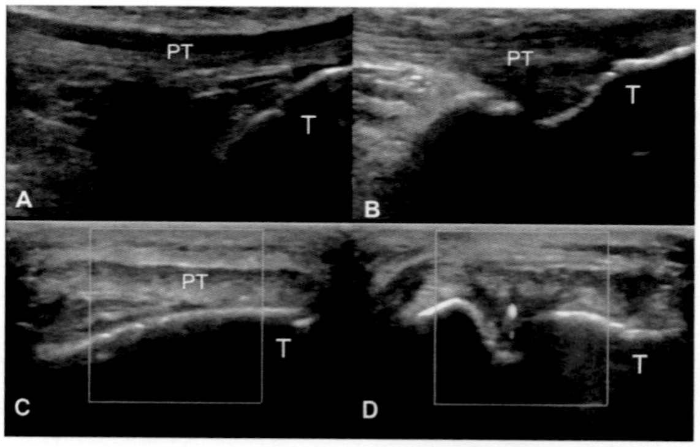

**Figure 9.15** Comparative patellar tendon (PT) imaging after bone-tendon-bone grafting. Longitudinal (A) and axial views of the normal side (C). On the operated side, the tendon is enlarged and edematous (B) and the cortical defect displays power doppler signal (D). T, tibia.

structure of the tendon [15]. In complete tears, ruptured muscle parts are separated from each other with rounded margins. Differentiation of the partial tears from complete tears is important since complete tears entail surgical intervention.

### Patellar tendon

Patellar tendon bridges the caudal aspect of the patella to the anterior tubercle of the tibia. Patellar tendinitis commonly ensues due to the repetitive use of knee extensor muscles. This condition, which is also known as `jumper's knee`, affects the proximal portion of the tendon at the apex of the patella. Jumper's knee is commonly seen in young active athletes e.g. long-distance runners and football players. In patellar tendinitis, the tendon may show multiple sites of hypoechoic thickening or may exhibit uniformly thickened and hypoechoic appearance (Figure 9.13 A). As mentioned above, chronic tendinitis process may show calcification in the tendon as well [3, 16].

Sinding-Larsen-Johansson (patellar apophysitis) and Osgood-Schlatter (tibial apophysitis) diseases are two conditions affecting the immature cartilage tendon junction in adolescents. The junction eventually becomes inflamed due to overloading. US imaging can readily demonstrate the abnormal echotexture, enlargement and the focal sharp-edged calcifications (Figure 9.13 C) [17]. Power Doppler examination can additionally show the ongoing inflammation (Figure 9.13 B).

Complete tears of the patellar tendon may result after direct trauma or following tendinopathies. The tear can be diagnosed by physical examination with a swollen knee, pain and tenderness on the infrapatellar region. However, US reveals separated tendon ends with an interrupted wavy tendon [18]. Incomplete tears are very rare [7] (Figures 9.14, 9.15).

Musculoskeletal Ultrasound in Physical and Rehabilitation Medicine

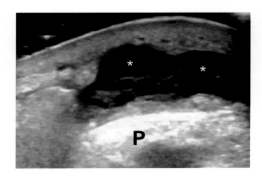

**Figure 9.16** Prepatellar bursitis (house-maid`s knee). The image demonstrates an-/hypo-echoic heterogenous fluid formation in the prepatellar bursa and thickening of the prepatellar subcutaneous tissue. P, patella.

## Bursitis

There are several bursae around the knee joint and any disease affecting the nearby structures may also involve the bursae, presenting as fluid accumulation. The prepatellar bursa is located in the subcutaneous tissue over the lower part of the patella. Prepatellar bursitis commonly known as `house-maid`s knee` occurs mainly due to trauma. On US, hypoechoic fluid formation and thickening of the prepatellar subcutaneous tissue are recognized [19] (Figure 9.16). In normal conditions, the prepatellar bursa cavity cannot be identified. Again, as the localization of the bursa is quite superficial, probe compression should be avoided during scanning for fluid. In acute conditions, power Doppler can exhibit excessive vascularization [4].

Infrapatellar bursa is deeply located between the patellar tendon and Hoffa`s fat pad. Aside from the overuse type of injuries, its is noteworthy that infrapatellar bursitis can accompany patholo-

gies of the entheseal region [20] (Figure 9.17 B). On the other hand, a small amount of fluid in the infrapatellar bursa can also be seen in healthy subject [7] (Figure 9.17 A).

### 9.3.2 Medial Knee

#### Medial collateral ligament

The medial collateral ligament (MCL) displays a tri-laminar appearance; two hyperechoic zones (superficial and deep) and a hypoechoic layer of connective tissue in between [9]. The deep layer is more prone to ruptures [21] and when there is an isolated tear in the deep layer, the superficial layer can displace laterally because of the accumulation of fluid or blood. MCL tear is usually seen together with medial meniscus and anterior cruciate ligament ruptures [1]. A thick or calcified ligament can represent an old injury [21]. Pellegrini-Stieda disease is a kind of heterotopic ossification within the upper part of the ligament which may appear with chronic partial avulsion of the MCL from the femoral origin (Figure 9.18). It is usually related with a chronic injury of valgus stress [3].

#### Pes anserinus

The pes anserine bursa may not be seen in normal subjects; however inflammation of the tendons, bursitis and ganglion formations can be the relevant pathologies commonly seen in this area (Figure 9.19). Hypoechoic mass in the anteromedial knee arising between the pes anserine tendons and the MCL represents bursitis. Power Doppler evaluation can help discriminate acute and chronic bursitis [3].

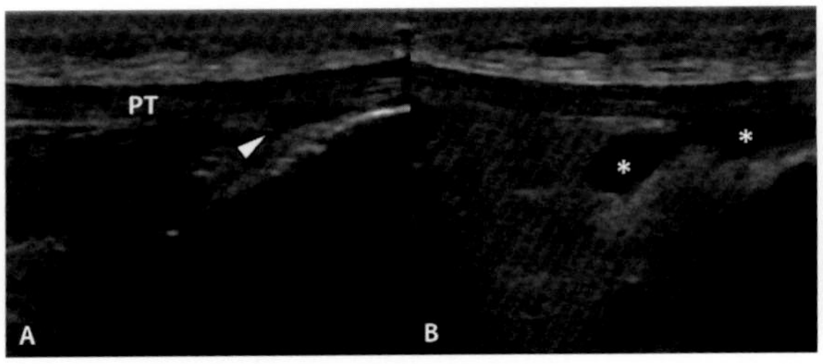

**Figure 9.17** Longitudinal US images of the infrapatellar region. The bursa is seen on the normal side (arrowhead) (A). Abnormal fluid accummulation (asterisks) is observed on the symptomatic side, consistent with infrapatellar bursitis. PT, patellar tendon.

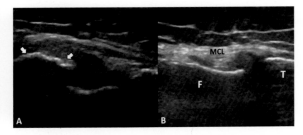

**Figure 9.18** Pellegrini-Stieda disease. Cloudy appearance of the heterotopic ossification (arrows) within the proximal portion of the medial collateral ligament (MCL) is observed (A). Normal side (B). T, tibia; F, femur.

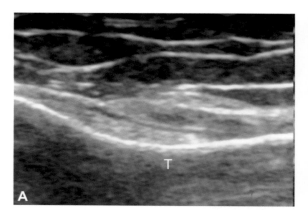 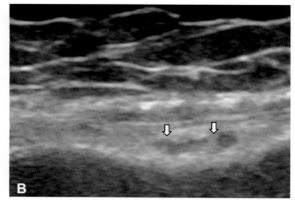

**Figure 9.19** Pes anserinus bursitis. Longitudinal image demonstrates abnormal fluid collection (arrows) between the blurred tendons and the tibia (T) (B). Normal side (A).

### 9.3.3 **Lateral Knee**

#### *Lateral collateral ligament*

Lateral collateral ligament (LCL) lesions are less commonly encountered than MCL. They are usually associated with varus stress injury of the knee [22]. On US, LCL is seen more hypoechoic, enlarged and thickened in a fusiform fashion in partial tears (Figure 9.20). Complete tear of the LCL is quite uncommon [3]. Although avulsion of the LCL at fibular insertion is also unusual, when it occurs, the biceps femoris tendon injury accompanies as well. Chronic friction type injury can cause bursitis between LCL and the popliteus tendon and exhibits an irregular fluid collection on US [3].

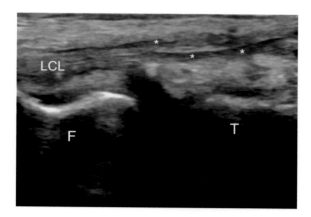

**Figure 9.20** Partial tear of the lateral collateral ligament (LCL) is diagnosed with intrasubstance heterogenous areas (asterisks) inside the thickened ligament. T, tibia; F, femur.

#### *Iliotibial band*

The most common pathology of ITB is the ITB friction syndrome [3]. This is often seen after strenuous physical activity causing chronic local impingement of the ITB against the lateral condyle [7]. This pathology is known as the 'runner's knee'. The ITB becomes thickened and inflamed, and a bursa may be seen between the ITB and the femoral condyle [3]. On US, the band loses clarity in its outer margin; becomes hypoechoic and thickened in a fusiform shape [3]. Dynamic evaluation by flexion and extension of the knee may help confirm the diagnosis of ITB friction syndrome.

#### *Lateral and medial menisci*

Although magnetic resonance imaging is the gold standard modality [23] to evaluate the meniscal lesions, US can be useful for patients with suspected internal knee derangement who cannot undergo the MRI exam because of claustrophobia, obesity and an incompatible implant [9].

Meniscal tears usually include anechoic or hypoechoic linear clefts within the meniscus but also hyperechoic tears have been identified [9]. Peripheral and posterior tears are better visualized and small internal or medial tears can be missed. Degeneration of the menisci may appear with swollen menisci with decreased echogenity on US [1]. The menisci often bulge out of the joint space and may include small cysts as well (Figure 9.21). Linear hyperechoic appearance can stem from meniscal chondrocalcinosis [2, 24].

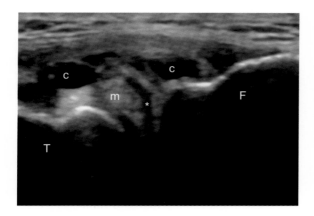

Figure 9.21 Medial longitudinal image of the knee joint demonstrating an extruded meniscus (m) with a horizontal tear (asterisk) and cyst (c) formation. T, tibia; F, femur.

Meniscal cysts (more on the lateral side) are encapsulated lesions, full of synovial-like fluid. These cysts can accompany horizontal tears, often containing septa or debris and visualized as hypoechoic or partially anechoic structures [1, 3, 25]. Meniscal cysts are more commonly seen in the lateral meniscus [25].

## Cruciate ligament pathology

Hyperflexion of the knee is required for evaluation of the distal ACL fibers. However, in an injured knee, this causes more stress on the joint and may be difficult. Herewith, detection of some indirect signs such as fluid, mass, or hematoma can be useful (3). A hypoechoic collection on the lateral wall of the intercondylar notch is regarded as proximal ACL hematoma, representing acute ACL rupture [26].

Posterior cruciate ligament (PCL) injuries are less common than the ACL injuries [3]. PCL ruptures are usually associated with other pathologies such as ACL and collateral ligament injuries. Hyperrotation, hyperextension or direct trauma to a flexed knee are the most common causes of PCL injury [3]. On US, PCL rupture can be visualized as the loss of normal shape, becoming hypoechoic and thickened to more than 10 mm [27].

## Femoral cartilage

The distal femoral cartilage is best evaluated in a hyperflexed knee at the patellar level [20]. Loss of clarity and sharp contour, margin irregularities

are the signs of cartilage pathology [28]. While asymmetrically thinned cartilage is seen in osteoarthritis, the type of involvement is more symmetrical in other diseases like rheumatoid arthritis [20]. Osteophytes can also be seen in patients with osteoarthritis. The tibiofemoral joint is the best place to visualize those osteophytes i.e. step-up bony prominences at the edges of the bony borders of joint margins [20].

### 9.3.4 Posterior Knee

#### Baker`s cyst

Baker`s cyst results from distension of the gastrocnemius-semimembranous bursa on the medial side of the popliteal fossa (Figure 9.22 A). Normally, little or no fluid is seen between these two structures on US (Figure 9.22 B). The bursa has communication with the knee joint and flexion causes uni-directional fluid accummulation inside it [7]. Baker's cyst can result from any disease that increases fluid in the joint e.g. inflammatory arthropathies, villonodular synovitis,

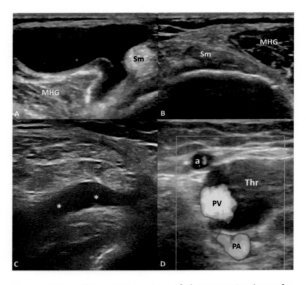

Figure 9.22 Comparative view of the posterior knee for Baker`s cyst (A). Normal side (B). Note the anechoic fluid between the medial head of the gastrocnemius muscle (MHG) and the semimembranosus tendon (Sm). Free fluid (asterisks) spreading into the fascial layers of the gastrocnemius muscle represents a ruptured Baker`s cyst (C). Power Doppler imaging for an aneurysmal dilatation (a) of the popliteal vein (PV) possibly due to a thrombus (Thr) (D). Although being more laterally localized, aneurysms of the popliteal artery (PA) or vein can easily be misinterpreted as a Baker's cyst.

osteonecrosis, meniscal tears and loose bodies [3, 29-31]. The bursa may appear septated and compartmentalized.

Rupture of the bursa can also be seen whereby its rounded shape is lost and the fluid distends into the gastro-soleus complex (Figure 9.22 C). This presents as sharp angulated anechoic zones within the muscle [32], and clinically painful swelling and tenderness over the calf. Sometimes this complication (also referred as pseudothrombophlebitis) may produce inflammatory changes that mimic thrombophlebitis. Inflammation of the surrounding tissues around the ruptured cyst may cause very little anechoic fluid left in the cyst and may show ill-defined areas of echogenicity [9, 16, 33, 34].

The differential diagnosis of a Baker's cyst comprises popliteal aneurysms (Figure 9.22 D), variceal dilatations and soft tissue masses (e.g. myxoid sarcoma, meniscal cyst) especially in the absence of signs of fluid communication between semimembranosus and medial gastrocnemius [32].

## Ganglion and synovial cysts

Other cysts can be seen in atypical locations in the posterior knee such as between biceps femoris muscle and gastrocnemius lateral head or in the proximal tibiofibular joint. These cysts are not called as Baker's cyst [3]. Ganglion cysts contain viscous, mucinous-like material and they rarely communicate with a joint. On the other hand, synovial cysts arise from a tendon sheath, joint capsule (commonly the tibiofibular) or adjacent bursa and they appear as anechoic, uni-/multilocular masses [24].

## Popliteal aneurysms

True aneurysm of the popliteal artery (all layers of the arterial wall are abnormally dilated) is the most common peripheral artery aneurysm. It is very important to diagnose the aneurysm because of the risk of severe thrombotic complications [35]. Moreover popliteal aneurysms are bilateral and have a high coexistence with abdominal aortic aneurysms. The aneurysm is usually found in older males. If it is large, the popliteal aneurysm can cause extrinsic compression to the popliteal vein resulting in leg swelling and deep venous thrombosis [7]. US is very convenient to depict the presence/patency of an aneurysm and the presence of a thrombus. Further, Doppler US can help differentiate between an aneurysm and other popliteal mass lesions (e.g. Baker's cyst; Figure 9.22 D). US can also identify popliteal pseudoaneurysms which are caused by osseous abnormalities such as osteochondromas [36].

## Popliteal artery entrapment syndrome

Popliteal artery entrapment syndrome is an uncommon cause of limb claudication resulting from abnormal anatomical relationship of the musculotendinous structures around the popliteal artery. The abnormal position causes deviation and compression of the popliteal artery. It is mostly encountered in young sports participants leading to calf hypertrophy, which unmasks the anatomical abnormality [37]. During physical examination, the popliteal and pedal pulses should be checked with passive dorsiflexion and forced plantar flexion of the ankle [38, 39]. Dynamic Doppler imaging during different maneuvers can be beneficial for the diagnosis.

# REFERENCES

1) Friedman L, Finlay K, Jurriaans E. Ultrasound of the knee. Skeletal Radiol. 2001; 30: 361-77.

2) Grobbelaar N, Bouffard JA. Sonography of the knee, a pictorial review. Semin Ultrasound CT MR. 2000; 21: 231-74.

3) Lee D, Bouffard JA. Ultrasound of the knee. Eur J Ultrasound. 2001; 14: 57-71.

4) Paczesny L, Kruczynski J. Ultrasound of the knee. Semin Ultrasound CT MRI. 2011; 32: 114-24.

5) Kane D, Balint PV, Sturrock RD. Ultrasonography is superior to clinical examination in the detection and localization of knee joint effusion in rheumatoid arthritis. J Rheumatol. 2003; 30: 966-71.

6) Jong IL, Song IS, Jung YB, Young GK, Wang CH, Hyun Y, et. al. Medial collateral ligament injuries of the knee: ultrasonographic findings. J Ultrasound Med. 1996; 15: 621-5.

7) Martinoli C, Bianchi S. Knee. In: Bianchi S, Martinoli C, editors. Ultrasound of the Musculoskeletal System. Berlin: Springer; 2007. p. 637-744.

8) Iagnocco A, Coari G, Zoppini A. Sonographic evaluation of femoral condylar cartilage in osteoarthritis and rheumatoid arthritis. Scand J Rheumatol. 1992; 21: 201-3.

9) van Holsbeeck M, Introcaso JH. Musculoskeletal ultrasound. St Louis: Mosby-Year Book; 2001.

10) De Maeseneer M, Vanderdood K, Marcelis S, Shabana W, Osteaux M. Sonography of the medial and lateral tendons and ligaments of the knee: The use of bony landmarks as an easy method for identification. AJR Am J Roentgenol. 2002; 178: 1437-44.

11) Suzuki S, Kasahara K, Futami T, Iwasaki R, Ueo T, Yamamuro T. Ultrasound diagnosis of pathology of the anterior and posterior ligaments of the knee joint. Arch Orthop Trauma Surg. 1991; 110: 200-3.

12) Delaunoy I, Feipel V, Appelboom T, Hauzeur JP. Sonography detection threshold for knee effusion. Clin Rheumatol. 2003; 22: 391-2.

13) Wakefield RJ, Balint PV, Szkudlarek M, Filippucci E, Backhaus M, D'Agostino MA, et al. OMERACT 7 Special Interest Group. Musculoskeletal ultrasound including definitions for ultrasonographic pathology. J Rheumatol. 2005; 32: 2485-7.

14) Wang SC, Chhem RK, Cardinal E, Cho KH. Joint sonography. Radiol Clin North Am. 1999; 37: 653-68.

15) La S, Fessell DP, Femino JE, Jacobson JA, Jamadar D, Hayes C. Sonography of partial-thickness quadriceps tendon tears with surgical correlation. J Ultrasound Med. 2003; 22: 1323-9.

16) Gibbon W. Musculoskeletal ultrasound. Baillieres Clin Rheumatol. 1996; 10: 561.

17) De Flaviis L, Nessi R, Scaglione P, Balconi G, Albisetti W, Derchi LE. Ultrasonic diagnosis of Osgood-Schlatter and Sinding-Larsen-Johansson diseases of the knee. Skeletal Radiol. 1989; 18: 193-7.

18) Carr JC, Hanly S, Griffin J, Gibney R. Sonography of the patellar tendon and adjacent structures in pediatric and adult patients. AJR Am J Roentgenol. 2001; 176: 1535-9.

19) Myllymäki T, Tikkakoski T, Typpö T, Kivimäki J, Suramo I. Carpet-layer's knee. An ultrasonographic study. Acta Radiol. 1993; 34: 496-9.

20) Vlad V, Iagnocco A. Ultrasound of the knee in rheumatology. Med Ultrason. 2012; 14: 318-25.

21) Strome GM, Bouffard JA, van Holsbeeck M. Knee. Clin Diagn Ultrasound. 1995; 30: 201-19.

22) Chernye S. Disorders of the knee. In: Dee R, et al., editors. Principles of orthopedic practice, Vol. 2. New York: McGraw Hill; 1989.

23) Azzoni R, Cabitza P. Is there a role for sonography in the diagnosis of tears of the knee menisci? J Clin Ultrasound. 2002; 30: 472-6.

24) Ptasznik R. Ultrasound in acute and chronic knee injury. Radiol Clin North Am. 1999; 37: 797-830.

25) Rutten MJ, Collins JM, van Kampen A, Jager GJ. Meniscal cysts: detection with high-resolution sonography. AJR Am J Roentgenol. 1998; 171: 491-6.

26) Ptasznik R, Feller J, Bartlett J, Fitt G, Mitchell A, Hennessy O. The value of sonography in the diagnosis of traumatic rupture of the anterior cruciate ligament of the knee. AJR Am J Roentgenol. 1995; 164: 1461-3.

27) Cho KH, Lee DC, Chhem RK, Kim SD, Bouffard JA, Cardinal E, et al. Normal and acutely torn posterior cruciate ligament of the knee at US evaluation: Preliminary experience. Radiology. 2001; 219: 375-80.

28) Balint PV, Kane D, Wilson H, McInnes IB, Sturrock RD. Ultrasonography of entheseal insertions in the lower limb in spondyloarthropathy. Ann Rheum Dis. 2002; 61: 905-10.

29) Yeh H, Rabinowitz J. Ultrasonography of the extremities and pelvic girdle and correlation with computed tomography. Radiology. 1982; 143: 519.

30) Moss G, Dishuk W. Ultrasound diagnosis of osteochondromatosis of the popliteal fossa. J Clin Ultrasound. 1984; 12: 232.

31) Kaufman R, Towbin R, Babcock D, Crawford AH. Arthrosonography in the diagnosis of pigmented villonodular synovitis. AJR Am J Roentgenol. 1982; 139: 396-8.

32) Ward EE, Jacobson JA, Fessell DP, Hayes CW, van Holsbeeck M. Sonographic detection of Baker's cysts: Comparison with MR imaging. AJR Am J Roentgenol. 2001; 176: 373-80.

33) Wylie E. Musculoskeletal and small parts ultrasound. Aust Fam Physician. 1995; 24: 562.

34) McDonald D, Leopold G. Ultrasound B-scanning

in the differentiation of Baker's cyst and thrombo-phlebitis. Br J Radiol. 1972; 45: 729.

35) Wright LB, Matchett WJ, Cruz CP, James CA, Culp WC, Eidt JF, et al. Popliteal artery disease: diagnosis and treatment. Radiographics. 2004; 24: 467-79.

36) Vanhegan IS, Shehzad KN, Bhatti TS, Waters TS. Acute popliteal pseudoaneurysm rupture secondary to distal femoral osteochondroma in a patient with hereditary multiple exostoses. Ann R Coll Surg Engl. 2012; 94: e134–e136.

37) Roche-Nagle G, Wong KT, Oreopoulos G. Vascular claudication in a young patient: popliteal entrapment syndrome. Hong Kong Med J. 2009; 15: 388-90.

38) Pham TT, Kapur R, Harwood MI. Exertional leg pain: teasing out arterial entrapments. Curr Sports Med Rep. 2007; 6: 371-5.

39) Gourgiotis S, Aggelakas J, Salemis N, Elias C, Georgiou C. Diagnosis and surgical approach of popliteal artery entrapment syndrome: a retrospective study. Vasc Health Risk Manag. 2008; 4: 83-8.

# Ultrasound Evaluation of the Ankle and Foot

## 10

Erhan ÇAPKIN, Murat KARKUCAK

## 10.1 INTRODUCTION

Although routine radiography is still important in the evaluation and diagnosis of foot and ankle problems, the use of ultrasonography (US) in evaluating joint, tendon, ligament, nerve and other soft tissue pathologies is getting more and more common.

Before starting the US examination, similar to the other regions, the sonographer should be aware of the patient's detailed medical history including sports and daily activities. Having a knowledge of the entire mechanism of an injury will help determine what structures might have been affected. Additionally, focusing on a certain part will shorten the length of the examination and allow the anatomic structures to be evaluated more accurately.

## 10.2 THE ANKLE

### 10.2.1 Examination Technique

A standard US examination of an ankle starts with the anterior part of the joint, then continues with the medial and lateral parts and ends with examination of the posterior ankle structures. Linear transducers at a frequency range of 5-15 MHz will be sufficient in order to examine the ankle and the surrounding soft tissues. While it is necessary to adjust according to the varying depths of different compartments (e.g. anterior superficial and posterior deep), it may also be beneficial to use a thin free pad to maintain total contact between the probe and skin during stress maneuvers [1].

*Anterior ankle*

While the patient is in a sitting position or lying on his/her back, the examination of the ante-

rior part of the ankle is best performed by bending the knee to 45°, so that the plantar surface of the foot is placed in a flat position on the examination table. The main anatomical structures to be examined are the extensor tendons, the anterior tibial artery, and the anterior synovial recess of the ankle-joint (Figure 10.1).

Longitudinal imaging is used for assessing tibiotalar joint fluid. On axial imaging, the tibialis anterior tendon (the most medial one) is almost twice as large as the other extensor tendons and the extensor digitorum longus (the most lateral one) can be distinguished as a single tendon separating into four cords going to the toes, as the probe is moved from proximal to distal. The synovial sheath of the ankle tendons can be distinguished with a high-frequency transducer. The anterior tibial artery is in a deeper position, located lateral to the extensor hallucis longus tendon. It can be determined easily with Doppler imaging or with its anechoic appearance and pulsatility. Longitudinal scans can also be used thereafter to verify the axial imaging findings (Figure 10.2).

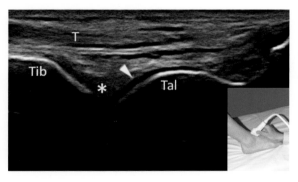

**Figure 10.1** Anterior ankle (longitudinal view). The tibialis anterior tendon (T), anechoic articular cartilage (arrowhead) and anterior recess of the ankle joint (asterisk) are seen. Tib, tibia; Tal, talus.

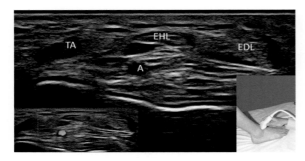

**Figure 10.2** Anterior ankle (axial view). Tendons of tibialis anterior (TA), extensor hallucis longus (EHL) and extensor digitorum longus (EDL) muscles and the anterior tibial artery (A) are observed. Below is the Doppler image of the same area showing the anterior tibial artery.

## Lateral ankle

In order to examine the lateral part of the ankle, the patient is asked to turn the front part of his/her foot slightly inward. The anatomical structures to be scanned in the lateral part comprise the peroneal tendons, lateral ligamentous complex, anterior tibiofibular ligament and the related bony structures. In the analysis of lateral ligaments, the tip of the lateral malleolus is the main landmark and particular care must be taken to place the transducer as parallel as possible to the analyzed ligament. Passive/active ankle movements can additionally be applied [2-4].

The anterior talofibular ligament appears in the form of a flat fibrillary band that connects the anterior part of the malleolar tip to the anterior talar neck (Figure 10.3). The probe is kept at 4 o'clock position for the right and at 8 o'clock position for

the left ankle. The calcaneofibular ligament can be examined by placing the transducer in coronal plane (at 6 o'clock position). In short axis, the calcaneofibular ligament has an elliptical shape and may sometimes resemble an intra-articular disconnected form compared to the peroneal tendons, particularly when it is surrounded by liquid. Due to its deep location, the posterior talofibular ligament cannot be readily evaluated by US. The anterior tibiofibular ligament is examined by placing the transducer obliquely upwards and medially from the anterior part of the lateral malleolus tip.

The supramalleolar, retromalleolar and inframalleolar parts of the peroneal tendons can be evaluated accurately by US. Like in other parts of the ankle, axial imaging would be initially preferred for better orientation. Possible anterior subluxation or dislocation of the tendons can be visualized during ankle dorsiflexion or eversion.

## Medial ankle

The patient lies on his/her back or sits down while the plantar surface of the foot is bent outwards or positioned like a "frog's leg". The medial ligamentous complex of the ankle, generally referred as the deltoid ligament, is best imaged by placing the probe as parallel as possible to the alignment of the ligament. It appears as a hypoechoic structure bridging the medial malleolus and talus (Figure 10.4). The tibialis posterior tendon can also be evaluated when the patient is lying face down and the plantar aspect of the foot is suspended from the side of the examination table in the flexion position [5]. In case of instability,

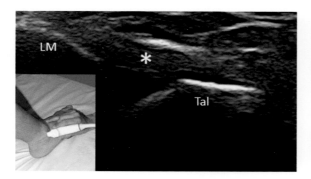

**Figure 10.3** The anterior talofibular ligament (asterisk) is visualized as a thin hyperechoic band that connects the anterior border of the talus (Tal) with the lateral malleolus (LM).

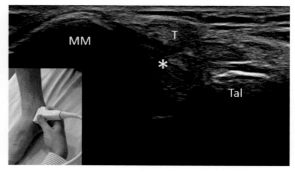

**Figure 10.4** The deltoid ligament (asterisk) is seen as a thick hypoechoic band bridging the anterior border of the tibia and the medial malleolus (MM). T, tibialis posterior tendon.

Musculoskeletal Ultrasound in Physical and Rehabilitation Medicine

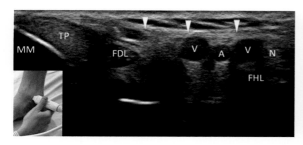

**Figure 10.5** Posterior to the medial malleolus (MM), the structures passing through the tarsal tunnel and the overlying flexor retinaculum (arrowheads) are observed. N, tibial nerve; A, posterior tibial artery; V, posterior tibial vein; TP, tibialis posterior tendon; FDL, flexor digitorum longus tendon; FHL, flexor hallucis longus tendon.

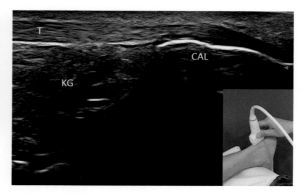

**Figure 10.6** Posterior ankle (longitudinal view). T, Achilles tendon; KG, Kager fat space; Cal, calcaneus.

this tendon can also be scanned posterior to the medial malleolus when the feet are in a dorsiflexion-inversion position. The tibialis posterior, the flexor digitorum longus and the flexor hallucis longus tendons are examined through short and long-axial scans in the supra/inframalleolar region. Usually, the tibialis posterior tendon has a diameter of 4-6 mm [6] and an elliptical hyperechoic structure. The flexor digitorum longus tendon is positioned posterior and slightly lateral to the tibialis posterior. US evaluation of the flexor hallucis longus tendon is more difficult due to its deep location (more posterior and inferior as well). Posterior tibial artery/vein, the tibial nerve and its distal braches can also be visualized posterior to the flexor digitorum longus tendon and superficial to the flexor hallucis longus tendon (Figure 10.5).

### Posterior ankle

For optimal assessment of the posterior ankle, the patient lies in prone position and suspending his/her feet freely from the side of the examination table. The Achilles tendon should be analyzed starting from the myotendinous junction to the calcaneal insertion through short and long-axial scanning. Its average thickness is approximately 5-6 mm [7]. Herein, it should be kept in mind that thickness measurements of ovoid structures can be measured correctly in axial planes [8]. The insertion of the Achilles tendon on the calcaneus is nearly 1 cm long and the tendon fibers follow an oblique course that may lead to hypoechoic appearance, imitating tendinous disease (Figure 10.6). As such, in order to evaluate this region promptly, and to distinguish the narrow band of

hypoechoic fibrocartilage connecting the tendon to the bone, changes need to be made in the angle of the US beam in general. The plantaris tendon in the medial part of the Achilles tendon can also be identified as a small elliptical hypoechoic structure in transverse scans [9]. There are two bursae close to the insertion of the Achilles tendon on the calcaneus, the retroachilles and the retrocalcaneal bursae. While the former is located between the skin and the tendon, the latter lies between the tendon insertion and the posterosuperior angle of the calcaneus. The retroachilles bursa is generally not visualized under normal conditions, whereas the retrocalcaneal bursa may be seen as a hypoechoic structure in the shape of a comma during plantar and dorsal flexion of the foot [10]. As fluid can be observed within the retrocalcaneal bursa also in asymptomatic patients, its anteroposterior diameter being <3 mm is regarded as normal [5]. The Kager fat pad, which is located deep to the Achilles tendon, appears as a soft-tissue region full of fat lobules. The small/tiny saphenous vein and the sural nerve pass along the subcutaneous tissue throughout the posterolateral region of the ankle. By determining the vein, the small sural nerve (located medial to it) can easily be identified.

## 10.3 THE FOOT

### 10.3.1 Examination Technique

#### The dorsal side

Standard US examination of the foot starts from the dorsal part. The patient lies in supine position, with the knee at 90° of flexion and the foot flat on the examination table. The extensor hallucis and extensor digitorum tendons can readily be scanned in axial and longitudinal planes until their distal insertions. The extensor hallucis brevis and extensor digitorum brevis muscles are located in a deeper position immediately below the branching bands of the extensor digitorum longus. By using transverse planes, medial branch of the dorsalis pedis artery and the deep peroneal nerve can be detected proximally. While moving distally, it should be kept in mind that a small amount of effusion in the dorsal recesses of the metatarsophalangeal or interphalangeal joints is normal and should not be interpreted as synovitis.

### The plantar side

Ultrasound examination of the plantar part of the foot is comfortably performed as the patient sits or lies in the supine position. Generally, plantar fascia is the first structure to assess. The probe is placed on the calcaneal tuberosity in the long axis, while the distal part of the probe is more medial than its distal part. The plantar fascia is observed as a distinctive hyperechoic fibrillary band similar to a tendon lying parallel to the skin (Figure 10.7). As the transducer is moved distally, it gradually thins out and becomes superficial. The strongest cord of the plantar fascia exists on the surface of the flexor digitorum brevis muscle [11, 12]. By bringing the transducer to a more lateral position, the thinner external part of the

plantar fascia over the abductor digiti minimi muscle can be evaluated. The medial cord of the aponeurosis, which is in an inferior position to the abductor hallucis muscle, appears as the thinnest part. In a deeper position, the second muscle layer containing the quadratus plantae muscle, lumbricals and flexor hallucis longus and flexor digitorum longus tendons can be visualized. Active/passive movements of the toes would indisputably help recognize each structure. It is a good landmark to identify the flexor digitorum longus tendon passing superficially and the flexor hallucis longus tendon passing below. The medial and lateral plantar neurovascular bundles pass in close relationship with the long flexor tendons and can be identified in axial view. Likewise, the interosseous muscles and the extrinsic tendons can be evaluated axially at the metatarsal level. Distally on the great toe, care should be given not to misinterpret the sesamoids as avulsion/fracture. In this regard, while sonopalpation may aid in the differential diagnosis, in case of sesamoiditis, it may not be much contributory [13].

## 10.4 ANKLE & FOOT PATHOLOGIES

### 10.4.1 Tendon Pathologies

The most common tendon pathologies of the ankle are those involving the Achilles tendon and they can substantially be visualized using US [14]. Achilles tendinopathy may be used as a general term to encompass tendinitis, tendinosis and

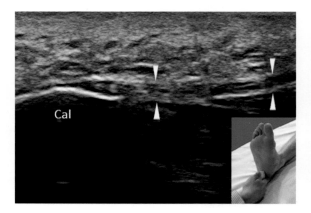

**Figure 10.7** Plantar foot (longitudinal view). The origin of the plantar fascia (arrowheads) from the calcaneal tuberosity (Cal) appears as a thin hypoechoic band.

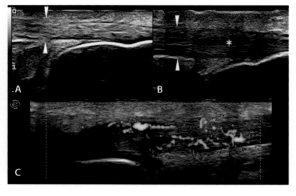

**Figure 10.8** Achilles tendinopathy. A - Normal side. B - Hypoechoic, thicker and edematous appearance of the tendon (asterisk). C - Power Doppler activity suggests active inflammation.

paratendinitis. Tenosynovitis is not encountered, due to the absence of a true synovial sheath surrounding the Achilles tendon and therefore inflammation may develop secondary to the involvement of the retrocalcaneal bursa [15]. On US, tendinitis is seen as a hypoechoic, thicker and edematous tendon. Power Doppler activity can be exhibited in the acute stage. In paratendinitis, US examination may reveal a normal intratendinous structure, peritendinous effusion, irregularities and adhesions around the tendon margins (Figure 10.8) [16].

The Achilles tendon is among the most frequently affected structures from metabolic disorders. Urate tophi deposition in gout can lead to intratendinous nodules and diffuse thickening in the tendon. In heterozygous familial hypercholesterolemia, bilateral tendon swelling and loss of fibrillar modulin together with structural heterogeneity and focal/diffuse hypoechoic areas (intratendinous xanthomas) may be seen in US [17]. Calcifications may also be found in the Achilles tendon, but they cannot be always linked to tendon degeneration. Broad diameter plaque-like ossifications may appear in the Achilles tendon following repeated trauma [18] (Figure 10.9). Calcaneal entesophytes are the most common osseous anomalies at the tendon insertion. These are commonly seen in athletes and may be painful. On US examination, irregular hyperechoic spur formations may be detected in the posterior calcaneus.

Degenerative processes in the Achilles tendon may lead to partial interstitial tears, particularly as a result of hypoxic and myxoid type tendon degeneration. These are more common in males (aged 40-50 years); and eccentric loading and explosive plyometric contractions during physical activities (e.g. jumping, running and agility activities) are the main cause of these injuries. The region of rupture is typically at a distance of 2-6 cm proximal to the calcaneal insertion, known as the hypovascularity "critical" zone [19]. However, the myotendinous junction and the bony insertion sites must be evaluated as well. Complete rupture of the Achilles tendon is observed as a focal defect between the margins of the torn ends, which may be blunted and retracted or jagged, giving rise to refractile shadowing (Figure 10.10). Tear separation may be revealed at dynamic exa-mination with passive plantar flexion or by squeezing the calf muscles.

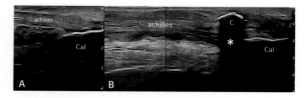

**Figure 10.9** Achilles tendinopathy. A - Normal side. B - Intratendinous calcification (C) and its acoustic shadowing (asterisk) can be seen within the tendon that is thickened and heterogenous. Cal, calcaneus.

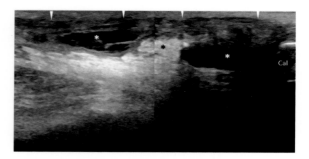

**Figure 10.10** Split screen longitudinal view of an Achilles tendon rupture demonstrates torn (white asterisks) and fibrotic (black asterisk) areas. Cal, calcaneus.

This will assist for differentiation of partial-thickness and full-thickness tears. In this sense, US has been shown to have 100% sensitivity and 83% specificity in the assessment of Achilles tendon tears [20].

Among the other tendon pathologies, tibialis anterior tendon problems may be encountered most commonly in the anterior compartment. US shows hypoechoic changes and swelling in tendinopathies and again ruptures are more common in young people and athletes, while spontaneous ruptures occur at advanced ages [21]. Other extensor tendon pathologies are rare. On the lateral side, peroneal tendons will have anechoic fluid collection (in the common sheath) in tenosynovitis. Their subluxation/dislocations together with the injury of the retinaculum accompany chronic ankle sprains [22]. The tibialis posterior tendon is the most frequently injured tendon in the medial compartment of the ankle. Inflammatory diseases commonly involve this tendon causing tendinitis, tenosynovitis (Figure 10.11) or ruptures [23]. In most cases, tears of the tibialis posterior tendon occur around the medial malleolus or in the navicular insertion [24, 25].

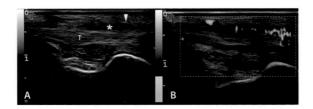

**Figure 10.11** Active tenosynovitis of the tibialis posterior tendon. Long-axis A. gray-scale and B. power Doppler images over the infra-malleolar area show effusion (asterisk) within the synovial sheath (arrowhead) of the tibialis posterior tendon (T).

### 10.4.2 Ligament Injuries

Dynamic assessment with US is paramount for ligament injuries [26] which are usually classified as: grade I, minimal stretching without disruption or instability; grade II, partial tears; grade III, complete tear.

The anterior talofibular ligament is the most commonly affected ligament in traumatic ankle injuries. At US examination, partial tears may appear as focal or diffuse hypoechoic areas (Figure 10.12). A hypoechoic space reflecting hematoma may also be detected between the free (retracted and wavy) ends of the severed ligament. Stress tests intended to determine joint laxity can assist during scanning [27, 28].

Deltoid ligament injuries usually occur during severe eversion associated with lateral malleolus fractures and lateral displacement of the talus.

Full thickness ruptures are rare and US findings usually comprise diffuse or focal hypoechoic ligament thickening and intraligamental linear defects (partial tears). Difficulty to visualize the ligament may also indicate rupture [29].

### 10.4.3 Bone and Soft Tissue Pathologies

*Ganglion cyst*

After the wrist/hand, ganglion cysts are commonly seen in the foot and they are rarely symptomatic [30]. They generally develop in the tarsal sinus and tarsal tunnel, around the Lisfranc joint and in the dorsal part of the metatarsophalangeal joints [31]. On US, ganglion cysts appear as round, oval and lobular anechoic lesions (Figure 10.13). The differential diagnosis includes abscess, seroma and varicosities. In particular, when the ganglion is large and surrounds the tendons, care must be taken to distinguish it from tenosynovitis.

*Plantar fasciitis*

Plantar fasciitis is the most common cause of heel pain. It develops due to excessive tension applied or to excessive exercise (jumping and running); but also has been found to be in relation with increasing weight [32]. Local micro-tears followed by reactive inflammatory changes at the calcaneal junction of the plantar fascia are hy-

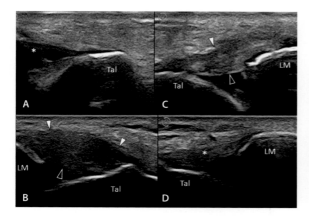

**Figure 10.12** Two different cases with intact but partially torn anterior talofibular ligament injuries. Asterisks indicate normal ligaments (A, D). Hypoechoic, thicker and edematous appearances (arrowheads) are present on the symptomatic sides (B, C). Tal, talus; LM, lateral malleolus.

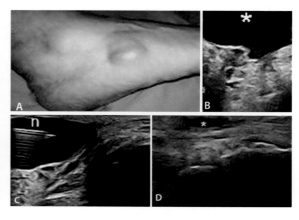

**Figure 10.13** Ganglion cyst. A - Photograph shows a stiff lump on the dorsolateral aspect of the midfoot. B - The well-marginated anechoic cystic lesion (asterisk). C - Ultrasound guided aspiration, needle (n). D - Post-aspiration image shows a very small remnant (asterisk).

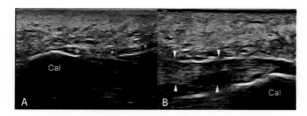

**Figure 10.14** Longitudinal plantar view demonstrating normal plantar fascia (asterisks) (A) and considerable swelling (arrowheads) with textural inhomogeneities, consistent with plantar fasciitis (B). Cal, calcaneus.

pothesized in the pathogenesis. Numerous studies have reported the appearance of the plantar fascia at US [33-35]. The region where pathological changes are most commonly seen is the posterior part of the fascia close to the insertion on the medial tubercle. The main sonographic findings are fascial thickening, hypoechoic texture with loss in the fibrillar pattern, opacification of the superficial and deep margins of the fascia and, rarely, perifascial effusion (Figure 10.14). US can be used effectively to guide local therapeutic procedures (e.g. injection, extracorporeal shock wave therapy) as well [36, 37].

### Degenerative osteoarthritis

The ankle and the first metatarsophalangeal joint are most widely affected by degenerative osteoarthritis. Neuropathic osteoarthropathy (particularly seen in diabetes mellitus) usually affects the middle tarsal and tarsometatarsal joints. Although radiographs may display a nice general overview; edema/hyperemia in the soft tissues, joint effusion, cortical irregularities and bone fragmentation can be promptly detected with US [38].

### Occult fractures

Small fractures (commonly seen in the lateral part of the talus) may frequently be overlooked in normal radiographs. Since patients present with nonspecific symptoms such as swelling, pain and sensitivity in the ankle, it is difficult to diagnose these fractures. Especially with the use of sonopalpation, focal interruption in the bony cortex sometimes with concomitant ligamentous injuries can easily be detected with US. Some authors have even emphasized that assessment of the lateral process of the talus with US in post-traumatic situations, particularly when fluid effusion is determined in the posterior subtalar joint, should be a routine part of ankle examination [39].

### Stress fractures

Stress fractures are more commonly seen in women in the postmenopausal period, and typically after protracted walking. Runners, dancers and soldiers (march fracture) are at high risk of metatarsal stress fractures [40]. The symptoms are generally non-specific and standard radiographs taken in the acute stages may fail to delineate the fracture. Although magnetic resonance imaging and scintigraphy are sensitive for the diagnosis, US is also used to visualize likely fluid accumulation, hypoechoic thickening in the periosteum and a hypervascular pattern around the bone [41].

### Morton's neuroma

Morton's neuroma is quite common among middle aged women. Several etiological theories have been suggested i.e. chronic repetitive trauma, ischemia, entrapment and intermetatarsal bursitis. Histopathologically, Morton's neuroma is not a genuine neuroma, because it consists of a perineural fibrotic mass associated with vascular proliferation and axonal degeneration [42]. It is frequently seen in the third, and to a much lesser extent in the fourth, interdigital nerve. Several reasons have been proposed for this involvement; first, the third digital nerve is thicker than the other digital nerves since it consists branches from the medial and lateral plantar nerves. Second, the nerve is closer to the head of the third metatarsal. Additionally, there is greater motility between the third and fourth metatarsal bones and the space in between is narrower compared to other areas [43].

While clinical examination is important in its diagnosis, dynamic US examination (dorsal and plantar approach) is of significant assistance to the physician, with 100% sensitivity and 83% specificity [43]. All intermetatarsal areas must be investigated with care since Morton's neuromas may be multiple. Morton's neuroma appears in the form of an ovoid hypoechoic mass between the metatarsal heads (Figure 10.15) but they can be anechoic or with mixed echogenicity as well [44]. Movement of the neuroma -with or without a clicking sound- during Mulder's test (sonographic Mulder's sign) is quite typical for the diagnosis

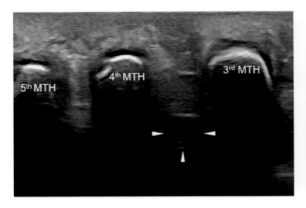

**Figure 10.15** Axial view at the level of the metatarsal heads (MTH) shows the hypoechoic Morton's neuroma (arrowheads) in the 3rd intermetatarsal space.

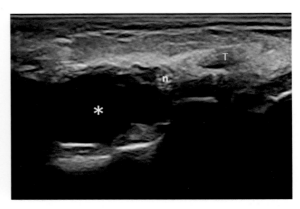

**Figure 10.16** Tarsal tunnel syndrome. Ganglion cyst in the tarsal tunnel (asterisk) adjacent to the tibial nerve (n) and the flexor tendon (T) is seen.

[45]. The normal plantar nerve is 1-2 mm in diameter at the level of the metatarsal heads and not easily visualized under US. Majority of the symptomatic neuromas exceed 5 mm in diameter, but its size and symptoms are not strictly correlated [44]. Of note, interdigital bursitis should be considered in the differential diagnosis.

### Tarsal tunnel syndrome

Tarsal tunnel syndrome develops as the result of the main body and/or branches of the tibial nerve becoming entrapped in the medial part of the ankle. US is beneficial for unmasking the possible cause of entrapment e.g. flexor tenosynovitis, subtalar joint related ganglions, lipomas, varicous enlargement of posterior tibial veins, accessory tendon or muscles (flexor digitorum accessorius longus) (Figure 10.16). The use of sono-tinel can significantly facilitate the US assessment [46].

### Bursitis

Retrocalcaneal bursa is the most commonly involved bursa in the foot and ankle. Retrocalcaneal bursitis may present with chronic posterior ankle pain (intensified by ankle dorsiflexion) and generally accompanies inflammatory disorders or Achilles tendinopathy. US examination reveals a swollen anechoic or hypoechoic structure in the shape of a comma between the Achilles tendon and the posterosuperior part of the calcaneus. It may also have a hypervascular appearance at Doppler imaging [47]. Retroachilles bursitis generally manifests as painful and sensitive subcutaneous swelling over the Achilles tendon. On US examination, it appears as localized fluid accumulation and thickening in the subcutaneous tissue immediately superficial to the retrocalcaneal part of the Achilles tendon. The subcalcaneal bursa extends between the plantar fascia and the

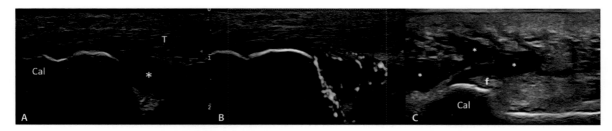

**Figure 10.17** Retrocalcaneal and subcalcaneal bursitis. Longitudinal gray-scale image reveals hypoechoic swelling of the retrocalcaneal bursa (asterisk) deep to a thickened Achilles tendon (T) (A). The peribursal area appears hypervascular at color Doppler imaging (B). Fluid accummulation (asterisks) over the calcaneus (cal) and plantar fascia (f) is consistent with subcalcaneal bursitis (C).

plantar fat pad. Degeneration of these structures may be associated with development of subcalcaneal bursitis (Figure 10.17).

## Soft tissue masses

Soft tissue masses in the ankle are rare. They may be asymptomatic or leading to pain, swelling, peripheral nerve and joint disorders [48]. US imaging provides information about the content, origin, vascularity of the mass and its relations with the nearby tissues [14]. Most soft tissue masses in the ankle are benign e.g. ganglion cysts, lipomas, bursitis, foreign body granuloma, plantar fibromatosis, pigmented villonodular synovitis, and giant cell tumor in a tendon sheath. Lipomas are non-malignant tumors made up of aggregates of mature adipocytes. On US, they exhibit variable echogenicity, frequently ovoid and well defined and the largest dimension lying parallel to the skin. The intraarticular form of pigmented villonodular synovitis may appear as a single nodule or a diffuse villonodular mass, generally seen as a monoartricular disorder in the ankle and posterior foot [49]. Giant cell tumor in the tendon sheath in the forefoot tends to appear in the regions between the toes. On US, giant cell tumor appears as a painless solid hypoechoic nodule in a hypervascular model alongside or surrounding the tendon. Plantar fibromatosis is a non-malignant fibroblastic proliferation of the plantar fascia and appears as a fusiform, hypoechoic or mixed echogenic mass. Schwannomas and neurofibromas are other mass lesions that can be observed in the ankle/foot. Among the malignant mass lesions, synovial sarcoma is the most common tumor and is mainly seen in adolescents and young adults [50].

The involvement of ankle and foot in *inflammatory disease* has been discussed in Chapter 13 - "Ultrasound Imaging in Rheumatic Diseases".

## REFERENCES

1) Sobel M, Levy ME, Bohne WH. Congenital variations of the peroneus quartus muscle: an anatomic study. Foot Ankle. 1990; 11: 81-8.
2) Campbell DG, Menz A, Isaacs J. Dynamic ankle ultrasonography. A new imaging technique for acute ankle ligament injuries. Am J Sports Med. 1994; 22: 855-8.
3) Brasseur JL, Luzzati A, Lazennec JY, Guérin-Surville H, Roger B, Grenier P. Ultrasonoanatomy of the ankle ligaments. Surg Radiol Anat. 1994; 16: 87-91.
4) Milz P, Milz S, Putz R, Reiser M. 13 MHz high-frequency sonography of the lateral ankle joint ligaments and the tibiofibular syndesmosis in anatomic specimens. J Ultrasound Med. 1996; 15: 277-84.
5) Nazarian LN, Rawool NM, Martin CE, Schweitzer ME. Synovial fluid in the hindfoot and ankle: detection of amount and distribution with US. Radiology. 1995; 197: 275-8.
6) Miller SD, van Holsbeeck M, Boruta PM, Wu KK, Katcherian DA. Ultrasound in the diagnosis of posterior tibial tendon pathology. Foot Ankle Int. 1996; 17: 555-8.
7) Weinfeld SB. Achilles tendon disorders. Med Clin North Am. 2014; 98: 331-8.
8) Fornage BD. Achilles tendon: US examination. Radiology. 1996; 159: 759-64.
9) Wening JV, Katzer A, Phillips F, Jungbluth KH, Lorke DE. Detection of the tendon of the musculus plantaris longus: diagnostic imaging and anatomic correlate. Unfallchirurgie. 1996; 22: 30-5.
10) Mathieson JR, Connell DG, Cooperberg PL, Lloyd-Smith DR. Sonography of the Achilles tendon and adjacent bursae. AJR Am J Roentgenol. 1988; 151: 127-31.
11) Gibbon WW, Long G. Ultrasound of the plantar aponeurosis (fascia). Skeletal Radiol. 1999; 28: 21-6.
12) Walther M, Radke S, Kirschner S, Ettl V, Gohlke F. Power Doppler findings in plantar fasciitis. Ultrasound Med Biol. 2004; 30: 435-40.
13) Frankel JP, Harrington JZ. Symptomatic bipartite sesamoids. J Foot Surg. 1990; 29: 318-23.

14) Ozcakar L, Tok F, De Muynck M, Vanderstraeten G. Musculoskeletal ultrasonography in physical and rehabilitation medicine. J Rehabil Med. 2012; 44: 310-8.

15) Wijesekera NT, Calder JD, Lee JC. Imaging in the assessment and management of Achilles tendinopathy and paratendinitis. Semin Musculoskelet Radiol. 2011; 15: 89-100.

16) Martinoli C, Bianchi S, Derchi LE. Tendon and nerve sonography. Radiol Clin North Am. 1999; 37: 691-711.

17) Kainberger F, Seidl G, Traindl O, Trattnig S, Breitenseher M, Schneider B, et al. Ultrasonography of the Achilles tendon in hypercholesterolemia. Acta Radiol. 1993; 34: 408-12.

18) Yu JS, Witte D, Resnick D, Pogue W. Ossification of the Achilles tendon: imaging abnormalities in 12 patients. Skeletal Radiol. 1994; 23: 127-31.

19) Hess GW. Achilles tendon rupture: a review of etiology, population, anatomy, risk factors, and injury prevention. Foot Ankle Spec. 2010; 3: 29-32.

20) Hartgerink P, Fessell DP, Jacobson JA, van Holsbeeck MT. Full-versus partial-thickness Achilles tendon tears: sonographic accuracy and characterization in 26 cases with surgical correlation. Radiology. 2001; 220: 406-12.

21) Dooley BJ, Kudelka P, Menelaus MB. Subcutaneous rupture of the tendon of tibialis anterior. J Bone Joint Surg. 1980; 62: 471-2.

22) Rosenberg ZS, Bencardino J, Astion D, Schweitzer ME, Rokito A, Sheskier S. MRI features of chronic injuries of the superior peroneal retinaculum. AJR Am J Roentgenol. 2003; 181: 1551-7.

23) Johnson K. Tibialis posterior tendon rupture. Clin Orthop Relat Res. 1983; 177: 140-7.

24) Jacobson JA, Andresen R, Jaovisidha S, De Maeseneer M, Foldes K, Trudell DR, et al. Detection of ankle effusions: comparison study in cadavers using radiography, sonography, and MR imaging. AJR Am J Roentgenol. 1998; 170: 1231-8.

25) Nallamshetty L, Nazarian LN, Schweitzer ME, Morrison WB, Parellada JA, Articolo GA, et al. Evaluation of posterior tibial pathology: comparison of sonography and MR imaging. Skeletal Radiol. 2005; 34: 375-80.

26) Van Dijk CN, Mol BW, Lim LS, Marti RK, Bossuyt PM. Diagnosis of ligament rupture of the ankle joint: physical examination, arthrography, stress radiography and sonography compared in 160 patients after inversion trauma. Acta Orthop Scand. 1996; 67: 566-70.

27) Peetrons P, Creteur V, Bacq C. Sonography of Ankle Ligaments. J Clin Ultrasound. 2004; 32: 491-9.

28) Carli AB, Akarsu S, Tekin L, Kıralp MZ. Sonographic diagnosis of recurrent peroneal tendon subluxation. Wien Klin Wochenschr. 2013; 125: 717-8.

29) Mansour R, Jibri Z, Kamath S, Mukherjee K, Ostlere S. Persistent ankle pain following a sprain: a review of imaging. Emerg Radiol. 2011; 18: 211-25.

30) Waldt S, Rechl H, Rummeny EJ, Woertler K. Imaging of benign and malignant soft tissue masses of the foot. Eur Radiol. 2003; 13: 1125-36.

31) Woertler K. Soft-tissue masses in the foot and ankle: characteristics on MR Imaging. Semin Musculoskelet Radiol. 2005; 9: 227-42.

32) Kane D, Greaney T, Shanahan M, Duffy G, Bresnihan B, Gibney R, et al. The role of ultra-sonography in the diagnosis and management of idiopathic plantar fasciitis. Rheumatology. 2001; 40: 1002-8.

33) McNally EG, Shetty S Plantar fascia: imaging diagnosis and guided treatment. Semin Musculoskelet Radiol. 2010; 14: 334-43.

34) Cardinal E, Chhem RK, Beauregard CG, Aubin B, Pelletier M. Plantar fasciitis: sonographic evaluation. Radiology. 1996; 201: 257-9.

35) Walther M, Radke S, Kirschner S, Ettl V, Gohlke F. Power Doppler findings in plantar fasciitis. Ultrasound Med Biol. 2004; 30: 435-40.

36) Tsai WC, Wang CL, Tang FT, Hsu TC, Hsu KH, Wong MK. Treatment of proximal plantar fasciitis with ultrasound-guided steroid injection. Arch Phys Med Rehabil. 2000; 81: 1416-21.

37) Hyer CF, Vancourt R, Block A. Evaluation of ultrasound-guided extracorporeal shock wave therapy (ESWT) in the treatment of chronic plantar fasciitis. J Foot Ankle Surg. 2005; 44: 137-43.

38) Ashman CJ, Klecker RJ, Yu JS. Forefoot pain involving the metatarsal region: differential diagnosis with MR imaging. Radiographics. 2001; 21: 1425-40.

39) Bonvin F, Montet X, Copercini M, Martinoli C, Bianchi S. Imaging of fractures of the lateral process of the talus, a frequently missed diagnosis. Eur J Ultrasound. 2003; 47: 64-70.

40) Shindle MK, Endo Y, Warren RF, Lane JM, Helfet DL, Schwartz EN, et al. Stress fractures about the tibia, foot, and ankle. J Am Acad Orthop Surg. 2012; 20: 167-76.

41) Bodner G, Stöckl B, Fierlinger A, Schocke M, Bernathova M. Sonographic findings in stress fractures of the lower limb: preliminary findings. Eur Radiol. 2005; 15: 356-9.

42) Jain S, Mannan K. The diagnosis and management of Morton's neuroma: a literature review. Foot Ankle Spec. 2013; 6: 307-17.

43) Levitsky KA, Alman BA, Jevsevar DS, Morehead J. Digital nerves of the foot: anatomic variations and implications regarding the pathogenesis of interdigital neuroma. Foot Ankle. 1993; 14: 208-14.

44) Quinn TJ, Jacobson JA, Craig JG, van Holsbeeck MT. Sonography of Morton's neuromas. AJR Am J Roentgenol. 2000; 174: 1723-8.

45) Torriani M, Kattapuram SV. Technical innovation. Dynamic sonography of the forefoot: the sonographic Mulder sign. AJR Am J Roentgenol. 2003; 180: 1121-3.

46) Martinoli C, Bianchi S, Gandolfo N, Valle M, Simonetti S, Derchi E. Ultrasound of nerve entrapments in osteofibrous tunnels. Radiographics. 2000; 20: 199-217.

47) Checa A, Chun W, Pappu R. Ultrasound-guided diagnostic and therapeutic approach to Retrocalcaneal Bursitis. J Rheumatol. 2011; 38: 391-2.

48) Ozdemir HM, Yildiz Y, Yilmaz C, Saglik Y. Tumors of the foot and ankle: analysis of 196 cases. J Foot Ankle Surg. 1197; 26: 403-8.

49) Kerimoglu S, Aynaci O, Saraçoglu M, Cobanoglu U. Synovial chondromatosis of the subtalar joint: a case report and review of the literature. J Am Podiatr Med Assoc. 2008; 98: 318-21.

50) Pham H, Fessell DP, Femino JE, Sharp S, Jacobson JA, Hayes CW. Sonography and MR imaging of selected benign masses in the ankle and foot. AJR Am J Roentgenol. 2003; 180: 99-107.

# Ultrasound Use in Physical and Rehabilitation Medicine

# Ultrasound Imaging in Sports Medicine

Fatih TOK

**11**

The growing emphasis on the health and fitness over the years has resulted in increases in both the number and kind of sports-related injuries. Paralleling this surge in various types of injuries, the need for prompt imaging has also mounted. Overall, musculoskeletal ultrasound (MSUS) and magnetic resonance imaging (MRI) have been the mainstay of sports-injury imaging armamentarium [1, 2]. Further, the improvements in ultrasound (US) technology and the production of portable machines that can be carried to the stadium/playing field have enhanced the interest concerning the use of MSUS in sports medicine [1, 3-6].

Aside from being less expensive and more widely accessible, US has many other advantages e.g. real time dynamic imaging, high resolution, simultaneous comparison, sonopalpation when compared with MRI [7-10]. Of note, the use of US for close treatment monitoring or for guidance during an immediate intervention are paramount for the management of sports injuries [11-14]. Lastly, MSUS can also be beneficial for fitness assessment via measuring the thickness and cross-sectional area of the muscles [15-18]. On the other hand, there are some drawbacks of MSUS, i.e. user-dependency and incomplete evaluation of the whole anatomy due to its inability to visualize structures/pathologies inside the bony tissues [1].

This chapter will focus on exemplary US findings as regards various sport-related injuries that are commonplace in daily practice.

## 11.1 EXAMINATION TECHNIQUE

As usual, US examination begins with a thorough clinical history taking and physical examination. Indisputably, simple steps to avoid patient discomfort should be taken for an efficacious examination. Careful scanning of the symptomatic region in longitudinal and transverse planes is crucial. Comparison with the normal side as well as dynamic [passive or active] imaging should be performed where necessary. Imaging systematically from origin to insertion or some other related structures (e.g. synergistic muscles) can sometimes be necessary/contributory in light of the history and physical examination. Power Doppler imaging may also help evaluate the vascularity of the pathology.

## 11.2 ULTRASOUND OF MUSCLES

Skeletal muscle is the largest tissue mass in the human body, accounting for almost 50% of the weight of an average person [24]. Its injury is common in athletes, both during training and in competition; but it also occurs frequently in the general population as more individuals try to increase their level of fitness [25]. Overall, muscle injuries account for approximately one-third of all sports-related injuries [26, 27]. Although imaging work-up may not always be necessary for minor lesions, confirming the diagnosis or defining the exact location and the extent of the injury can definitely guide the decision-making in case of a professional athlete [28-30].

US examination of a muscle injury should begin with a short history, with the patient identifying the site of maximal symptoms. Palpation of the injured muscle both in the relaxed position and during contraction is also contributory. Lesions are mostly discovered by a careful and slow examination of the entire muscle including the enthesis, musculotendinous junction, intramuscular septa, and epimysium are performed. Other useful information includes localization of the injury relative to nearby neurovascular bundles and joints as well.

Sonographic palpation, i.e. trying to find the point of maximal tenderness during the examination by a gentle but firm compression of the probe on the skin, is a very valuable tool. Herewith, this can also let the patient guide the examination. Of note, dynamic imaging and comparison with the other limb is mandatory and especially when looking for a muscle hernia, the probe must be placed very smoothly on the skin because the hernia could disappear with too much compression.

Evaluation in both the longitudinal and transverse planes is performed using a high multifrequency probe. Occasionally, depending on patient size and the depth of muscle involved, a lower frequency (5-7 MHz) linear or even a low-frequency (2-4 Hz) curvilinear probe may be required (e.g. for imaging priformis muscle). However, with frequency reduction, spatial resolution and the ability to detect low-grade or small injuries diminishes rapidly. Compound imaging and tissue harmonic imaging are software adjustments that may further improve lesion conspicuity [31-33]. Power Doppler is of use in identifying hyperemia associated with acute injuries. Extended field-of-view imaging is very helpful in assessing the length of muscle strain injury or gap following muscle tear. However in many cases, where lesions are localized and focally symptomatic, this technique may be of limited utility.

## 11.2.1 Normal Sonographic Anatomy

Muscle fibers -the fundamental building blocks of a skeletal muscle- form into bundles or fascicles but they are beyond the resolution of US. Fascicles that are surrounded by the perimysium, fine septated fibroadipose tissue arranged in parallel bands, whose orientation gives the "pennation" of the muscle. These septa form the tendons by joining at each end of the muscle. Surrounding the entire muscle and separating one muscle from another is the aponeurosis (Figure 11.1). On US, the muscle fibers themselves are hyporeflective and the connective tissue that invests groups of muscle fibers is hyper-reflective. As such, on long-axis view, the echotexture of a normal skeletal muscle appears as hyperechoic septae, thin, bright, linear bands ("veins on a leaf"). On short-axis views, the muscle bundles appear as spot echoes with short, curvilinear, bright lines spread throughout the hypoechoic background ("starry night") [1, 34]. The epimysium and muscle ten-

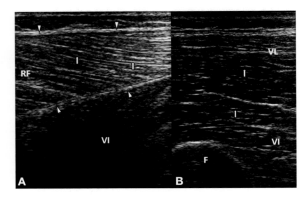

**Figure 11.1** A - Longitudinal image of normal rectus femoris muscle. Longitudinal striations are seen within the muscle representing the obliquely oriented perimysium (arrows) which converge towards the muscle aponeurosis (arrowheads) - the typical configuration of "veins on a leaf". B - Axial images of normal vastus lateralis. The perimysium is seen as dots and lines representing the "starry sky" appearance. RF, rectus femoris; VI, vastus intermedius; VL, vastus lateralis; F, femur.

dons are hyperechoic structures that fuse as the tendon emerges from the muscle belly. The tendons are fibrillar structures appearing as multiple hyperechoic stripes, prone to anisotropy artifact. Similarly, anisotropy artifact can also be seen (to a small extent) in the muscle fibers i.e. the endomyseal and perimyseal fibers.

## 11.2.2 Muscle Injuries

Muscle trauma may be divided into acute and chronic injury. Muscle contusions and muscle strains or tears account for the vast majority of acute skeletal muscle injuries, most commonly seen in athletes. Compartment syndrome can also ensue as a serious consequence of acute trauma. On the other hand, chronic injuries include muscle scar, hernia and myositis ossificans.

*Acute muscle injuries*

The goal of imaging acute muscle tears is to estimate the severity of injury and to determine if surgical repair is necessary. Another important question is, for sure, whether/when the professional athlete can play [25, 35]. The overwhelming majority of acute muscle pathologies is traumatic in origin, either being specific to a particular sports play or due to inappropriate exercise training [1, 36]. Those injuries can be divided into two main groups as extrinsic and intrinsic. The former group takes place after an external trauma, either a contusion or a penetrating injury, and the lesion is usually located under the site of trauma. The latter group stems from a contraction or simultaneous elongation of a muscle. Both types generally end up with hemorrhage and haematoma, mostly seen in the myotendinous junction which is the weakest portion of the muscle-tendon-bone unit [37].

*Muscle contusion* results most commonly from a direct blunt impact, particularly during contact sports. After a contusion, microscopical disruption of capillaries and muscle fibers occur, with hemorrhage lying between the torn fibers and infiltrating around the intact fibers [38]. Sonographically, a contusion is seen as an ill-defined area of hyperechogenicity in the muscle, which may cross fascial planes. However, a hematoma appears as a hypoechoic fluid collection and may contain debris [25, 39]. In the first 24 hours following injury, a focal hematoma can actually have a variable appearance from anechoic or hypoechoic to hyperechoic [31]. This appearance will change over the next 2 to 3 days, becoming hypoechoic or anechoic. Finally, a hematoma will show increasing echogenicity with fluid-fluid levels. Over the following weeks, a hematoma will become more organized and can develop a focal scar [40]. Occasionally, acute on chronic changes can also occur (Figure 11.2).

Although the diagnosis of a muscle contusion can rely on history and physical examination, US imaging has an additional role in its management, particularly in athletes (Figure 11.2). It helps to exclude the presence of a significant muscle tear. Yet, in the absence of a significant tear, immobilization for a short interval (e.g. 48 hours) and anti-inflammatory agents are used before graded reintroduction of activities. With an associated muscle tear, consideration may be given to longer rehabilitation or operative repair [38].

*Muscle strains, tears and lacerations* typically occur near the musculotendinous junction which is the weakest link within the muscle. The musculotendinous junction includes not only the vicinity where the tendon emerges from the muscle belly but has a long intramuscular component where muscle tissue lies in close proximity to the intramuscular central tendon. Another important junctional zone would be the area beneath the epimysium and where muscles are attached to periosteum [31].

Factors predisposing to muscle strain injuries include eccentric contraction (active muscle contraction in the presence of forced muscle elongation), complex muscle internal architecture [24], increased proportion of fast twitch fibers and muscles that cross two joints [31, 41]. Muscles that have previously been injured are also more susceptible to recurrent injuries [24]. Symptoms are similar to those of contusion injuries; however, a history of extreme muscle exertion/activity is typical. In addition, signs may be more localized, with point tenderness and palpable tissue defects. Similar to contusions, the diagnosis can be made on clinical grounds, and US imaging is used to confirm the diagnosis and demonstrate the pattern and grade of injury [31, 42]. Likewise, several clinical and imaging grading systems for muscle strain injuries have been described that are relevant for prognosis and patient rehabilitation [43].

On US, grade I muscle strains (elongation injury) may have a normal appearance or show focal or general areas (5%) of increased echogenicity [25, 39] (Figure 11.3 A and B). Perifascial fluid and flame-shaped, hypoechoic cavities in the muscle belly may be seen as well. Examination in multiple

**Figure 11.2** A, B - A 22-year-old man with an old total rupture of the gastrocnemius (G) muscle following a non-penetrating direct trauma. Ultrasound image (axial view) demonstrates the anechoic gap (arrows) between the two heads of the muscle (A). Note the areas of skin depression at the rupture site (B). C - A 21-year-old man with chronic rectus abdominis (RA) laceration after being stabbed. Ultrasound image (axial view) shows the ruptured area as an anechoic gap (arrows).

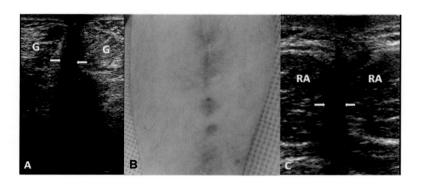

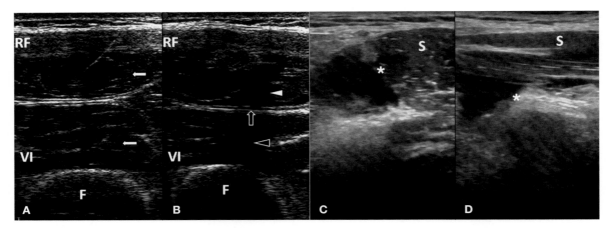

**Figure 11.3**  A, B - A 21-year-old man with a grade 1 strain lesion in the rectus femoris muscle (RF). Axial images show hypoechoic and deteriorated structural pattern (white arrowhead) on the injured side (B) and the "starry-sky appearance" (white arrows) on the normal side (A). Note the "mirror image artifact" (black arrowhead) -due to the highly reflective surface of muscle aponeurosis (black arrow)- in the vastus intermedius muscle (VI). C, D - A 22-year-old man with a grade 2 strain lesion at the proximal myotendinous junction of the sartorius muscle (S). There is a large anechoic area -consistent with hematoma- which lies close to the insertion of the muscle (white asterisk). Axial view (C). Longitudinal view (D).

planes is crucial to differentiate subtle lesions from artifacts. Grade 1 injury usually occurs when a muscle is stretched to its elastic limit and the patient reports severe pain throughout the muscle without point tenderness, making this entity clinically indistinguishable from cramps [44].

Grade II muscle strains (partial muscle rupture) show discontinuity of muscle fibers with hypervascularity around them [39] and loss of perimysial striation adjacent to the musculotendinous junction [31] (Figure 11.3 C and D). A hypoechoic gap is indentified within the muscle substance. Fragments of torn muscle originating from the walls of the cavity can be identified within the hematoma filling the gap. It involves more than 5% of muscle substance but less than the entire muscle cross section. An intramuscular fluid collection may be seen with a surrounding hyperechoic halo. Of note, a hematoma at the myotendinous junction is pathognomonic for a grade 2 injury [31] (Figure 11.4). The tendon fibers are also irregular and thinned. Gentle pressure can be applied with the transducer in order to demonstrate the hematoma and the torn muscle fragments. Immediately after the injury, patients often describe a "snap" accompanied by the sudden onset of sharp focal pain [44]. Unlike grade I strain, point tenderness, focal swelling and ecchymosis are present. Herewith, the ecchymotic area does not necessarily indicate the exact localiza-

tion of the injury; therefore thorough US scanning for relevant compartments should remain as a prerequisite.

Grade III muscle strains (complete muscle rupture) show complete discontinuity of muscle fibers and associated hematoma [39]. Often there is retraction of the tendon ends, making the diagnosis more obvious. The evaluation of the injured muscle can be limited secondary to extensive acute edema and hemorrhage. On US, it may sometimes be difficult to determine whether there is a partial or complete tear due to blood and edema filling the defect between the torn muscles. Real-time dynamic imaging may help in such cases. When the muscle is superficially located, the gap between the retracted ends of the ruptured muscle can be palpated. Ecchymosis is also common (see figure 11.3).

The initial extent of injury and the degree of separation are good predictors of recovery and return to normal function. In this sense, owing to its convenient use, serial US evaluations can also be very beneficial in the follow-up of athletes with muscle strains. The amount of intramuscular scar formation is inversely proportional to the ability of a muscle to produce tension, and directly proportional to the risk of recurrent injury [1, 44, 45]. Low-grade injuries heal within 1 to 2 weeks, whereas high-grade injuries may require 4 to 8 weeks [31, 46, 47]. Herewith, structural follow-up

Musculoskeletal Ultrasound in Physical and Rehabilitation Medicine

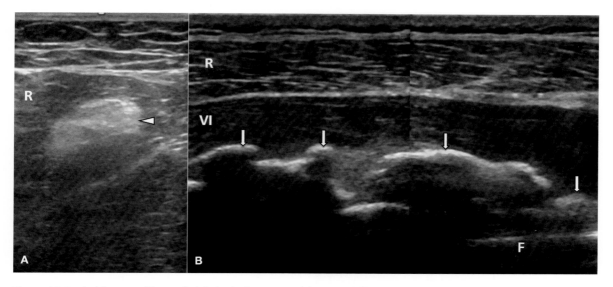

**Figure 11.4** A - Ultrasound image (axial view) of a 23-year old man with fibrous scar (arrowhead) -possibly due to recurrent injuries- in the rectus femoris muscle (R). B - Myositis ossificans following massive hemorrhage within the vastus intermedius muscle (VI) in a rugby player. Longitudinal split screen sonogram shows widespread calcifications (arrows) paralleling the femoral shaft (F).

(with US imaging) would not preclude functional/physical assessment in elite athletes -especially for the decision of return to sports.

*Muscle laceration* is a form of partial muscle tear that arises from direct penetrating trauma, involving the epimysium and the underlying muscle tissue. Clinical and US findings are similar to grade II strains, where as ecchymosis is much more common.

*Acute compartment syndrome* most commonly arises following trauma due to raised intracompartmental pressures (caused generally by hematoma and edema). When edema supervenes after a muscle injury, the muscle swells and capillary compression occurs. At this point, decreased blood flow leads to tissue hypoxia, and this in turn leads to further muscle injury, swelling, and eventually to muscle necrosis [31]. In severe cases, the scenario may end up with rhabdomyolysis, renal failure, and even death. Capillary closure pressure is reached before mean arterial pressure is exceeded; consequently the assessment of distal arterial flow would be a poor and late marker for the syndrome. The diagnosis should be suspected clinically, however US may be helpful in identifying the possible underlying cause or demonstrating the increased size and echotextural changes of the pertinent muscle compartment [1]. Imaging features range from tissue swelling and increased

muscle reflectivity with milder injuries to more heterogeneous appearances with muscle tissue that has already undergone ischemic necrosis. Focal collections may signal an underlying cause for the syndrome, allowing a more minimally invasive compartment decompression. Doppler arterial and venous flow studies will remain normal until gross changes have occurred by the time the diagnosis is clinically apparent [24].

## Chronic muscle injuries

Return to normal is not exceptional but takes time. Muscle regeneration occurs if the sarcolemnal sheaths are not involved in the rupture. Most acute injuries resolve usually over a period of weeks to months, leaving no residual sonographic abnormality. Although rehabilitation of muscle sprain or tear in athletes is determined on clinical grounds, resolution of sonographic changes can be considered for return to sporting activity [1, 47, 48].

An *intramuscular scar* appears as a linear or irregular echogenic structure that may be surrounded by a hypoechoic zone or halo, typically found within the muscle or the myotendinous junction [31, 40, 43]. Scar formation is usually seen when the injury is large, recurrent or if the resumption of sporting activities was too early. It is poorly symptomatic and actually itself predisposes to recurrent tears. Accordingly, the presence of a scar tissue may pose significant challenges for elite athletes [40, 42, 49, 50]. Although very rare, *post-traumatic cysts* can also ensue after muscle tears and can stay for months, sometimes necessitating interventions as well (see figure 11.4).

Post-traumatic *myositis ossificans* (MO) is a more common complication with an incidence of 9-17% following a direct blow to a muscle; however many patients will not give a history of antecedent trauma [51]. Its pathophysiology is unclear and it may be asymptomatic or painful. As it can occur secondary to very minor muscle trauma, clinical diagnosis is difficult. It is seen most frequently in young adults, typically within large bulky muscles, especially the quadriceps. When it presents with a painful mass, differentiation from a soft-tissue tumor is also required. In this sense, US imaging plays a pivotal role especially in the early period or during follow-up of its different stages [43]. Yet, the transition between the noncalcified and calcified stages is detected much earlier by US than other imaging techniques [31]. On US, MO appears as a hypoechoic, heterogeneous mass with Doppler signal prominent at its periphery [47, 52]. Over time, as the lesion matures, peripheral ossification produces acoustic shadowing.

*Muscle hernia* is an uncommon benign condition that results from acquired focal defect by a direct trauma to the muscle within the investing fascial layers of muscle (epimysium). Although the diagnosis is often suggested clinically, with its dynamic imaging, US is the ideal modality to confirm the diagnosis. While a typical painless soft-tissue lump is palpable with contraction of the underlying muscle, US displays normal muscle tissue extending through a focal epimysial defect. Long-axis images will show perimysium bowed or "bulging" into the defect [31]. Minimal pressure should be applied with the US probe as the hernia can inadvertently be reduced and consequently missed with too much pressure. Multiple herniations may also indicate an underlying chronic compartment syndrome.

## 11.3 ULTRASOUND OF TENDONS

Tendons pathologies are common conditions in daily sports medicine practice. Although clinical evaluation remains the mainstay for the early and accurate diagnosis of a tendon pathology, post-traumatic local edema and severe pain can limit physical examination, and even complete tears can be missed. But as early diagnosis can reduce patient discomfort and guide prompt management, imaging modalities are necessary. MSUS and MRI are competing modalities in that sense; however due to the nature of the tendons (which include few mobile protons), MRI does not show the internal architecture as well as US. Moreover, given the recent developments in high-frequency broadband transducers, diagnostic capacity of US in visualizing internal tendon arrangement and peritendinous structures such as retinacula and synovial bursae have further improved.

Tendons consist of linear fibrils of type 1 collagen embedded in an extracellular matrix and are charecterized by high tensile strength, similar to that of bone. The fibrils are oriented in a direction specific to the forces applied during the interaction between a tendon and its muscle and skeletal attachment. Endotendineum and peritendineum -composed of loose connective tissue, elastic fibers and small vessels- envelop the collagen bundles and are in continuity with the epitendineum, a dense connective tissue layer tightly bound to the outer tendon surface [53-55]. In its immediate environment, a tendon can be enclosed or surrounded by a synovial sheath (e.g. biceps tendon, wrist and ankle tendons) or a paratenon of loose vascular areolar connective tissue (e.g. patellar and Achilles tendons) [56-57]. The synovial sheath is a complex structure composed of two interconnecting layers: an internal, visceral one covering the epitendineum and an external, parietal layer in continuity with the adjacent connective spaces. The sheath is infolded by the tendon, so that both visceral and parietal layers are connected by mesotendon, providing a route for the blood supply. The virtual cavity formed by these layers contains a small amount of fluid that facilitates frictionless gliding of the tendon inside the sheath. Herewith, as some of those sheaths directly communicate with the adjacent joints (e.g. proximal biceps, flexor hallucis longus), care should be given before a diagnosis of a tendinopathy (instead of joint effusion) is erroneously made [56]. Lastly, some tendons also have adjacent bursae (e.g. rotator cuff and iliopsoas) and overuse injuries can produce bursitis often before tendinitis.

Majority of the tendons are superficial and can be assessed with a high frequency linear transducer with a thick layer of coupling gel. Small portable US scanners are also available for examining patients immediately after injury, even on the sports field. Similar to muscle injuries, US examination starts with history taking and physical examination. Particular attention should be paid for anisotropy artifact; while it may significantly challenge tendon imaging, its prompt recognition can also facilitate the diagnostic approach. Again, dynamic scanning is of great diagnostic value for assessing a tear, subluxation and adhesion. Interrogation with power Doppler technique can sensitively be used to display inflammation or healing neovascularity [58, 59]. During Doppler assessment, the tendon should be in a relaxed position, contrary to the tensed position in which tendons are typically evaluated for tears and tendinopathy.

## 11.3.1 Normal Sonographic Anatomy

Longitudinal sonograms of tendons show an internal network made up of many fine, tightly packed parallel echoes that resemble a fibrillar pattern. The linear internal fibrillar echoes correspond not to the tendon bundles but to the interfaces between them and the peritendineum [60, 61]. Transverse images depict tendons as hyperechoic structures that appear as an internal homogeneous structure made by multiple small echogenic dots packed together (Figure 11.5). The peritenon appears as a hyperechoic line at the superficial and deep aspect of the tendon. The thin synovial sheath can not be seen even with high-

resolution transducers, unless there is fluid surrounding the tendon. Under normal circumstances, color and power Doppler do not show flow signals inside tendons; however thin vessels can be detected running adjacent to tendons representing vessels of synovial sheaths or peritenon.

## 11.3.2 Tendon Injuries

Similar to muscle lesions, the spectrum of tendon pathologies detectable with US is quite wide and heterogenous.

### Tendinosis

Tendon degeneration, often referred to as "tendinosis", is not characterized by an inflammatory response but rather infiltration of fibroblasts and vessels [62]. Tendinosis is a common pathology in sports medicine practice and it is generally considered to be due to repetitive microtrauma with an ongoing chronic cycle of degeneration - repair resulting in a weakened tendon. From the clinical point of view, tendinosis typically presents with tendon swelling, tenderness, absent or moderate pain aggravated by activities [57].

On US, early tendinosis appears as tendon thickening whereby observation of changes in the normal contour and echotexture would be more practical than relying on absolute measurements. Since these findings may be subtle comparison with the

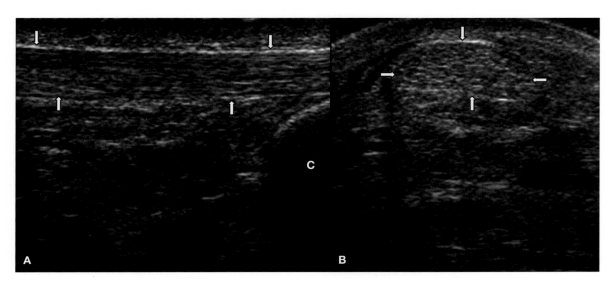

**Figure 11.5** Normal Achilles tendon. Longitudinal view (A) demonstrates the tendon (with typical hyperechoic fibrillar pattern) inserting on the calcaneus (C). Axial image (B) shows the tendon as an ovoid structure with intrinsic punctiform appearance.

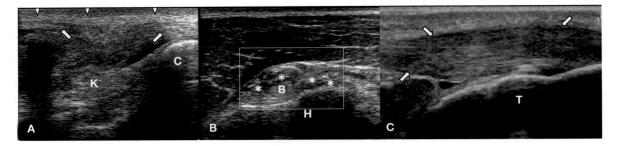

**Figure 11.6**  A- A 22-year-old runner with partial-thickness tear of the Achilles tendon after a pentathlon accident. While the superficial part of the tendon (arrowheads) is intact, the ruptured ends (arrows) seem to be retracted. C, calcaneus; K, Kager's fat pad. B - A 21-year-old man (hammer thrower) with chronic tenosynovitis of the long head of biceps muscle. Axial image shows synovial hypertophy (asterisks) and positive doppler signals. B, biceps tendon; H, humerus. C - A 23-year-old man with patellar tendinosis. Longitudinal image shows convex tendon thickening (arrows), edema and partial loss of the fibrillar pattern at its distal insertion. T, tibia.

asymptomatic side is invaluable. As tendinosis progresses, the fibrillar pattern is lost and replaced by hypoechoic changes with further swelling [56, 63]. These features can be focal or can progress to involve the full tendon thickness, sometimes with calcifications as well. Power Doppler interrogation can give idea for active inflammation (Figure 11.6).

### Tears

Tears of normal tendons are extremely rare and are usually part of severe acute injury. Of note, preceding tendinosis might indisputably predispose to tears. Partial tears (partial- or full-thickness) are detected by hypoechoic or anechoic focal defects involving either the surface or substance of the tendon [64]. Continuous fibers are seen adjacent to a partial tear, and retraction is not a significant hallmark. With the presence of tendon heterogeneity on US images, differentiation between tendinosis and a partial tear becomes quite challenging [61]. Sometimes, they may also coexist with overlapping findings [65].

The clinical diagnosis of complete tendon tears is usually less challenging than that of partial tendon tears. However, owing to the compensation of other tendons or soft tissue edema obliterating the tendon defect, physical examination might be equivocal. Moreover, as tendons retract with time, making retrieval and reattachment more complicated; US examination is paramount not only for prompt diagnosis but also for the onward management [66]. On US imaging, full-thickness distruption of the tendon with retraction of the torn edges, usually accompanied by a hematoma, is the main finding [66]. When the tendon sheaths are also ruptured accompanied hematoma is usually larger and has irregular and indistinct margins [61, 66]. As a result of sound-beam refraction at the frayed tendon ends, posterior acoustic shadowing at the site of tendon tear or behind the retracted tendon stump may be an associated finding.

Another way to better visualize all these types of injuries is definitely to use the dynamic imaging feature of US whereby active and passive motions would open up the gap in the tendon. This sign is especially useful if the gap is otherwise filled with echogenic fluid or debris masquerading the discontinuity of the tendon during static imaging. The size of the gap can be measured and this may also be useful in determining whether a lesion is amenable to non-surgical management [67].

### Tendinitis and tenosynovitis

The spectrum of US findings depends on the type of the tendon involved, as well as on the associated changes occuring in the tendon enveloped and the associated synovial bursae. The inflammatory process can result in "peritendinitis" for tendons invested by paratenon and "tenosynovitis" for tendons invested by synovial sheath. Tendinitis is always possible in both clinical conditions.

Tendons without a synovial sheath can be frequent targets in sport-related injuries mainly because they usually originate from the most powerful muscles in the human body. For instance, the involvement of the Achilles tendon -one of the most frequently involved tendons in several sports activities [7]- may typically yield fluid accumula-

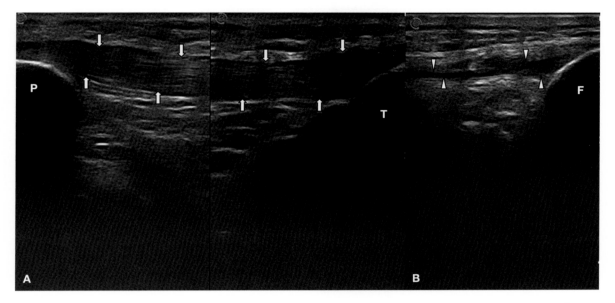

**Figure 11.7**  A - Patellar tendinosis (jumper's knee) in a 22-year-old basketball player. Split-screen longitudinal image demonstrates diffuse thickening of the patellar tendon with areas of hypoechogenicity (arrows). P, patella; T, tibia. B - Longitudinal image of a 23-year-old football player with hypoechoic and irregular iliotibial band (arrowheads) at its insertion. F, fibula.

tion and patchy thickenings in the paratenon, irregularities of tendon margins and adhesions.

Tenosynovitis is detected with hypoechoic or anechoic fluid distending the tendon sheath, with inflammatory changes of the related tendon proper as well [i.e. edema and heterogenous hypoechoic swelling]. Synovial proliferation of the tendon sheath can be seen, thus confirming concurrent synovitis. Doppler US imaging may be helpful to further evaluate the inflammatory process inside/around the tendon [1, 6].

Some typical/common examples of sports related tendon injuries could be listed as rotator cuff problems, runner's knee, jumper's knee and Achilles tendinopathies [68-72] (Figure 11.7).

## 11.4 ULTRASOUND OF LIGAMENTS

Traumatic injuries of the ligaments are quite common, mainly seen in athletes participating in contact sports. Although clinical examination is the mainstay for diagnosis of ligament lesions, imaging modalities is important for precise diagnosis. Due to the lack of immediate/reliable detection of the ligaments, joint sprains can often be undertreated, resulting in chronic pain, muscular weakness, instability, and/or impingement syn-

dromes, sometimes requiring surgical ligament reconstruction [73].

US is an effective method to evaluate the integrity of the ligaments [49, 74]. Ligaments are categorized as intra-articular or extra-articular. While US assessment of the intra-articular ligaments is not always easy due to acoustic barriers, extra-articular ligaments can effectively be imaged with US, similar to the tendons [67]. Ligaments are composed of dense, regular connective tissue similar to that of tendons and demonstrate a bright, echogenic and linear structure. They are best identified by placing the probe between the two bones that they connect. To differentiate between the surrounding hyperechoic fat, the anisotropic characteristics of the ligaments may be used.

Ligament injuries are ultrasonographically classified in three categories [75]. In a mild acute sprain, the ligament may be normal or slightly thickened, and its hyperechoic fibrillar structure may be slightly altered. In a moderate to severe (partial) tear, there is partial interruption in the midsubstance or insertion of the ligament manifested by an anechoic area, but the ligament remains taut during dynamic examination. In a more severe (complete) ligamentous tear, there is complete interruption or avulsion of fibers manifested by a hypoechoic gap;

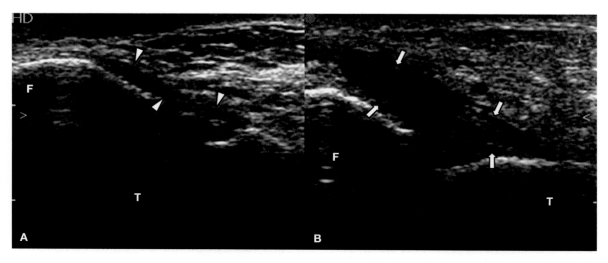

**Figure 11.8** Anterior talofibular ligament sprain in a 24-year-old soccer player. While the normal ligament (arrowheads) is seen as a thin band extending between the talus (T) and fibula (F) (A), the injured ligament is observed as intact but edematous (arrows) (B).

the ligament may be wavy and does not tauten with dynamic stress [73]. The gap allows a hemorrhagic effusion to extrude outside the joint, into the subcutaneous soft tissues or within a neighboring tendinous sheath. Bony avulsion at a ligamentous insertion can be another manifestation of a severe sprain [76, 77]. With chronic tears, US shows thickening of the ligament, and ossifications can be found within its substance [49].

A few typical/common examples of sports related ligament injuries would be goalkeeper's thumb, climber's finger and ankle sprains (anterior talofibular, deltoid, calcaneofibular ligament injuries) (Figure 11.8).

## 11.5 ULTRASOUND OF JOINTS

Based on their anatomy, joints can be divided into three main groups as fibrous, cartilaginous and synovial. Synovial joints have the highest degree of motion and they are the most commonly injured joints in athletes. They are formed by articulating bone surfaces, fibrous capsule and ligaments, synovium and other intra-articular structures (menisci, labra, ligaments, fat pads, etc.).

In general, US examination of a joint reveals two interrupted sharp hyperechoic lines (bones) covered with a thin hyperechoic capsule and often with anechoic smooth linear band of hyaline cartilage on the opposing bony surfaces. A small

amount of fluid can normally be found in the synovial recesses [78]. The synovial tissue lining the joint is immeasurably thin, with smooth, regular contours and a clearly identifiable hyperechoic line defines the joint capsule.

Ultrasound may be helpful in distinguishing simple effusions from other types. In a simple effusion, the fluid seems hypoechoic or anechoic, compressible, devoid of Doppler flow and is bounded by the joint capsule. If the amount of fluid is small, examination of the contralateral joint may be helpful. In hemarthrosis or infection, there may be a diffuse increase in the echogenicity of the fluid, often with layering of fluid or particulate debris. But US cannot always differentiate accurately whether the fluid collection is inflammatory, infectious or hematogenous. But, in such cases, it can definitely facilitate precise aspiration for further analysis. Besides, it can also give a basic estimate of fluid viscosity, aiding selection of the appropriate gauge size of the needle for aspiration. Additionally, in certain conditions with dense fluid collection or collections filled with synovial hypertrophy, US may even refrain from aspiration, avoiding a likely dry tap. On the other hand, fluid can also accumulate in the bursae (normally observed as thin anechoic bands) causing bursitis. Simple bursitis may be characterized by anechoic fluid with or without septations, whereas chronic bursitis often displays moderately echogenic bursal thickening attributable to

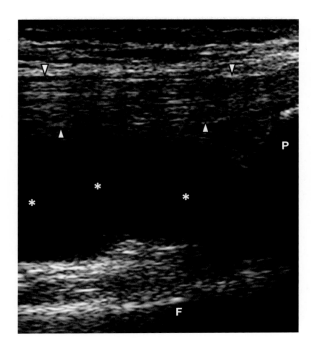

**Figure 11.9** Suprapatellar longitudinal view of the knee shows extensive joint fluid in the suprapatellar recess (asterisks) beneath the quadriceps tendon (arrowheads). P, patella; F, femur.

layering of cells (haematocrit effect), quite similar to hematoma. Due to the presence of corpuscular content, hemorrhagic fluid collections are in fact homogeneously echogenic within the first 2-3 days. After the third day, the hemarthrosis shows a progressive reduction in echogenicity due to lytic enzymes' release.

Eventually, US shows echogenic branches, corresponding to fibrinous clots, crossing the anechoic appearing zone. Many joints contain fibrocartilaginous structures, including menisci in the knee, labra in the hip and shoulder, triangular fibrocartilage in the wrist, and volar/plantar plates in the hand/foot. Because of their deep location and close contact with the bone, these structures can partly be evaluated with US. Tears (anechoic clefts) or associated cysts of the posterior labrum of the shoulder and anterior labrum of the hip joints can be readily detected with static/dynamic US [9, 80].

Concerning meniscal lesions, US is able to show mainly the peripheral portions -which are in fact areas that are poorly evaluated with artroscopy. Again, meniscal tears (extending to the outer layers) or concomitant lesions/cysts can be visualized during knee US [78, 81].

chronic impingement or overuse [1, 79] (Figura 11.9).

At US, haemarthrosis may appear as a joint effusion with or without internal echoes depending on the duration of the haemorrhage and with

## 11.6 ULTRASOUND OF ENTHESES

Enthesopathy, i.e. the inflammation at tendon, ligament and capsule insertions (enthesis), is one the common clinical conditions in sports medicine

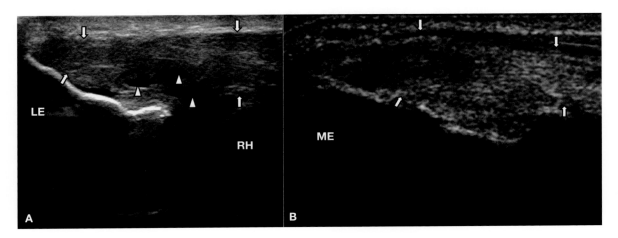

**Figure 11.10** A - Lateral epicondylitis. Ultrasound image (longitudinal view) of the lateral elbow depicts a swollen common extensor tendon origin (arrows) with a partial tear (arrowheads) in its deep portion. B - Medial epicondylitis. Longitudinal image shows a thickened and inhomogeneous common flexor tendon (arrows). LE, lateral epicondyle; RH, radial head; ME, medial epicondyle.

practice. The functioning enthesis dissipates stress over a wide area, including the insertion, immediately adjacent to the tendon and the adjacent bone. Soft tissue components of entheses are traditionally evaluated by clinical examination based on the presence of tenderness and/or swelling while x-rays are used to assess associated bony changes.

The accuracy of these methods are uncertain, though. As such, similar to the tendons and ligaments (due the various aforementioned advantages), US imaging is noteworthy for assessing entheseal regions as well.

Enthesopathy in sports injury, is an inflammatory-degenerative problem usually caused by the overload/use of entheseal region. Typical examples would be golfer's elbow (medial epicondylitis), tennis elbow (lateral epicondylitis) and plantar fasciitis.

US imaging yields findings pertaining to both the bony cortex (periosteal thickening or irregular bony contours e.g. erosions, spurs and enthesophytes) and the related soft tissues (edema, thickening, decreased echogenicity, calcification, bursitis)]. Increased vascularity (consistent with inflammation) on Doppler imaging would also be contributory. Further, especially for bony lesions, sonographic palpation may be very helpful in depicting even small lesions that are not visible on radiographs [82, 83] (Figure 11.10).

## 11.7 MISCELLANEOUS LESIONS

Exercise induced lower leg pain, often termed as shin splint is a major problem that affects athletes, especially runners and jumpers. American

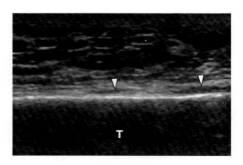

**Figure 11.11** Shin splint. Longitudinal ultrasound image of the medial side of tibia (T) shows periosteal edema (arrowheads) consistent with periostitis.

Medical Association's standard nomenclature defines shin splints as "pain and discomfort in the legs due to repetitive running on hard surfaces or forceful excessive use of the foot flexors". The patients typically present with pain and tenderness lateral to the tibia or along the posteromedial border of the middle to lower tibia [1]. Focal thickenings at the anchor points of the muscle compartments to the periosteum (a sort of periostitis) along the posteromedial and lateral borders of the tibia may be observed on US imaging (Figure 11.11). Doppler US may also show inflammatory findings [44].

Overall, US provides multiplanar views with real-time functional assessment delivered by a cheap, reproducible, and well-tolerated examination, which can also be carried to the playing field or elsewhere. Besides, together with the modern technology, US appears to be a highly sensitive imaging modality/alternative for prompt evaluation of acute and chronic sport related injuries.

# REFERENCES

1) Tok F, Özçakar L, De Muynck M, Kara M, Vanderstraeten G. Musculoskeletal ultrasound for sports injuries. Eur J Phys Rehabil Med. 2012; 48: 651-63.

2) Sofka CM, Pavlov H. Sports injury update: imaging features. Curr Probl Diagn Radiol. 2001; 30: 174-87.

3) Hashefi M. Ultrasound in the diagnosis of noninflammatory musculoskeletal conditions. Semin Ultrasound CT MR. 2011; 32: 74-90.

4) Hashefi M. Ultrasound in the diagnosis of noninflammatory musculoskeletal conditions. Ann N Y Acad Sci. 2009; 1154: 171-203.

5) Klauser A, Bodner G, Frauscher F, Gabl M, Zur Nedden D. Finger injuries in extreme rock climbers. Assessment of high-resolution ultrasonography. Am J Sports Med 1999; 27: 733-7.

6) Ozçakar L, Tok F, De Muynck M, Vanderstraeten G. Musculoskeletal ultrasonography in physical and rehabilitation medicine. J Rehabil Med. 2012; 44: 310-8.

7) Filippucci E, Meenagh G, Delle Sedie A, Riente L, Iagnocco A, Bombardieri S, et al. Ultrasound imaging for the rheumatologist XII. Ultrasound imaging in sports medicine. Clin Exp Rheumatol. 2007; 25: 806-9.

8) Grassi W, Filippucci E, Farina A, Cervini C. Sonographic imaging of tendons. Arthritis Rheum. 2000; 43: 969-76.

9) Jacobson JA. Ultrasound in sports medicine. Radiol Clin North Am. 2002; 40: 363-86.

10) Romagnoli C, Chhem RK, Cardinal E. Muscle and fascia. In: Chhem RK, Cardinal E, editors. Guidelines and gamuts in musculoskeletal ultrasound. New York: Wiley-Liss; 1999. p. 247-79.

11) Tok F, Demirkaya E, Özçakar L. Musculoskeletal ultrasound in pediatric rheumatology. Pediatr Rheumatol Online J. 2011; 9: 25.

12) Rees JD, Wılson AM, Wolman RL. Current concepts in the management of tendon disorders. Rheumatology. 2006; 45: 508-21.

13) Öhberg L, Lorentzon R, Alfredson H. Eccentric training in patients with chronic Achilles tendinosis: normalised tendon structure and decreased thickness at follow-up. Br J Sports Med. 2004; 38: 8-11.

14) Ozçakar L, Carli AB, Tok F, Tekin L, Akkaya N, Kara M. The utility of musculoskeletal ultrasound in rehabilitation settings. Am J Phys Med Rehabil. 2013; 92: 805-17.

15) Gill NW, Mason BE, Gerber JP. Lateral abdominal muscle symmetry in collegiate single-sided rowers. Int J Sports Phys Ther. 2012; 7: 13-9.

16) McCreesh K, Egan S. Ultrasound measurement of the size of the anterior tibial muscle group: the effect of exercise and leg dominance. Sports Med Arthrosc Rehabil Ther Technol. 2011; 3: 18.

17) Hyde J, Stanton WR, Hides JA. Abdominal muscle response to a simulated weight-bearing task by elite Australian Rules football players. Hum Mov Sci. 2012; 31: 129-38.

18) Jansen JA, Mens JM, Backx FJ, Stam HJ. Changes in abdominal muscle thickness measured by ultrasound are not associated with recovery in athletes with longstanding groin pain associated with resisted hip adduction. J Orthop Sports Phys Ther. 2009; 39: 724-32.

19) Ozçakar L, Carli AB, Tok F, Tekin L, Akkaya N, Kara M. The utility of musculoskeletal ultrasound in rehabilitation settings. Am J Phys Med Rehabil. 2013; 92: 805-17.

20) Ozçakar L, Tok F, Kesikburun S, Palamar D, Erden G, Ulaşli A, et al. Musculoskeletal sonography in physical and rehabilitation medicine: results of the first worldwide survey study. Arch Phys Med Rehabil. 2010; 91: 326-31.

21) Imamura M, Özçakar L, Fregni F, Hsing WT, Battistella LR. Exploring a long-term global approach for musculoskeletal ultrasound training: WORLD-MUSCULUS. J Rehabil Med. 2012; 44: 991-2.

22) Ozçakar L, De Muynck M, Imamura M, Vanderstraeten G. Musculoskeletal ultrasound in PRM. From EURO-MUSCULUS towards WORLD-MUSCULUS. Eur J Phys Rehabil Med. 2012; 48: 649-50.

23) Ozçakar L, Tunç H, Oken O, Unlü Z, Durmuş B, Baysal O, et al. Femoral cartilage thickness measurements in healthy individuals learning, practicing and publishing with TURK-MUSCULUS. J Back Musculoskelet Rehabil. 2014; 27: 117-24.

24) Woodhouse JB, McNally EG. Ultrasound of skeletal muscle injury: an update. Semin Ultrasound CT MR. 2011; 32: 91-100.

25) Blankenbaker DG, Tuite MJ. Temporal changes of muscle injury. Semin Musculoskelet Radiol. 2010; 14: 176-93.

26) Kirkendall DT, Garrett WE Jr. Clinical perspectives regarding eccentric muscle injury. Clin Orthop Relat Res. 2002; 81: 9.

27) Best TM. Soft-tissue injuries and muscle tears. Clin Sports Med. 1997; 16: 419-34.

28) Sallay PI, Friedman RL, Coogan PG, Garrett WE. Hamstring muscle injuries among water skiers. Functional outcome and prevention. Am J Sports Med. 1996; 24: 130-6.

29) Pomeranz SJ, Heidt RS Jr. MR imaging in the prognostication of hamstring injury. Work in progress. Radiology. 1993; 189: 897-900.

30) Heiser TM, Weber J, Sullivan G, Clare P, Jacobs RR. Prophylaxis and management of hamstring muscle injuries in intercollegiate football players. Am J Sports Med. 1984; 12: 368-370.

31) Koh ES, McNally EG. Ultrasound of skeletal muscle injury. Semin Musculoskelet Radiol. 2007; 11: 162-73.

32) Entrekin RR, Porter BA, Sillesen HH, Wong AD, Cooperberg PL, Fix CH. Real-time spatial compound imaging: application to breast, vascular, and musculoskeletal ultrasound. Semin Ultrasound CT MR. 2001; 22: 50-64.

33) Tranquart F, Grenier N, Eder V, Pourcelot L. Clinical use of ultrasound tissue harmonic imaging. Ultrasound Med Biol. 1999; 25: 889-94.

34) Pinzon EG, Moore RE. Musculoskeletal ultrasound. A brief overview of diagnostic and therapeutic applications in musculoskeletal medicine. Pract Pain Manege. 2009; 1: 34-43.

35) El-Khoury GY, Brandser EA, Kathol MH, Tearse DS, Callaghan JJ. Imaging of muscle injuries. Skeletal Radiol. 1996; 25: 3-11.

36) Jarvinen TAH, Jarvinen TLN, Kaariainen M, Kalimo H, Jarvinen M. Muscle injuries: biology and treatment. Am J Sports Med. 2005; 33: 745-64.

37) Zamorani MP, Valle M. Muscle and Tendon. In: Bianchi S, Martinoli C, editors. Ultrasound of the musculoskeletal system. 1st ed. Berlin: Springer; 2007. p. 45-96.

38) Beiner JM, Jokl P. Muscle contusion injuries: current treatment options. J Am Acad Orthop Surg. 2001; 9: 227-37.

39) Lee JC, Healy J. Sonography of lower limb muscle injury. AJR Am J Roentgenol. 2004; 182: 341-51.

40) Fornage BD. The case for ultrasound of muscles and tendons. Semin Musculoskelet Radiol. 2000; 4: 375-91.

41) Bianchi S, Martinoli C, Waser NP, Bianchi-Zamorani MP, Federici E, Fasel J. Central aponeurosis tears of the rectus femoris: sonographic findings. Skeletal Radiol. 2002; 31: 581-6.

42) Cross TM, Gibbs N, Houang MT, Cameron M. Acute quadriceps muscle strains: magnetic resonance imaging features and prognosis. Am J Sports Med. 2004; 32: 710-9.

43) McNally E. Practical Musculoskeletal Ultrasound. Edinburgh, UK: Churchill Livingstone; 2004.

44) van Holsbeeck MT, Introcaso JH. Sonography of muscle. In: Bralow L, editor. Musculoskeletal ultrasound. 2nd ed. St Louis, MO: Mosby Inc.; 2001. p. 23-75.

45) Chew K, Stevens KJ, Wang TG, Fredericson M, Lew HL. Introduction to diagnostic musculoskeletal ultrasound: part 2: examination of the lower limb. Am J Phys Med Rehabil. 2008; 87: 238-48.

46) Noonan TJ, Garrett WE. Muscle strain injury: diagnosis and treatment. J Am Acad Orthop Surg 1999; 7: 262-9.

47) Campbell RSD, Wood J. Ultrasound of muscle. Imaging. 2002; 14: 229-40.

48) Brittenden J, Robinson P. Imaging of pelvic injuries in athletes. Br J Radiol. 2005; 78: 457-68.

49) Peetrons P, Creteur V, Bacq C. Sonography of ankle ligaments. J Clin Ultrasound. 2004; 32: 491-9.

50) Cross TM, Gibbs N, Houang MT, Cameron M. Acute quadriceps muscle strains: magnetic resonance imaging features and prognosis. Am J Sports Med. 2004; 32: 710-19.

51) Beiner JM, Jokl P. Muscle contusion injury and myositis ossificans traumatica. Clin Orthop Relat Res. 2002; 403 Suppl: S110-9.

52) Peck RJ, Metreweli C. Early myositis ossificans: a new echographic sign. Clin Radiol. 1988; 39: 586-8.

53) Zamorani MP, Valle M. Muscle and Tendon. In: Bianchi S, Martinoli C, editors. Ultrasound of the musculoskeletal system. 1st ed. Berlin: Springer; 2007. p. 45-96.

54) Towers JD, Russ EV, Golla SK. Biomechanics of tendons and tendon failure. Semin Musculoskelet Radiol. 2003; 7: 59-65.

55) Brinckmann P, Frobin F, Leivseth G. Musculoskeletal biomechanics. New York, NY: Thieme, 2002.

56) Robinson P. Sonography of common tendon injuries. AJR Am J Roentgenol. 2009; 193: 607-18.

57) Bianchi S, Martinoli C, Abdelwahab IF. Ultrasound of tendon tears. Part 1: general considerations and upper extremity. Skeletal Radiol. 2005; 34: 500-12.

58) Alfredson H, Ohberg L, Forsgren S. Is vasculoneural ingrowth the cause of pain in chronic Achilles tendinosis? An investigation using ultrasonography and colour Doppler, immunohistochemistry, and diagnostic injections. Knee Surg Sports Traumatol Arthrosc. 2003; 11: 334-8.

59) Ohberg L, Alfredson H. Effects on neovascularisation behind the good results with eccentric training in chronic mid-portion Achilles tendinosis? Knee Surg Sports Traumatol Arthrosc. 2004; 12: 465-70.

60) Bertolotto M, Perrone R, Martinoli C, Rollandi GA, Patetta R, Derchi LE. High resolution ultrasound anatomy of normal Achilles tendon. Br J Radiol. 1995; 68: 986-91.

61) Martinoli C, Bianchi S, Derchi LE. Ultrasound of tendon and nerves. Radiol Clin North Am. 1999; 37: 691-711.

62) Connell DA, Ali KE, Ahmad M, Lambert S, Corbett S, Curtis M. Ultrasound-guided autologous blood injection for tennis elbow. Skeletal Radiol. 2006; 35: 371-7.

63) Campbell RS, Grainger AJ. Current concepts in imaging of tendinopathy. Clin Radiol. 2001; 56: 253-67.

64) J acobson JA. Ultrasound in sports medicine. Radiol Clin North Am. 2002; 40: 363-86.

65) Torriani M, Kattapuram SV. Musculoskeletal ultrasound: an alternative imaging modality for sports-related injuries. Top Magn Reson Imaging. 2003; 14: 103-11.

66) Allen GM, Wilson DJ. Ultrasound in sports medicine--a critical evaluation. Eur J Radiol. 2007; 62: 79-85.

67) Kijowski R, De Smet AA. The role of ultrasound in the evaluation of sports medicine injuries of the upper extremity. Clin Sports Med. 2006; 25: 569-90.

68) Wohlwend JR, van Holsbeeck M, Craig J, Shirazi K, Habra G, Jacobsen G, et al. The association between irregular greater tuberosities and rotator cuff tears: a sonographic study. AJR Am J Roentgenol. 1998; 171: 229-33.

69) Zanetti M, Metzdorf A, Kundert HP, Zollinger H, Vienne P, Seifert B et al. Achilles tendons: clinical relevance of neovascularization diagnosed with power Doppler US. Radiology. 2003; 227: 556-60.

70) Hollenberg GM, Adams MJ, Weinberg EP. Sonographic appearance of nonoperatively treated Achilles tendon ruptures. Skeletal Radiol. 2000; 29: 259-64.

71) Blankenbaker DG, De Smet AA. The role of ultrasound in the evaluation of sports injuries of the lower extremities. Clin Sports Med. 2006; 25: 867-97.

72) Khoury V, Guillin R, Dhanju J, Cardinal E. Ultrasound of ankle and foot: overuse and sports injuries. Semin Musculoskelet Radiol. 2007; 11: 149-61.

73) Brasseur JL, Luzzati A, Lazennec JY, Guerin-Surville H, Roger B, Grenier P. Ultrasono-anatomy of the ankle ligaments. Surg Radiol Anat. 1994; 16: 87-91.

74) Morvan G, Mathieu P, Busson J, Wybier M. Ultrasonography of tendons and ligaments of foot and ankle. J Radiol. 2000; 81: 361-80.

75) Morvan G, Busson J, Wybier M, Mathieu P. Ultrasound of the ankle. Eur J Ultrasound. 2001; 14: 73-82.

76) Campbell DG, Menz A, Isaacs J. Dynamic ankle ultrasonography. A new imaging technique for acute ankle ligament injuries. Am J Sports Med. 1994; 22: 855-8.

77) van Holsbeeck MT, Introcaso JH. Sonography of large synovial joints. In: Bralow L, editor. Musculoskeletal ultrasound. 2nd ed. St Louis, MO: Mosby Inc.; 2001. p. 235-75.

78) Chew K, Stevens KJ, Wang TG, Fredericson M, Lew HL. Introduction to diagnostic musculoskeletal ultrasound: part 2: examination of the lower limb. Am J Phys Med Rehabil. 2008; 87: 238-48.

79) Hammar MV, Wintzell GB, Aström KG, Larsson S, Elvin A. Role of us in the preoperative evaluation of patients with anterior shoulder instability. Radiology. 2001; 219: 29-34.

80) Blankenbaker DG, De Smet AA. The role of ultrasound in the evaluation of sports injuries of the lower extremities. Clin Sports Med. 2006; 25: 867-97.

81) Miller TT, Shapiro MA, Schultz E, Kalish PE. Comparison of sonography and MRI for diagnosing epicondylitis. J Clin Ultrasound. 2002; 30: 193-202.

82) Sofka CM. Ultrasound in sports medicine. Semin Musculoskelet Radiol. 2004; 8: 17-27.

# Ultrasound Imaging for Peripheral Nerve Problems

## 12

Murat KARA

## 12.1 INTRODUCTION

Peripheral nerve problems are commonplace in physical and rehabilitation medicine daily practice and they can readily mimic various musculoskeletal disorders. Although the combination of a substantial physical examination and a following electrodiagnostic study is used for the diagnosis of peripheral nerve pathologies, they cannot directly localize the exact site of injury and cannot uncover the morphological changes within a nerve or the likely underlying cause. In addition, during electrodiagnostic studies, electrophysiologists may encounter various confusing clinical scenarios or equivocal/contradictory results, especially in cases with technical difficulties during sensory assessments with surface electrodes (even with near-nerve needle techniques) and during the assessment of certain focal lesions e.g. tarsal tunnel syndrome, meralgia paraesthetica and Morton's neuroma [1]. In this regard, direct visualization of nerve and/or relevant accompanying soft tissue abnormalities with an imaging modality -i.e. ultrasound (US) or magnetic resonance imaging (MRI)- may enhance the diagnosis and the surgical outcome.

With the advent of high-frequency probes and enhanced software US provides several advantages over MRI; it has a superior spatial resolution (250-400 μm at a depth of about 0.5-1.5 cm from the skin), it is more convenient and cost-effective [2-5]. Further, due to its additional advantages such as dynamic real-time nature and availability of simultaneous comparisons with normal structures as well as better patient tolerance, US has become an established and widespread first-line imaging method for the evaluation of peripheral nerve disorders. In this regard, physiatrists can scan several peripheral nerves along their anatomical courses immediately after clinical examination. Of note, "sonopalpation" can be used as "sono-Tinel" for peripheral nerves [6]. In short, US can help discover a possible underlying/concomitant etiology, precisely guide an onward intervention (i.e. planning for injection or surgery) and follow-up.

Further, developments in power Doppler and Doppler sensitivity have made it possible to evaluate vascular changes within a major nerve segment. In challenging cases, it can even be an essential diagnostic tool rather than being only an adjunct to electrodiagnostics or contribute to the eventual diagnosis via muscle imaging for denervation signs e.g. denervation edema or chronic fatty atrophy. On the other hand, US imaging of peripheral nerve problems definitely requires knowledge of the anatomy/topography being examined, specific training, long-term experience, and most importantly, close clinical correlation with the patient's neurologic and electrodiagnostic findings [7].

Morphologically, a peripheral nerve has a round or flattened structure with complex internal architecture. It consists of nerve fibers (made of axons with/without myelin sheaths and Schwann cells), and together with its surrounding connective tissue (endoneurium), these fibers form the nerve fascicles. In turn, each nerve fascicle is surrounded by the perineurium which comprises connective tissue, vessels and lymphatics. Multiple nerve fascicles are enclosed by epineurium which is a relatively thicker membrane compared to the endoneurium and perineurium, and which contains of loose areolar tissue with some elastic fibers and perineural vessels.

## 12.2 EXAMINATION TECHNIQUE

The preference of transducer for evaluating peripheral nerve US depends on the regional anatomy to be examined. High-frequency linear probes (10-18 MHz) and related soft tissue contrast-enhancing are required for peripheral nerve imaging. With improved performance of the transducers/machines, almost all major peripheral nerves (median, ulnar, radial, femoral, fibular and tibial nerves), many small ones (e.g. musculocutaneous, posterior interosseous, palmar cutaneous branch of the median nerve, sural, saphenous, lateral femoral cutaneous) (Figure 12.1) and even digital nerves have become visible with US imaging [8, 9]. Some cranial nerves (i.e. optic, facial, vagus and spinal accessory nerves) at several levels along their courses, cervical nerve roots at paravertebral levels and the brachial plexus can also be scanned (Figure 12.2). On the other hand, some deeply located nerves and those which are hidden by intervening bones (sympathetic chain and splanchnic nerves) can hardly be seen with US. In addition, perineural structures (e.g. differentiation with fat may be difficult) greatly influence peripheral nerve imaging, especially when the nerve runs deeply as in obese patients. In general, peripheral nerves course deeper in the lower extremities than in the upper extremities; thus necessitating a lower frequency (2-7 MHz) transducers.

The evaluation of a peripheral nerve depends on the suspected diagnosis. While US imaging may fo-

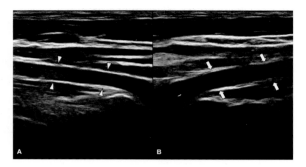

**Figure 12.2** Comparative US imaging (oblique coronal view) of the neck shows elongated hypoechoic cervical roots (arrowheads) exiting the neural foramina (A), and diffuse enlargement (arrows) on the side of radiculopathy (B).

cus on a particular region of interest for entrapment syndromes, complete scanning throughout the course of a peripheral nerve might be essential for widespread involvement. Although axial (short-axis) and longitudinal (long-axis) views are always coupled during the examination, axial imaging is more convenient and prompt for long distance nerve scanning. In short-axis plane, the nerve is seen like a "honeycomb" pattern with hypoechoic neuronal fascicle groups and hyperechoic interfascicular perineurium and outer epineurium. On the other hand, long-axis imaging (seen as multiple hypoechoic lines divided by hyperechoic bands) can be performed at any location where the tubular structure of the nerve is to be visualized. Of note, this hypo-/hyper-echoic pattern relates to the nerve itself, anatomical location (superficial or deep) and frequency of the transducer. Some nerves (e.g. ulnar nerve at the cubital tunnel, radial nerve at the spiral groove) often appear as one/several large hypoechoic fascicle(s), while small nerves (e.g. superficial radial or posterior interosseous nerve) can be seen as a single hypoechoic fascicle with an oval shape [10]. Moreover, nerves tend to become hyperechoic as they reside deeper within muscle compartments (Figure 12.3).

During imaging, nerves should be distinguished from other major tubular structures (tendons, arteries and veins) for proper identification. Tendons are fibrillar, incompressible, mobile and give significant anisotropy. Nerves are fascicular, more compressible, less mobile and give less anisotropy. Peripheral nerves usually travel very close to vessels. As such, initial recognition of an anechoic vessel can actually be used for better identification of an accompanying nerve. Arteries can be detected with their pulsations and veins

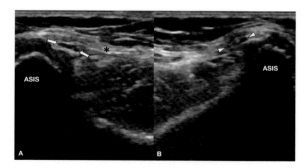

**Figure 12.1** Comparative US imaging (axial view) of the lateral femoral cutaneous nerve in a patient with meralgia paresthetica. A - On the entrapped side, the nerve seems to be swollen and hypoechoic (notched arrows) where it passes medial to the anterior superior iliac spine (ASIS) and below the inguinal ligament (asterisk); B - On the normal side, the nerve shows a relatively normal hyperechoic appearance (arrowheads) at the same level.

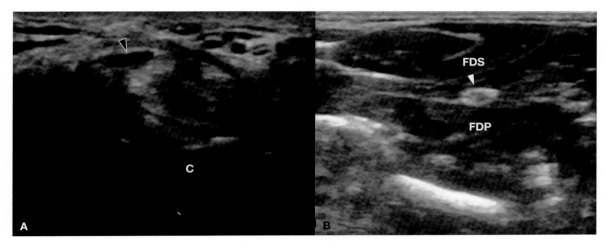

**Figure 12.3** US imaging (axial views) shows hypoechoic median nerve (black arrowhead) in a superficial location at the level of the carpal bones (A), which becomes hyperechoic (white arrowhead) as it runs deeper within the flexor muscle compartments (B). (C, carpal bones, FDS, flexor digitorum superficialis, FDP, flexor digitorum profundus).

with their easy collapse even with mild compression. Additionally, Doppler imaging can also be used for confirmation of a vascular structure.

## 12.3 ASSESSMENT

### 12.3.1 Size and Shape

Enlargement of a nerve/fascicle is the most common US finding in case of chronic neuropathies. Selective enlargement of fascicle(s) within the nerve can be found in some types of Charcot-Marie-Tooth disease and chronic inflammatory demyelinating polyradiculoneuropathy [11-14]. On the other hand, in compressive syndromes, abnormal pressure leads to local disruption in microcirculation and venous congestion, and then epi/endoneurial edema develops. Therefore, the nerve becomes flattened/pinched at the site of compression, and enlarged proximally (sometimes distally as well) [2]. The most common diagnostic measurements are cross sectional area (CSA) and swelling ratio in the short-axis images. The probe should be angled perpendicular to the nerve with minimal pressure at the site of maximum enlargement.

Cross sectional area (CSA) should be measured just inside of the epineurium (hyperechoic rim) while the extremity is kept in a constant position [15]. Values higher than 2 standard deviations above the mean reference value or ≥1.5 times higher than an unaffected portion of the same nerve are commonly considered as nerve enlargement [16, 17]. The swelling ratio (CSA at the maximal enlargement site/CSA at an unaffected site) may improve the diagnosis in case of nerve variations or diffuse nerve enlargement due to a coexisting polyneuropathy [18].

### 12.3.2 Echogenicity and Vascularity

In pathological conditions, the typical honeycomb pattern of the nerve can become homogeneously hypoechoic with loss of the fascicular pattern due to increased intraneural edema and with reduced echogenicity of the epineurium. Several studies have demonstrated increased hypoechogenicity in entrapment syndromes and diabetic polyneuropathy [19-21].

Normally, endo/perineural blood flow in a healthy nerve can not be observed with Doppler US. However, when there is inflammation (like in chronic compressive syndromes or certain inflammatory neuropathies), power Doppler imaging may yield positive signals [22-29]. Since these inflammatory findings may indicate further nerve fiber damage in different neuropathies, their detection/quantification might be noteworthy [22-24].

### 12.3.3 Mobility

Although nerve mobility has been measured for median nerve at the carpal tunnel and for ulnar nerve at the elbow, its evaluation may also be contributory in other nerve syndromes/lesions. Nerve mobility has been found as decreased in carpal tunnel syndrome (CTS) [30, 31] and as possibly increased in ulnar neuropathy at the elbow [32]. To evaluate nerve mobility in CTS, patients are asked to simultaneously move their fingers while the probe is positioned longitudinally at the distal wrist crease level. The median nerve glides slightly (less than the tendons) in the distal-proximal direction with finger movements. Decreased mobility can be quantified in both lateral and distal-proximal planes in patients with CTS [30, 31]. The ulnar nerve at the elbow can move to the tip of the medial epicondyle (subluxation) or completely relocate over the medial epicondyle (dislocation) during the elbow flexion.

## 12.4 IMAGING FOR ENTRAPMENT SYNDROMES

Entrapment problems are quite common peripheral nerve diseases. Peripheral nerves can be compressed especially at certain anatomic sites where they run through an osseofibrous canal or under an abnormal muscle/fibrous band, or a space-occupying lesion (i.e. ganglion, tenosynovitis, synovial cyst, lipoma). Ganglion cysts are the 2nd most common cause of a peripheral nerve entrapment following the typical entrapment syndromes in osseofibrous tunnels. They can be divided into intraneural (rarely seen) or extraneural (joint capsule, muscle, tendon and peritendinous structures) ganglia [33-38]. At US examination, extraneural ganglia appear as a grapelike, echo-free, polycystic and non-vascularized structure with/without septations. Table 12.1 shows the commonly seen nerve entrapment syndromes.

Abnormal US findings related with compressive neuropathies include fusiform enlargement of the nerve proximal to the site of compression, changes in the shape (an abrupt sudden flattening of the nerve at the site of compression), decreased echogenicity, increased vascularity and changes in mobility of the nerve (Figures 12.4 and 12.5). Although the underlying mechanism is unclear,

**Table 12.1** Ultrasonographic CSA (mm²) reference and cut-off values for the commonly seen nerve entrapment syndromes

| Nerve | CSA (normal) | Syndrome | Compression site | CSA (cut-off) | Sensitivity (%) | Specificity (%) |
|---|---|---|---|---|---|---|
| Median nerve | 8.4±2.0[17] | Carpal tunnel syndrome | Carpal tunnel | ≥9.0 [40] | 87 | 83 |
| Ulnar nerve | 6.6 (99% CI; 6.1-7.1)[76] | Cubital tunnel syndrome | Cubital tunnel | ≥10.0 [73] | 88 | 88 |
| Ulnar nerve | 5.9 (99% CI; 5.4-6.4)[76] | Guyon's canal syndrome | Guyon's canal | - | | |
| Radial nerve | 3.2±1.5[17] | Spiral groove syndrome | Spiral groove | - | | |
| Fibular nerve | 7.5 (95% CI; 7.0-7.9)[101] | Fibular neuropathy | Fibular head | >8.0 [101] | 86 | 73 |
| Tibial nerve | 6.3±1.45[17] | Tarsal tunnel syndrome | Tarsal tunnel | - | | |
| Interdigital nerve | * | Morton's neuroma | 3rd/4th intermetatarsal space | - | | |
| LFCN | 1.0±0.4[8] | Meralgia paresthetica | Level of the inguinal ligament | - | | |
| PIN | 1.9[9] | PIN syndrome | Supinator area at the elbow | - | | |

CSA; cross-sectional area, CI; confidence interval, LFCN; lateral femoral cutaneous nerve, PIN; posterior interosseous nerve, * ~2 mm in diameter.

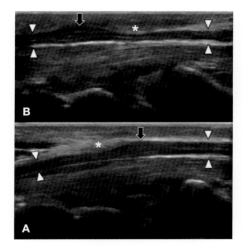

**Figure 12.4** Median nerve (white arrowheads) ultrasonography (longitudinal view) in a patient with bilateral carpal tunnel syndrome. When compared with the entrapment sites (asterisks), the swollen areas (black arrows) are the distal side on the operated hand (A), and the proximal side on the non-operated side (B).

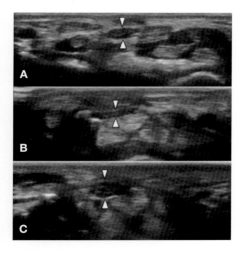

**Figure 12.5** US imaging (axial view) of the median nerve (white arrowheads) in a patient with previously operated carpal tunnel syndrome. The median nerve is seen normal proximal to the carpal tunnel (A), flattened at the level of the tunnel (B), swollen and more hypoechoic distal to the tunnel (C).

nerve enlargement can be caused by increased chronic pressure on the nerve which results in intraneural edema, venous congestion, and impaired axoplasmic flow [39]. In this regard, experimental studies have demonstrated inflammation, demyelination, remyelination, fibrosis and thickening of the connective tissues due to chronic nerve compression [40, 41]. US can also be useful to identify or rule out possible (aforementioned) secondary causes (Figures 12.6 and 12.7).

## 12.4.1 Carpal Tunnel Syndrome

Carpal tunnel syndrome (CTS) is the most common entrapment neuropathy with a prevalence ranging from 1% to 5% in the general population (up to 14.5% in certain occupational groups) whereby more than three-quarters are women [42-44]. It is mostly idiopathic or related with some occupations or systemic diseases (i.e. diabetes mellitus, hypothyroidism, pregnancy or obe-

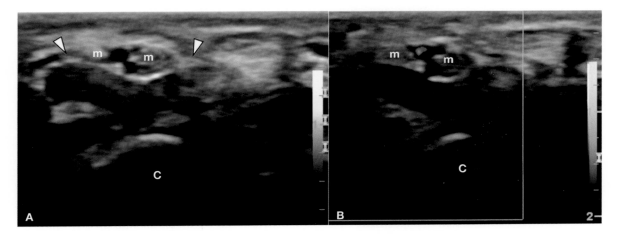

**Figure 12.6** US imaging (axial view) of the median nerve (m) in a patient with carpal tunnel syndrome. A) The bifid median nerve is seen in its normal position under the flexor retinaculum (white arrowheads); B) power Doppler ultrasound shows that the bifid median nerve is also accompanied by a persistent median artery. (C, carpal bones).

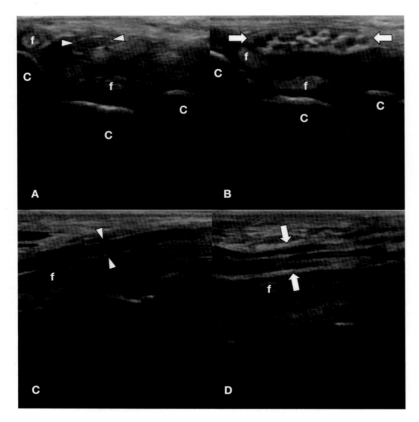

**Figure 12.7** Comparative US imaging of the median nerves at the level of the carpal bones (c) in a patient with fibrolipomatous hamartoma. On the normal side, the median nerve shows a relatively normal hypoechoic appearance (arrowheads) at axial (A) and longitudinal (C) views. On the pathologic side, enlarged median nerve (arrows) with multiple anechoic fascicles and hyperechoic connective tissue are observed on axial (B) and longitudinal (D) images. f, flexor tendon.

sity). Although electrodiagnostic testing is the gold standard for its diagnosis, US can also be used as a first-line screening/confirmatory tool in the diagnostic algorithm [5]. Measurement of the nerve CSA at proximal carpal tunnel (pisiform bone level) is the most sensitive and specific US finding for the diagnosis of CTS [45-49].

Other US findings include hypoechogenicity, reduced mobility and increased vascularity. Although the electrodiagnostic studies have an accuracy of 85-90% [50, 51], they are less accurate in the early stage when symptoms are mild [52]. In addition, morphologic changes of the median nerve may not occur either in the early stage of CTS when increased vascularity might be the only pathologic finding. Therefore, evaluating vascularity can increase the sensitivity/specificity of US in the diagnosis of CTS, especially in patients with a negative nerve conduction test. In this regard, hypervascularity within the nerve on Doppler US

can be an additional diagnostic parameter due to its high accuracy (95%) for CTS [26].

The usefulness of US findings in the diagnosis of CTS has been widely discussed in the literature (see table 12.1). The diagnostic accuracy of US is as high as that of electrodiagnostic studies [45-49, 53-59]. A recent evidence-based guideline [49] showed that US assessment of median nerve CSA at the wrist is accurate and may be suggested as a diagnostic test for CTS (strength level A). In addition, US should be considered to screen for structural abnormalities in patients with CTS (strength level B). On the other hand, as they do not assess the same parameters, electrophysiological studies and US should be considered as complementary methods, improving diagnostic accuracy.

Ultrasound (US) can also be used to discover possible underlying causes in patients with secondary CTS. Screening for an abnormality leading CTS is especially important in patients with atypical symptoms, trauma, unilateral or sudden onset findings [33, 60]. Median nerve can be entrapped under the flexor retinaculum due to some predisposing factors related with space-occupying lesions (i.e. ganglion cyst, fibrolipomatous hamartoma, tendon sheath fibroma, amyloid deposits), or anatomic variants (i.e. bifid median nerve, persistent median artery, presence of an accessory tendon/muscle) within the tunnel (Figures 12.6 and 12.7) [33, 46, 60-64]. For instance, having a higher CSA than a normal median nerve, a bifid median nerve can be an independent risk factor for the development of CTS [62]. Yet, bifid median nerve was detected in 2-13% [62-64], persistent median artery in 9-13% [62, 63], tenosynovitis in 6% and accessory muscles in 3% of patients with CTS [63]. In a study evaluating patients with unilateral CTS, US detected occult ganglia causing CTS in 25% of the patients' affected wrists [33]. Therefore, clinicians should be aware of such variants not only for the diagnosis but also for the onward interventions (injection or surgery). Of note, US can also guide those procedures or even thereafter i.e. follow-up for scar tissue, hematoma, abscess or iatrogenic nerve injuries. Likewise, significant decreases in CSA together with improvements in symptoms and electrodiagnostic findings have been reported after carpal tunnel release surgery [64-67].

Ultrasound (US) findings may also give information about the severity of CTS [46, 68-71]. Increased CSA has been reported to be related with severity parameters such as clinical scales, hand function and electrophysiological findings [69-71]. Interestingly, Lee et al. [71] found an association between the CSA and the severity of electrophysiologic findings, and they suggested 15 mm$^2$ as the cut-off value to undergo surgical decompression. With treatment, improvements in CSA ensue after improvement in symptoms, often taking 12 to 18 months to normalize [72]. On the other hand, hypervascularity visualized by color Doppler US was also found to be correlated with the severity of CTS detected by electrodiagnostic testing [24, 25].

## 12.4.2 Cubital Tunnel Syndrome

Ulnar neuropathy at the elbow is the 2$^{nd}$ most common entrapment syndrome only after CTS (about 1/13$^{th}$ as common as CTS in the same population) and more than two-thirds of the pa-

tients are men [44, 73]. Ulnar nerve runs through an osseofibrous passage way formed by a condylar groove between the medial epicondyle and olecranon bridged by the cubital tunnel retinaculum. Then, it enters to a narrow tunnel between the two heads of the flexor carpi ulnaris muscle covered by the arcuate ligament (proper cubital tunnel). Ulnar nerve can be entrapped either at the condylar groove or at the edge of the arcuate ligament -called as cubital tunnel syndrome (CuTS). Patients with CuTS may present with medial elbow pain, sensory symptoms in the 4$^{th}$ and 5$^{th}$ fingers, and in chronic stages, weakness of the ulnar-innervated muscles.

Ulnar nerve measurement at the condylar groove depends on different factors including patient's age, weight, gender, race and elbow position [74]. The ulnar nerve may be examined with the elbow flexed between 15 to 90 degrees [15]. Normally, the nerve appears more hypoechoic due to the curved route (anisotropy artifact) and it is slightly enlarged at the condylar groove (6.8 mm$^2$) when compared with the distal (5.7 mm$^2$) and proximal forearm (6.2 mm$^2$) CSA measurements [75]. Entrapment of the ulnar nerve under the arcuate ligament results in focal enlargement with loss of fascicular pattern just proximal to the compression site, at the condylar groove (Figure 12.8). This swelling is the major diagnostic finding for CuTS, with >80% of sensitivity (see table 12.1) [15, 18, 76, 77]. US can also increase the sensitivity of electrodiagnostic testing up to 98% in CuTS [78]. In this regard, comparison with the healthy side (if possible) can be helpful and should also be performed.

While enlarged CSA of the ulnar nerve was found to be correlated with the electrophysiological findings [77, 79, 80], US can also be useful to localize the ulnar nerve injury, especially in patients with absent motor or sensory responses. Additionally, it can be helpful for determining the severity and prognosis of CuTS as well. Furthermore, like in other entrapment syndromes, US can visualize different anatomical variations and/or pathologic changes in the nerve surroundings i.e. ganglion, spur, shallow condylar groove, cubitus valgus, heterotopic ossification or accessory anconeus epitrochlearis muscle [81, 82]. For sure, dynamic imaging can readily help demonstrate particular problems like subluxation or dislocation of the ulnar nerve during elbow flexion or snapping medial head of the triceps mus-

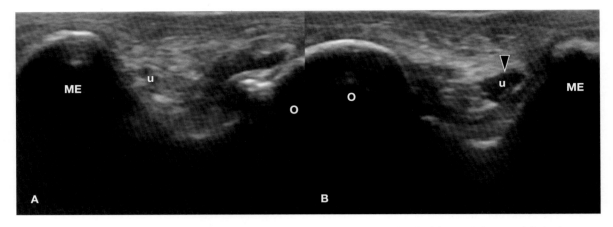

**Figure 12.8** Comparative US imaging (axial view) of the ulnar nerves (u) at the level of the medial epicondyle (ME) in a patient with cubital tunnel syndrome. On the normal side (A), the nerve shows a relatively normal hypoechoic appearance (A), however it is seen as enlarged (arrowhead) on the symptomatic side (B). O, olecranon.

cle. Subluxation (often bilateral) can be seen in 24-47% of asymptomatic healthy subjects and it can lead to friction neuritis in some patients [83-85]. Finally, Doppler imaging can show the possible vascular pathologies (e.g. ulnar recurrent artery or aberrant veins) nearby/within the cubital tunnel [86].

### 12.4.3 Guyon's Canal Syndrome

Ulnar neuropathy at wrist (Guyon's canal syndrome) is a relatively uncommon condition whereby the nerve becomes compressed while passing through the Guyon's canal. The osteofibrotic canal is formed by pisiform (medial wall), hook of the hamate (lateral wall), transverse carpal ligament (floor), and palmar carpal ligament and palmaris brevis muscle (roof) [87]. Guyon's canal syndrome is commonly related with work or sport-based (e.g. in bicyclists) overuse, anatomic abnormalities (anomalous muscles, hypoplastic hamulus, multiple ulnar nerve branches and increased amount of fat tissue), and space-occupying lesions (ganglion cyst, aneurysms of the ulnar artery, lipoma or heterotopic ossification) [88-90]. In this regard, it has been reported that ganglion cysts caused ulnar nerve compression in about 30-40% of patients with Guyon's canal syndrome [38].

Guyon's canal syndrome can manifest with various sensory and/or motor symptoms depending on the location of the compression. At wrist (volar side), the ulnar nerve can be visualized axially as a round or oval structure just medial to the pulsatile ulnar artery. The probe is then moved proximally and distally 1 to 2 cm in each direction to detect the maximum enlargement site. The upper limit of normal CSA (mean + 2 standard deviation) for the ulnar nerve at the wrist level is 8.1 mm² [76], but the diagnostic accuracy of this cut-off value has not been tested (see table 12.1). US imaging of the pisiform bone and ulnar nerve just distal to the pisiform bone level is also important, as pathologies can arise from this location [91].

### 12.4.4 Spiral Groove Syndrome

Together with the deep brachial artery/vein, the radial nerve courses between the posterolateral aspect of the humeral shaft and the triceps muscle. After innervating the triceps and anconeus muscles, it wraps around the humerus at the spiral groove. At this level, radial nerve becomes quite susceptible to compression and trauma due to its close relationship with the bone and its fixity while it penetrates the lateral intermuscular septum [92]. The most common radial neuropathy develops at the spiral groove due to prolonged positioning of the arm on a hard surface during sleep, surgery or alcohol intoxication ("Saturday night palsy"), humeral shaft fracture and infarction from vasculitis [92, 93]. Wrist drop develops due to denervation of the forearm and hand extensors. Paresthesia and/or hypoesthesia can also occur over the lateral dorsal forearm and hand in

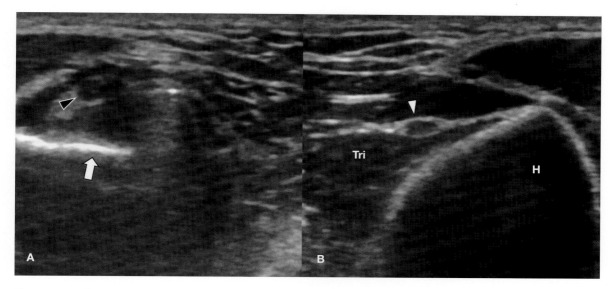

**Figure 12.9** Comparative US imaging (axial view) for the radial nerve entrapment. The nerve is seen as enlarged and hypoechoic (black arrowhead) due to a humeral fracture (white arrow) at the level of the spiral canal (A). The nerve (white arrowhead) is normal on the contralateral side. (H, humerus, Tri, triceps muscle).

the distribution of the superficial radial sensory nerve (Figure 12.9).

The radial nerve can be followed through its course in an axial plane with the patient seated, and arm in the neutral position, forearm pronated, and elbow moderately flexed [10]. At the spiral groove, radial nerve appears as an oval and well-defined fascicular structure whereby its CSA is about 3 to 4 mm² [94, 95]. In case of a spiral groove syndrome, the radial nerve becomes focally swollen, with a hypoechoic appearance and loss of the fascicular pattern [93]. Fragmented fractures of the humerus, constricting fibrous bands arising from the triceps muscle, hypertrophied callus, scar tissue, space-occupying masses and neurogenic tumors involving the radial nerve can be visualized by US [92, 93, 96].

## 12.4.5 Fibular Neuropathy at the Fibular Head

Entrapment of the common fibular nerve around the fibular head is the most common mononeuropathy of the lower extremity. The common fibular nerve arises from the sciatic nerve above the popliteal fossa and gives off the recurrent articular, superficial fibular and deep fibular nerves at the level of the fibular neck. It innervates ankle dorsiflexor and evertor muscles;

therefore its complete lesion results in foot drop, slapping gait and sensory disturbance over the anterolateral calf and dorsum of the foot. Fibular nerve can usually be compressed in a narrow area between the fibular bone and the fascia where the nerve winds around the fibular head. Due to its quite superficial course and relatively fixed location at the level of the fibular head, common fibular nerve is prone to stretch injury or trauma during knee varus-hyperextension. Main causes for fibular neuropathy (Figure 12.10) include habitual leg-crossing and squatting, dramatic weight loss, casting, direct trauma or an extrinsic compression due to either prolonged immobilization (deep sleep, coma, surgery, etc.) or space-occupying lesions (ganglion/synovial cysts, fractures, osteophytes, osteochondromas, tumors and varicosities) [97-100].

Ultrasound (US) imaging of the fibular nerve can be easy if followed from the sciatic bifurcation. The nerve should be followed distally, until it gives the superficial and deep fibular branches. As the nerve curves around the fibular head, it can be difficult to obtain an exact cross-sectional image but a few studies have shown the normal CSA of the fibular nerve at the fibular head (see table 12.1) [17, 101]. In case of a fibular neuropathy, US can primarily be used to visualize the enlargement of the nerve, decreased echogenici-

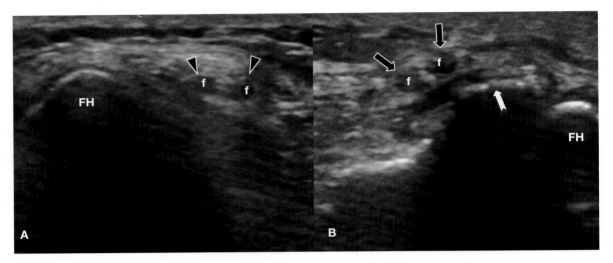

**Figure 12.10** Comparative US imaging (axial view) of the fibular nerves (f) in a patient with fibular nerve palsy. On the normal side (A), the nerve (black arrowheads) is seen next to the fibular head (FH). On the symptomatic side (B), the entrapped nerve is seen as enlarged and hypoechoic (black arrows) due to callus formation (white notched arrow).

ty, and the likely secondary causes (e.g. extensions of ganglia associated with the tibiofibular joint or common fibular nerve sheath) leading to entrapment [102, 103].

### 12.4.6 Tarsal Tunnel Syndrome

Tarsal tunnel is a fibroosseous canal through which the posterior tibial neurovascular bundle and three tendons (tibialis posterior, flexor digitorum longus and flexor hallucis longus) pass. Tarsal tunnel syndrome is caused by compression of the tibial nerve and/or its branches (medial and lateral plantar nerves, and a sensory medial calcaneal branch) in the posteromedial aspect of the ankle under the flexor retinaculum. It is characterized by poorly localized burning pain and paresthesia along the medial ankle radiating to the medial and/or plantar aspect of the foot and toes. In 80% of the cases, the entrapment occurs due to secondary causes including footwear or tight plaster casts (the most common reasons), trauma (i.e. calcaneal sprain or fracture), degenerative bone disease, local tenosynovitis, talocalcaneal coalition and space-occupying lesions (e.g. ganglion cysts, lipoma, varicose veins or accessory flexor digitorum muscle) [35, 104, 105]. The tibial nerve can be scanned (from proximal to distal) posterior to the flexor digitorum longus tendon and the accompanying posterior tibial artery/vein can be used for easy localization. Again, the typical

changes of a compressive neuropathy (local fusiform thickening together with loss of the normal fascicular pattern) and/or an underlying secondary cause can effectively be detected with US (see Chapter 10 - "Ultrasound Evaluation of the Ankle and Foot").

### 12.4.7 Morton's Neuroma

Morton's neuroma (interdigital neuritis) is a common entrapment syndrome which generally affects middle-aged women. The main causative factors are recurrent local compression of the interdigital nerves (especially the 2nd or 3rd) under the transverse intermetatarsal ligament, ischemia, and intermetatarsal bursitis. Patients generally present with local sharp pain (at the base of the involved web space radiating to the digits) which is aggravated by walking in high-heeled shoes with a narrow toe box and relieved by rest and/or removing the shoes.

Interdigital nerves have normally a small size of about 2 mm in diameter, therefore their visualization is difficult. Although the diagnosis of Morton's neuroma is usually made with clinical examination, imaging with US or MRI can be required for prompt management. Studies comparing US and MRI in its diagnosis have shown that US had slightly higher sensitivity than MRI (90-96% vs. 88%, respectively) [106, 107]. Via detection of the adjacent intermetatarsal vessels, Doppler imaging can be useful to localize these nerves. Morton's neuroma can be seen as a small, fusiform or ovoid hypoechoic nodule with US. Local tenderness with sonopalpation (sono-Tinel) or dynamic evaluation with provocative testing for a sonographic Mulder sign may further help in the diagnosis [108].

## 12.5 IMAGING FOR TRAUMATIC AND POSTOPERATIVE LESIONS

Traumatic peripheral nerve lesions (traction, penetrating trauma, contusion, or iatrogenic) are common in clinical practice. The most commonly injured nerves (in decreasing order) are radial, ulnar and median nerves in the upper limb and sciatic, fibular, tibial and femoral nerves in the lower limb [109]. The degree and type of injury are important to determine proper management in patients with traumatic nerve lesions. Although clinical examination and electrophysiological tests are usually the mainstay in that sense, they have limited ability to find out the exact location or for prompt morphological assessment, especially in the early post-injury period when electrophysiological tests are noncontributory. Therefore, US, which has a high negative predictive value for excluding peripheral nerve injury [5], may also be used as a first-line modality. For instance, it can distinguish severe axonotmesis and neurotmesis before reinnervation occurs, which is not possible by electrophysiological tests in the early period [110]. On the other hand, differentiating neuropraxia from axonotmesis would be difficult.

Ultrasound (US) can readily provide structural evaluation of the injured nerves (its fascicle, perineurium, epineurium and the surrounding tissues) (Figure 12.11). As such, US imaging is paramount for visualizing axonal swelling, partial/complete discontinuity of the nerve, neuroma, bone fragments, callus formation after fractures, foreign bodies and scar tissue either during the initial examination or follow-up [110-113]. A typical example would be traumatic stump neuroma which is the most severe chronic condition after a partially/completely injured nerve. Nonneoplastic proliferation of the proximal stump (terminal neuroma) can be seen as a clearly bordered, homogeneously hypoechoic and club-shaped lesion, especially with the help of "sonopalpation" [2].

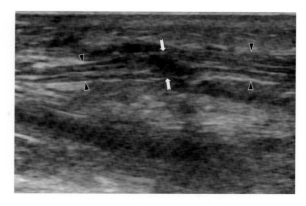

**Figure 12.11** US imaging (longitudinal view) of the ulnar nerve (arrowheads) at the level of the mid-forearm shows enlarged and hypoechoic nerve (notched arrows) due to a traumatic injury.

## 12.6 IMAGING FOR POLYNEUROPATHIES/ NEURONOPATHIES

The gold standard for diagnosis of polyneuropathy (PNP) includes a detailed neurological examination along with electrophysiological tests. However, decreased amplitudes (characteristic for axonal PNP) may be found in demyelinating PNP and reduced conduction velocity (typical for demyelinating PNP) in axonal PNP. Further, as many types of PNPs display both axonal and demyelinating characteristics, electrophysiological differentiation between axonal and demyelinating PNPs can often be unclear [114]. However, classification of the PNP to the myelin sheath and/or axon may be important for etiology and proper treatment. In this regard, nerve biopsy appears to be the most accurate method, but it is an invasive procedure.

Being a noninvasive convenient imaging technique, US can be useful for evaluating certain PNPs, including multifocal motor neuropathy, Charcot-Marie-Tooth disease (Figure 12.12), diabetes mellitus, vasculitic neuropathy, acromegaly, amyloidosis, and chronic inflammatory demyelinating PNP [14, 21, 115-119]. In these disorders, hypervascularity, hypoechogenicity and different size/site of enlargement can be seen in various peripheral nerves. Demyelinating PNPs usually display higher enlargement than axonal ones. In diabetic PNP, increased nerve CSA was found at entrapment sites [21, 117, 120] but not at non-entrapment sites [121, 122]. De- and remyelinating

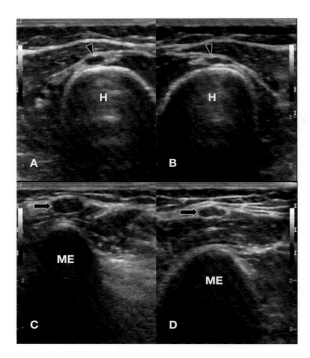

**Figure 12.12** Comparative US imaging (axial view) shows bilaterally enlarged radial (arrowheads) and ulnar nerves (arrows) at the level of the spiral groove (A, B) and at the level of the medial epicondyle (C, D) in a 14-year-old boy with Charcot-Marie-Tooth type 1A disease. H, humerus, ME, medial epicondyle.

processes may result in increased CSA of the peripheral nerves in association with histological onion bulbs [121]. US can also show increased CSA in immune-mediated -and more prominently in demyelinating- hereditary PNPs [13, 14, 115, 116, 123, 124]. Polysegmental nerve enlargements

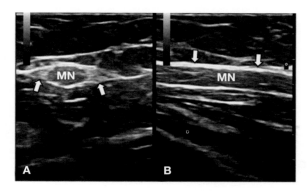

**Figure 12.13** US imaging of the median nerve (MN) proximal to the carpal tunnel in a patient with leprosy. Arrows demonstrate the thickened epineurium of the enlarged nerve on axial (A) and longitudinal (B) views.

of the cervical roots and distal nerve trunks can be visualized in chronic inflammatory demyelinating PNP and multifocal motor neuropathy [116, 119]. Of note, US imaging can also be a useful screening tool for other family members, especially in Charcot-Marie-Tooth type 1A neuropathy and neurofibromatosis syndromes.

Ultrasound has been reported to be superior to electromyography testing in detecting fasciculations [125, 126]. Yet, while needle electromyography clearly shows fasciculations, it is not practical/comfortable to scan each/every muscle. On the other hand, with US, one can easily image any muscle without any discomfort. With advancing disease, together with increased muscle echogenicity and decreased muscle thickness, decreased CSA in motor nerves in amyotrophic lateral sclerosis can develop [127]. Nerve atrophy can also be seen in sensory nerves of patients with post-herpetic neuralgia [128].

Ultrasound can also be useful in evaluating lepromatous neuropathy, a complication of an inflammatory neuropathy with significant worldwide prevalence and morbidity. Nerves are often enlarged (often palpable), especially in areas/tissues where they are superficial and cool (i.e. ulnar nerve at the elbow, the tibial nerve at the ankle, fibular nerve at the fibular head, and greater auricular nerve) [129]. Since leprosy is one of the most common treatable generalized PNP, its early detection is important for preventing life-long disability. Being able to detect subclinical involvement, US actually provides more information about the nerve abnormality than clinical/electrophysiological findings in lepromatous neuropathy [23, 29]. Increased nerve size (with thickened epineurium) and hypervascularity (inflammation) can be detected with US (Figure 12.13).

## 12.7 IMAGING TUMORS AND TUMOR-LIKE LESIONS

Peripheral nerve tumors are rare, accounting for nearly 12% of all benign and 8% of all malignant soft tissue tumors [14, 130]. They are mostly benign and include traumatic neuroma, Morton's neuroma, fibrolipomatous hamartoma of a nerve, nerve sheath ganglion, perineurioma, and benign/malignant peripheral nerve sheath tumors (PNST). Imaging methods usually do not allow definite evidence of the underlying histology. US can readily

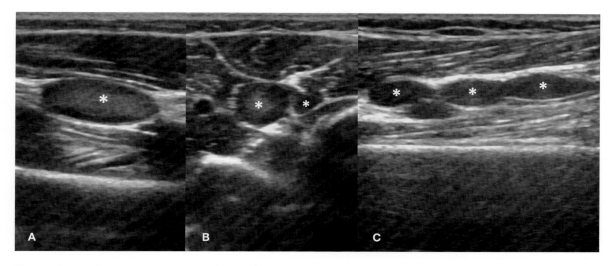

**Figure 12.14** US imaging in a patient with neurofibromatosis type 1. Neurofibromas (asterisks) are seen in the longitudinal (A) and axial (B) views of the median nerve (mid-forearm) and in the longitudinal view of the sciatic nerve (mid-thigh) (C).

be used to detect/classify these tumors (as intrinsic, extrinsic, or arising from the nerve sheath) or to provide information as regards their vascularity.

Benign PNST (neurofibromas and schwannomas) derive from Schwann cells. While neurofibromas infiltrate the nerve trunk and require resection and grafting, schwannomas usually dislocate the nerve fascicles and can be shelled out while preserving nerve contiguity [131, 132]. These tumors are usually ovoid/fusiform with well-defined borders in direct continuity with the nerves, containing heterogeneously hypoechoic cystic and solid soft tissue components in gray-scale (Figure 12.14) and increased vascularization in Doppler US [133]. Short-axis images are usually more helpful for evaluating the nerve/tumor relationship. Although a clear sonographic differentiation between schwannomas and neurofibromas is difficult, a nerve eccentrically entering the mass strongly suggests a diagnosis of schwannoma. When compared to neurofibromas, schwannomas often show more intratumor cystic components and hypervascular pattern at Doppler imaging (Figure 12.15) [5].

Neurofibromas most commonly develop in patients with 20-30 years of age with no sex predilection [134-136]. They can be divided into three forms as localized (90%), diffuse or plexiform. Localized neurofibroma is typically visualized as the "onion skin image" or the "target sign" which results from a centrally hyperechoic (fibrotic area) and peripherally hypoechoic mass (myxomatous

tissue) [103]. The diffuse type affects children and young adults and involves the subcutaneous tissue of the head and neck. The typical US image of a plexiform neurofibroma is described as "bag-of-worms" formed by diffuse tortuous nerve thickenings [137]. Malignant PNST are extremely rare and they often develop from sarcomatous transformation of a neurofibroma. Plexiform neurofibromas are pathognomonic for neurofibromatosis

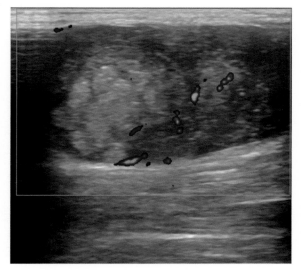

**Figure 12.15** Ultrasound imaging (axial view) shows a schwannoma in the median nerve at the level of the axilla. It is seen as globoid, hypoechoic, clearly demarcated and hypervascular.

**Table 12.2**   Clinical and US findings used to differentiate benign vs. malignant PNSTs

|  | Benign PNST | Malign PNST |
|---|---|---|
| Pain, sensory/motor deficits | Rare | Common |
| Growth pattern | Stable/slow | Rapid, with worsening of neurologic symptoms/signs |
| Size | Generally small | Usually larger (>5 cm) |
| US findings | Hypoechoic, commonly homogeneous | Hypoechoic, commonly heterogeneous |
| Borders | Well-defined | Ill-defined |
| Target sign* | Common | Rare |
| Doppler US findings | Peripheral hypervascular changes | Anarchic hypervascularization pattern with low perfusion resistances |

US, ultrasound; PNST, peripheral nerve sheath tumor
* Hyperechoic centre (fibrotic focus) within a peripheral hypoechoic rim (myxomatous tissue)

type 1 and over 65% of them have malignant potential [138]. Although it is not always easy to distinguish benign and malignant PNST, there are some key points for clinical and US findings [134] (Table 12.2). US can also be helpful for evaluating the extent of involvement which would especially be important for patients who are planned to undergo surgery.

Aside from aforementioned extraneural ganglions (commonly seen) causing peripheral nerve entrapments, intraneural ganglia are relatively rare and mainly located in the knee region [102, 130]. They occur within the nerve sheaths/fascicles and seem to be related to the superior tibiofibular joint and articular/capsular branches of the fibular or tibial nerves. They are one of the leading causes of fibular nerve entrapment at the level of the fibular head. They can cause local symptoms and/or nerve dysfunction (predominantly affecting the deep fibular branch) and have a high rate of postoperative recurrence. As an extension of the superior tibiofibular joint, they can be visualized as spindle-shaped intraneural cystic lesion within the nerve sheath causing peripheral displacement of the fascicles and fusiform thickening of the nerve. Guided with real-time US, needle aspiration can improve the patient's symptoms by lowering the intracystic pressure and then the pressure on the affected nerve.

Fibrolipomatous hamartoma is an uncommon, slow-growing developmental tumor-like lesion of the peripheral nerves characterized by fibrofatty proliferation of the peri- and epineural tissues. It often presents during early childhood or young adults with no familial and gender predisposition. It most commonly affects the upper extremity, predominantly the median nerve at the wrist level. Other nerves including radial, ulnar and sciatic nerves, the nerves of the foot or the cranial nerves can rarely be involved as well. In addition, diffuse enlargement of one or more fingers (lipomatous macrodactyly) can often accompany the scenario in up to two-thirds of the cases [130]. Affected nerve segments are substantially enlarged and the fatty fibrous tissue can be visualized as hyperechoic, surrounding the hypoechoic nerve fascicles (see figure 12.7) [37]. Of note, hypervascularization is never seen at Doppler US [12].

# REFERENCES

1) Özçakar L, Kara M, Yalçın B, Yalçın E, Tiftik T, Develi S, Yazar F. Bypassing the challenges of lower-limb electromyography by using ultrasonography. AnatoMUS-II. J Rehabil Med. 2013; 45: 604-5.

2) Kopf H, Loizides A, Mostbeck GH, Gruber H. Diagnostic sonography of peripheral nerves: indications, examination techniques and pathological findings. Ultraschall Med. 2011; 32: 242-63.

3) Stoll G, Wilder-Smith E, Bendszus M. Imaging of the peripheral nervous system. Handb Clin Neurol. 2013; 115: 137-53.

4) Özçakar L, Malas FU, Kara G, Kaymak B, Hasçelik Z. Musculoskeletal sonography use in physiatry: a single-center one-year analysis. Am J Phys Med Rehabil. 2010; 89: 385-9.

5) Fowler JR, Maltenfort MG, Ilyas AM. Ultrasound as a first-line test in the diagnosis of carpal tunnel syndrome: a cost-effectiveness analysis. Clin Orthop Relat Res. 2013; 471: 932-7.

6) Kara M, Özçakar L, De Muynck M, Tok F, Vanderstraeten G. Musculoskeletal ultrasound for peripheral nerve lesions. Eur J Phys Rehabil Med. 2012; 48: 665-74.

7) Ozçakar L, Yalçın B, Kara M, Yalçın E, Tiftik T, Gülbar S, Develi S, Yazar F. AnatoMUS-I: ultrasonographic imaging of the peripheral nerves of the upper limb. J Rehabil Med. 2012; 44: 381-2.

8) Zhu J, Zhao Y, Liu F, Huang Y, Shao J, Hu B. Ultrasound of the lateral femoral cutaneous nerve in asymptomatic adults. BMC Musculoskelet Disord. 2012; 13: 227.

9) Jelsing EJ, Presley JC, Maida E, Hangiandreou NJ, Smith J. The effect of magnification on sonographically measured nerve cross-sectional area. Muscle Nerve. 2014 May 3. [Epub ahead of print].

10) Won SJ, Kim BJ, Park KS, Yoon JS, Choi H. Reference values for nerve ultrasonography in the upper extremity. Muscle Nerve. 2013; 47: 864-71.

11) Martinoli C, Schenone A, Bianchi S, Mandich P, Caponetto C, Abbruzzese M, Derchi LE. Sonography of the median nerve in Charcot-Marie-Tooth disease. AJR Am J Roentgenol. 2002; 178: 1553-6.

12) Gruber H, Glodny B, Bendix N, Tzankov A, Peer S. High-resolution ultrasound of peripheral neurogenic tumors. Eur Radiol. 2007; 17: 2880-8.

13) Cartwright MS, Brown ME, Eulitt P, Walker FO, Lawson VH, Caress JB. Diagnostic nerve ultrasound in Charcot–Marie-Tooth disease type 1B. Muscle Nerve. 2009; 40: 98-102.

14) Sugimoto T, Ochi K, Hosomi N, Takahashi T, Ueno H, Nakamura T, et al. Ultrasonographic nerve enlargement of the median and ulnar nerves and the cervical nerve roots in patients with demyelinating Charcot-Marie-Tooth disease: distinction from patients with chronic inflammatory demyelinating polyneuropathy. J Neurol. 2013; 260: 2580-7.

15) Beekman R, Visser LH, Verhagen WI. Ultrasonography in ulnar neuropathy at the elbow: a critical review. Muscle Nerve. 2011; 43: 627-35.

16) Hobson-Webb LD, Massey JM, Juel VC, Sanders DB. The ultrasonographic wrist-to-forearm median nerve area ratio in carpal tunnel syndrome. Clin Neurophysiol. 2008; 119: 1353-7.

17) Kerasnoudis A, Pitarokoili K, Behrendt V, Gold R, Yoon MS. Cross sectional area reference values for sonography of peripheral nerves and brachial plexus. Clin Neurophysiol. 2013; 124: 1881-8.

18) Yoon JS, Walker FO, Cartwright MS. Ultrasonographic swelling ratio in the diagnosis of ulnar neuropathy at the elbow. Muscle Nerve. 2008; 38: 1231-5.

19) Tagliafico A, Tagliafico G, Martinoli C. Nerve density: a new parameter to evaluate peripheral nerve pathology on ultrasound. Preliminary study. Ultrasound Med Biol. 2010; 36: 1588-93.

20) Boom J, Visser LH. Quantitative assessment of nerve echogenicity: comparison of methods for evaluating nerve echogenicity in ulnar neuropathy at the elbow. Clin Neurophysiol. 2012; 123: 1446-53.

21) Watanabe T, Ito H, Sekine A, Katano Y, Nishimura T, Kato Y, et al. Sonographic evaluation of the peripheral nerve in diabetic patients: the relationship between nerve conduction studies, echo intensity, and cross-sectional area. J Ultrasound Med. 2010; 29: 697-708.

22) Ghasemi-Esfe AR, Khalilzadeh O, Vaziri-Bozorg SM, Jajroudi M, Shakiba M, Mazloumi M, Rahmani M. Color and power Doppler US for diagnosing carpal tunnel syndrome and determining its severity: a quantitative image processing method. Radiology. 2011; 261: 499-506.

23) Bathala L, Kumar K, Pathapati R, Jain S, Visser LH. Ulnar neuropathy in Hansen disease: clinical, high-resolution ultrasound and electrophysiologic correlations. J Clin Neurophysiol. 2012; 29: 190-3.

24) Mohammadi A, Ghasemi-Rad M, Mladkova-Suchy N, Ansari S. Correlation between the severity of carpal tunnel syndrome and color Doppler sonography findings. AJR Am J Roentgenol. 2012; 198: W181.

25) Evans KD, Roll SC, Volz KR, Freimer M. Relationship between intraneural vascular flow measured with sonography and carpal tunnel syn-

drome diagnosis based on electrodiagnostic testing. J Ultrasound Med. 2012; 31: 729-36.

26) Mallouhi A, Pülzl P, Trieb T, Piza H, Bodner G. Predictors of carpal tunnel syndrome: accuracy of gray-scale and color Doppler sonography. AJR Am J Roentgenol. 2006; 186: 1240-5.

27) Goedee HS, Brekelmans GJ, van Asseldonk JT, Beekman R, Mess WH, Visser LH. High resolution sonography in the evaluation of the peripheral nervous system in polyneuropathy-a review of the literature. Eur J Neurol. 2013; 20: 1342-51.

28) Lolge SJ, Morani AC, Chaubal NG, Khopkar US. Sonographically guided nerve biopsy. J Ultrasound Med. 2005; 24: 1427-30.

29) Elias J Jr, Nogueira-Barbosa MH, Feltrin LT, Furini RB, Foss NT, Marques W Jr, dos Santos AC. Role of ulnar nerve sonography in leprosy neuropathy with electrophysiologic correlation. J Ultrasound Med. 2009; 28: 1201-9.

30) Nakamichi K, Tachibana S. Restricted motion of the median nerve in carpal tunnel syndrome. J Hand Surg Br. 1995; 20: 460-4.

31) Hough AD, Moore AP, Jones MP. Reduced longitudinal excursion of the median nerve in carpal tunnel syndrome. Arch Phys Med Rehabil. 2007; 88: 569-76.

32) Filippou G, Mondelli M, Greco G, Bertoldi I, Frediani B, Galeazzi M, et al. Ulnar neuropathy at the elbow: how frequent is the idiopathic form? An ultrasonographic study in a cohort of patients. Clin Exp Rheumatol. 2010; 28: 63-7.

33) Nakamichi K, Tachibana S. Unilateral carpal tunnel syndrome and space-occupying lesions. J Hand Surg Br. 1993; 18: 748-9.

34) Inaparthy PK, Anwar F, Botchu R, Jahnich H, Katchburian MV. Compression of the deep branch of the ulnar nerve in Guyon's canal by a ganglion: two cases. Arch Orthop Trauma Surg. 2008; 128: 641-3.

35) Nagaoka M, Satou K. Tarsal tunnel syndrome caused by ganglia. J Bone Joint Surg Br. 1999; 81: 607-10.

36) Kara M, Yalçin S, Tiftik T, Özçakar L. Proximal median nerve entrapment caused by a distal biceps tendon cyst: an ultrasonographic diagnosis. Am J Phys Med Rehabil. 2013; 92: 942-3.

37) Kara M, Tiftik T, Yetişgin A, Ural G, Ozçakar L. Ultrasound in the diagnosis and treatment of posterior interosseous nerve entrapment: a case report. Muscle Nerve. 2012; 45: 299-300.

38) Elias DA, Lax MJ, Anastakis DJ. Musculoskeletal images. Ganglion cyst of Guyon's canal causing ulnar nerve compression. Can J Surg. 2001; 44: 331-2.

39) Rempel D, Dahlin L, Lundborg G. Pathophysiology of nerve compression syndromes: response of peripheral nerves to loading. J Bone Joint Surg Am. 1999; 81: 1600-10.

40) Powell HC, Myers RR. Pathology of experimental nerve compression. Lab Invest. 1986; 55: 91-100.

41) Lundborg G, Myers R, Powell H. Nerve compression injury and increased endoneurial fluid pressure: a "miniature compartment syndrome". J Neurol Neurosurg Psychiatry. 1983; 46: 1119-24.

42) Atroshi I, Gummesson C, Johnsson R, Ornstein E, Ranstam J, Rosen I. Prevalence of carpal tunnel syndrome in a general population. JAMA. 1999; 282: 153-8.

43) Roquelaure Y, Ha C, Pelier-Cady MC, Nicolas G, Descatha A, Leclerc A, et al. Work increases the incidence of carpal tunnel syndrome in the general population. Muscle Nerve. 2008; 37: 477-82.

44) Mondelli M, Giannini F, Giacchi M. Carpal tunnel syndrome incidence in a general population. Neurology. 2002; 58: 289-94.

45) Wiesler ER, Chloros GD, Cartwright MS, Smith BP, Rushing J, Walker FO. The use of diagnostic ultrasound in carpal tunnel syndrome. J Hand Surg Am. 2006; 31: 726-32.

46) Kaymak B, Ozcakar L, Cetin A, Candan Cetin M, Akinci A, Hascelik Z. A comparison of the benefits of sonography and electrophysiologic measurements as predictors of symptom severity and functional status in patients with carpal tunnel syndrome. Arch Phys Med Rehabil. 2008; 89: 743-8.

47) Tai TW, Wu CY, Su FC, Chern TC, Jou IM. Ultrasonography for diagnosing carpal tunnel syndrome: a meta-analysis of diagnostic test accuracy. Ultrasound Med Biol. 2013; 39: 1129-30.

48) Descatha A, Huard L, Aubert F, Barbato B, Gorand O, Chastang JF. Meta-analysis on the performance of sonography for the diagnosis of carpal tunnel syndrome. Semin Arthritis Rheum. 2012; 41: 914-22.

49) Cartwright MS, Hobson-Webb LD, Boon AJ, Alter KE, Hunt CH, Flores VH, et al. American Association of Neuromuscular and Electrodiagnostic Medicine. Evidence-based guideline: neuromuscular ultrasound for the diagnosis of carpal tunnel syndrome. Muscle Nerve. 2012; 46: 287-93.

50) Jablecki CK, Andary MT, Floeter MK, Miller RG, Quartly CA, Vennix MJ, et al. Practice parameter: electrodiagnostic studies in carpal tunnel syndrome-report of the American Association of Electrodiagnostic Medicine, American Academy of Neurology, and the American Academy of Physical Medicine and Rehabilitation. Neurology. 2002; 58: 1589-92.

51) Chang MH, Wei SJ, Chiang HL, Wang HM, Hsieh PF, Huang SY. Comparison of motor conduction techniques in the diagnosis of carpal tunnel syndrome. Neurology. 2002; 58: 1603-7.

52) Wilder-Smith EP, Seet RC, Lim EC. Diagnosing carpal tunnel syndrome: clinical criteria and ancillary tests. Nat Clin Pract Neurol. 2006; 2: 366-74.

53) Fowler JR, Gaughan JP, Ilyas AM. The sensitivity and specificity of ultrasound for the diagnosis of carpal tunnel syndrome: a meta-analysis. Clin Orthop Relat Res. 2011; 469: 1089-94.

54) Visser LH, Smidt MH, Lee ML. High-resolution sonography versus EMG in the diagnosis of carpal tunnel syndrome. J Neurol Neurosurg Psychiatry. 2008; 79: 63-7.

55) Klauser AS, Halpern EJ, Faschingbauer R, Guerra F, Martinoli C, Gabl MF, et al. Bifid median nerve in carpal tunnel syndrome: assessment with us cross-sectional area measurement. Radiology. 2011; 259: 808-15.

56) Kluge S, Kreutziger J, Hennecke B, Vogelin E. Inter- and intraobserver reliability of predefined diagnostic levels in high-resolution sonography of the carpal tunnel syndrome-a validation study on healthy volunteers. Ultraschall Med. 2010; 31: 43-7.

57) van Neck JW, de Kool BS, Hekking-Weijma JI, Walbeehm ET, Visser GH, Blok JH. Histological validation of ultrasound-guided neurography in early nerve regeneration. Muscle Nerve. 2009; 40: 967-75.

58) Wong SM, Griffith JF, Hui AC, Lo SK, Fu M, Wong KS. Carpal tunnel syndrome: diagnostic usefulness of sonography. Radiology. 2004; 232: 93-9.

59) Claes F, Meulstee J, Claessen-Oude Luttikhuis TT, Huygen PL, Verhagen WI. Usefulness of additional measurements of the median nerve with ultrasonography. Neurol Sci. 2010; 31: 721-5.

60) Kara M, Ozçakar L, Ekiz T, Yalçın E, Tiftik T, Akyüz M. Fibrolipomatous hamartoma of the median nerve: comparison of magnetic resonance imaging and ultrasound. PM R. 2013; 5: 805-6.

61) Erol O, Ozçakar L, Kaymak B. Bifid median nerve revisited: imaging and clinical aspects. Plast Reconstr Surg. 2004; 113: 1289-90.

62) Bayrak IK, Bayrak AO, Kale M, Turker H, Diren B. Bifid median nerve in patients with carpal tunnel syndrome. J Ultrasound Med. 2008; 27: 1129-36.

63) Padua L, Liotta G, Di Pasquale A, Granata G, Pazzaglia C, Caliandro P, et al. Contribution of ultrasound in the assessment of nerve diseases. Eur J Neurol. 2012; 19: 47-54.

64) Abicalaf CA, de Barros N, Sernik RA, Pimentel BF, Braga-Baiak A, Braga L, et al. Ultrasound evaluation of patients with carpal tunnel syndrome before and after endoscopic release of the transverse carpal ligament. Clin Radiol. 2007; 62: 891-4.

65) Kim JY, Yoon JS, Kim SJ, Won SJ, Jeong JS. Carpal tunnel syndrome: Clinical, electrophysiological, and ultrasonographic ratio after surgery. Muscle Nerve. 2012; 45: 183-8.

66) Smidt MH, Visser LH. Carpal tunnel syndrome: clinical and sonographic follow-up after surgery. Muscle Nerve. 2008; 38: 987-91.

67) Vögelin E, Nüesch E, Jüni P, Reichenbach S, Eser P, Ziswiler HR. Sonographic follow-up of patients with carpal tunnel syndrome undergoing surgical or nonsurgical treatment: prospective cohort study. J Hand Surg Am. 2010; 35: 1401-9.

68) Bayrak IK, Bayrak AO, Tilki HE, Nural MS, Sunter T. Ultrasonography in carpal tunnel syndrome: comparison with electrophysiological stage and motor unit number estimate. Muscle Nerve. 2007; 35: 344-8.

69) Lee CH, Kim TK, Yoon ES, Dhong ES. Correlation of high-resolution ultrasonographic findings with the clinical symptoms and electrodiagnostic data in carpal tunnel syndrome. Ann Plast Surg. 2005; 54: 20-3.

70) Padua L, Pazzaglia C, Caliandro P, Granata G, Foschini M, Briani C, Martinoli C. Carpal tunnel syndrome: ultrasound, neurophysiology, clinical and patient-oriented assessment. Clin Neurophysiol. 2008; 119: 2064-9.

71) Lee D, van Holsbeeck MT, Janevski PK, Ganos DL, Ditmars DM, Darian VB. Diagnosis of carpal tunnel syndrome. Ultrasound versus electromyography. Radiol Clin North Am. 1999; 37: 859-72.

72) Ziswiler HR, Reichenbach S, Vögelin E, Bachmann LM, Villiger PM, Jüni P. Diagnostic value of sonography in patients with suspected carpal tunnel syndrome: a prospective study. Arthritis Rheum. 2005; 52: 304-11.

73) Mondelli M, Giannini F, Ballerini M, Ginanneschi F, Martorelli E. Incidence of ulnar neuropathy at the elbow in the province of Siena (Italy). J Neurol Sci. 2005; 234: 5-10.

74) Thoirs K, Williams M, Phillips M. Ultrasonographic measurements of the ulnar nerve at the elbow. Role of confounders. J Ultrasound Med. 2008; 27: 737-43.

75) Okamoto M, Abe M, Shirai H, Ueda N. Diagnostic ultrasonography of the ulnar nerve in cubital tunnel syndrome. J Hand Surg Br. 2000; 25: 499-502.

76) Cartwright MS, Shin HW, Passmore LV, Walker FO. Ultrasonographic findings of the normal ulnar nerve in adults. Arch Phys Med Rehabil. 2007; 88: 394-6.

77) Volpe A, Rossato G, Bottanelli M, Marchetta A, Caramaschi P, Bambara LM, et al. Ultrasound evaluation of ulnar neuropathy at the elbow: correlation with electrophysiological studies. Rheu-

matology (Oxf). 2009; 48: 1098-101.

78) Beekman R, Van Der Plas JP, Uitdehaag BM, Schellens RL, Visser LH. Clinical, electrodiagnostic, and sonographic studies in ulnar neuropathy at the elbow. Muscle Nerve. 2004; 30: 202-8.

79) Bayrak AO, Bayrak IK, Turker H, Elmali M, Nural MS. Ultrasonography in patients with ulnar neuropathy at the elbow: comparison of cross-sectional area and swelling ratio with electrophysiological severity. Muscle Nerve. 2010; 41: 661-6.

80) Mondelli M, Filippou G, Frediani B, Aretini A. Ultrasonography in ulnar neuropathy at the elbow: relationships to clinical relationships to clinical and electrophysiological findings. Neurophysiol Clin. 2008; 38: 217-26.

81) Kara M, Kaymak B, Malas FU, Tiftik T, Yazar F, Erkin G et al. The purview of multifascicle ulnar nerves in cubital tunnel syndrome: single-case sonographic observation. Muscle Nerve. 2009; 40: 664-5.

82) Özçakar L, Cakar E, Kiralp MZ, Dinçer U. Static and dynamic sonography: a salutary adjunct to electroneuromyography for cubital tunnel syndrome. Surg Neurol. 2009; 72: 311-2.

83) Kim BJ, Date ES, Lee SH, Yoon JS, Hur SY, Kim SJ. Distance measure error induced by displacement of the ulnar nerve when the elbow is flexed. Arch Phys Med Rehabil. 2005; 86: 809-12.

84) Okamoto M, Abe M, Shirai H, Ueda N. Morphology and Dynamics of the ulnar nerve in the cubital tunnel. Observation by ultrasonography. J Hand Surg Br. 2000; 25: 85-9.

85) Bianchi S, Martinoli C. Elbow. In: Bianchi S, Martinoli C, editors. Ultrasound of the Musculoskeletal System. Berlin: Springer; 2007. p. 349-405.

86) Kılıç E, Ozcakar L. Ulnar nerve compression possibly due to aberrant veins: sonography is elucidatory for idiopathic cubital tunnel syndrome. Rheumatol Int. 2011; 31: 139-40.

87) Bachoura A, Jacoby SM. Ulnar tunnel syndrome. Orthop Clin North Am. 2012; 43: 467-74.

88) Pierre-Jerome C, Moncayo V, Terk MR. The Guyon's canal in perspective: 3-T MRI assessment of the normal anatomy, the anatomical variations and the Guyon's canal syndrome. Surg Radiol Anat. 2011; 33: 897-903.

89) Dodds GA III, Hale D, Jackson WT. Incidence of anatomic variants in Guyon's canal. J Hand Surg. 1990; 15: 352-5.

90) Coulier B, Goffin D, Malbecq S, Mairy Y. Colour duplex sonographic and multislice spiral CT angiographic diagnosis of ulnar artery aneurysm in hypothenar hammer syndrome. JBR-BTR. 2003; 86: 211-4.

91) Cartwright MS, Walker FO. Neuromuscular ultrasound in common entrapment neuropathies. Muscle Nerve. 2013; 48: 696-704.

92) Bodner G, Buchberger W, Schocke M, Bale R, Huber B, Harpf C, Gassner E, Jaschke W. Radial nerve palsy associated with humeral shaft fracture: evaluation with US-initial experience. Radiology. 2001; 219: 811-6.

93) Bodner G, Huber B, Schwabegger A, Lutz M, Waldenberger P. Sonographic detection of radial nerve entrapment within a humerus fracture. J Ultrasound Med. 1999; 18: 703-6.

94) Girtler MT, Krasinski A, Dejaco C, Kitzler HH, Cui LG, Sherebrin S, Gardi L, Chhem RK, Fenster A, Romagnoli C, De Zordo T. Feasibility of 3D ultrasound to evaluate upper extremity nerves. Ultraschall Med. 2013; 34: 382-7.

95) Foxall GL, Skinner D, Hardman JG, Bedforth NM. Ultrasound anatomy of the radial nerve in the distal upper arm. Reg Anesth Pain Med. 2007; 32: 217-20.

96) Peer S, Bodner G, Meirer R, Willeit J, Piza-Katzer H. Examination of postoperative peripheral nerve lesions with high resolution sonography. AJR Am J Roentgenol. 2001; 177: 415-9.

97) Kiliç E, Ozgüçlü E, Erol O, Özçakar L. Bilateral foot drop after intestinal surgery: peroneal neuropathy unabated in elderly patients. J Am Geriatr Soc. 2007; 55: 1897.

98) Kara M, Özçakar L, Erol O, Kaymak B. Peroneal neuropathy due to ground pad burn injury after a radiofrequency ablation surgery. Ann Surg Oncol. 2007; 14: 1243-4.

99) Erol O, Özçakar L, Kaymak B. Bilateral peroneal neuropathy after surgery in the lithotomy position. Aesthetic Plast Surg. 2004; 28: 254-5.

100) Özçakar L, Aknc A, Aksoy DY, Cetinkaya Y, Aydnl M. Peroneal neuropathy due to a popliteal aneurysm in a patient with infectious endocarditis. Ann Vasc Surg. 2004; 18: 115-7.

101) Visser LH, Hens V, Soethout M, De Deugd-Maria V, Pijnenburg J, Brekelmans GJ. Diagnostic value of high-resolution sonography in common fibular neuropathy at the fibular head. Muscle Nerve. 2013; 48: 171-8.

102) Visser LH. High-resolution sonography of the common peroneal nerve: detection of intraneural ganglia. Neurology. 2006; 67: 1473-5.

103) Chiou HJ, Chou YH, Chiou SY, Liu JB, Chang CY. Peripheral nerve lesions: role of high-resolution US. Radiographics. 2003; 23: e15.

104) Nagaoka M, Matsuzaki H. Ultrasonography in tarsal tunnel syndrome. J Ultrasound Med. 2005; 24: 1035-40.

105) Chen WS. Lipoma responsible for tarsal tunnel syndrome. A propos of 2 cases. Rev Chir Orthop Reparatrice Appar Mot. 1992; 78: 251-4.

106) Fazal MA, Khan I, Thomas C. Ultrasonography and magnetic resonance imaging in the diagnosis of Morton's neuroma. J Am Podiatr Med Assoc. 2012; 102: 184-6.

107) Pastides P, El-Sallakh S, Charalambides C. Morton's neuroma: A clinical versus radiological diagnosis. Foot Ankle Surg. 2012; 18: 22-4.

108) Symeonidis PD, Iselin LD, Simmons N, Fowler S, Dracopoulos G, Stavrou P. Prevalence of interdigital nerve enlargements in an asymptomatic population. Foot Ankle Int. 2012; 33: 543-7.

109) Taylor CA, Braza D, Rice JB, Dillingham T. The incidence of peripheral nerve injury in extremity trauma. Am J Phys Med Rehabil. 2008; 87: 381-5.

110) Tagliafico A, Altafini L, Garello I, Marchetti A, Gennaro S, Martinoli C. Traumatic neuropathies: spectrum of imaging findings and postoperative assessment. Semin Musculoskelet Radiol. 2010; 14: 512-22.

111) Karabay N, Toros T. Ultrasonographic evaluation of the iatrogenic peripheral nerve injuries in upper extremity. Eur J Radiol. 2010; 73: 234-40.

112) Lee FC, Singh H, Nazarian LN, Ratliff JK. High-resolution ultrasonography in the diagnosis and intraoperative management of peripheral nerve lesions. J Neurosurg. 2011; 114: 206-11.

113) Kömürcü E, Ozçakar L, Safaz I, Göktepe AS. A common peroneal neuroma due to a bony spur in a lower-limb amputee: a sonographic diagnosis. Am J Phys Med Rehabil. 2010; 89: 434-5.

114) Tankisi H, Pugdahl K, Johnsen B, Fuglsang-Frederiksen A. Correlations of nerve conduction measures in axonal and demyelinating polyneuropathies. Clin Neurophysiol. 2007; 118: 2383-92.

115) Hobson-Webb LD. Neuromuscular ultrasound in polyneuropathies and motor neuron disease. Muscle Nerve. 2013; 47: 790-804.

116) Beekman R, van den Berg LH, Franssen H, Visser LH, van Asseldonk JT, Wokke JH. Ultrasonography shows extensive nerve enlargements in multifocal motor neuropathy. Neurology. 2005; 65: 305-7.

117) Lee D, Dauphinee DM. Morphological and functional changes in the diabetic peripheral nerve: using diagnostic ultrasound and neurosensory testing to select candidates for nerve decompression. J Am Podiatr Med Assoc. 2005; 95: 433-7.

118) Resmini E, Tagliafico A, Nizzo R, Bianchi F, Minuto F, Derchi L, et al. Ultrasound of peripheral nerves in acromegaly: changes at 1-year follow-up. Clin Endocrinol (Oxf). 2009; 71: 220-5.

119) Rajabally YA, Morlese J, Kathuria D, Khan A. Median nerve ultrasonography in distinguishing neuropathy subtypes: a pilot study. Acta Neurol Scand. 2012; 125: 254-9.

120) Watanabe T, Ito H, Morita A, Uno Y, Nishimura T, Kawase H, et al. Sonographic evaluation of the median nerve in diabetic patients: comparison with nerve conduction studies. J Ultrasound Med. 2009; 28: 727-34.

121) Zaidman CM, Al-Lozi M, Pestronk A. Peripheral nerve size in normals and patients with polyneuropathy: an ultrasound study. Muscle Nerve. 2009; 40: 960-6.

122) Hobson-Webb LD, Massey JM, Juel VC. Nerve ultrasound in diabetic polyneuropathy: correlation with clinical characteristics and electrodiagnostic testing. Muscle Nerve. 2013; 47: 379-84.

123) Taniguchi N, Itoh K, Wang Y, Omoto K, Shigeta K, Fujii Y, Namekawa M, Muramatsu S, Nakano I. Sonographic detection of diffuse peripheral nerve hypertrophy in chronic inflammatory demyelinating polyradiculoneuropathy. J Clin Ultrasound. 2000; 28: 488-91.

124) Hobson-Webb LD, Cartwright MS. Nerve ultrasound in CIDP: Poly-parameters for polyneuropathies. Clin Neurophysiol. 2014; 125: 3-4.

125) Walker FO, Donofrio PD, Harpold GJ, Ferrell WG. Sonographic imaging of muscle contraction and fasciculations: a correlation with electromyography. Muscle Nerve. 1990; 13: 33-9.

126) Misawa S, Noto Y, Shibuya K, Isose S, Sekiguchi Y, Nasu S, et al. Ultrasonographic detection of fasciculations markedly increases diagnostic sensitivity of ALS. Neurology. 2011; 77: 1532-7.

127) Cartwright MS, Walker FO, Griffin LP, Caress JB. Peripheral nerve and muscle ultrasound in amyotrophic lateral sclerosis. Muscle Nerve. 2011; 44: 346-51.

128) Renna R, Erra C, Almeida V, Padua L. Ultrasound study shows nerve atrophy in post herpetic neuralgia. Clin Neurol Neurosurg. 2012; 114: 1343-4.

129) Rodrigues LC, Lockwood DNj. Leprosy now: epidemiology, progress, challenges, and research gaps. Lancet Infect Dis. 2011; 11: 464-70.

130) Murphey MD, Smith WS, Smith SE, Kransdorf MJ, Temple HT. From the archives of the AFIP Imaging of musculoskeletal neurogenic tumors: radiologic-pathologic correlation. Radiographics. 1999; 19: 1253-80.

131) Tsai WC, Chiou HJ, Chou YH, Wang HK, Chiou SY, Chang CY. Differentiation between schwannomas and neurofibromas in the extremities and superficial body: the role of high-resolution and color Doppler ultrasonography. J Ultrasound Med. 2008; 27: 161-6.

132) Beaman FD, Kransdorf MJ, Menke DM. Schwannoma: radiologic pathologic correlation. Radiographics. 2004; 24: 1477-81.

133) Reynolds DL Jr, Jacobson JA, Inampudi P, Jamadar DA, Ebrahim FS, Hayes CW. Sonographic characteristics of peripheral nerve sheath tumors. AJR Am J Roentgenol. 2004; 182: 741-3.

134) Abreu E, Aubert S, Wavreille G, Gheno R, Canella C, Cotten A. Peripheral tumor and tumor-like neurogenic lesions. Eur J Radiol. 2013; 82: 38-50.

135) Kara M, Yilmaz A, Ozel S, Ozçakar L. Sonographic imaging of the peripheral nerves in a patient with neurofibromatosis type 1. Muscle Nerve. 2010; 41: 887-8.

136) Kara M, Akyüz M, Yılmaz A, Hatipoğlu C, Ozçakar L. Peripheral nevre involvement in a neurofibromatosis type 2 patient with plexiform neurofibroma of the cauda equina: a sonographic vignette. Arch Phys Med Rehabil. 2011; 92: 1511-4.

137) Valle M, Zamorani MP. Nerve and blood vessels. In: Bianchi S, Martinoli C, editors. Ultrasound of the musculoskeletal system. Berlin: Springer; 2007. p. 97-136.

138) Riccardi VM. Von Recklinghausen neurofibromatosis. N Engl J Med. 1981; 305: 1617-27.

# Ultrasound Imaging in Rheumatic Diseases

## 13

Erkan KILIÇ, Özgür AKGÜL, Gamze KILIÇ, Salih ÖZGÖÇMEN

## 13.1 INTRODUCTION

Starting from early 70's (used for differentiating Baker's cysts from thrombophlebitis) and followed by imaging for synovitis a few years later, musculoskeletal ultrasound (US) has become an established and validated tool for the diagnosis and follow-up of rheumatic diseases in current practice [1-3]. Availability of high-resolution transducers as well as its other well-known advantages made US a paramount imaging tool in the daily life of rheumatologists [4-7]. While it significantly provides morphological data as regards disease progression and treatment response, US imaging also guides several therapeutic procedures such as joint aspiration, synovial or soft tissue biopsy, joint or tendon sheath injections [5].

On the other hand, as the US waves cannot penetrate through the bones, imaging for intraosseous pathologies (e.g. osteitis, bone marrow edema) and certain intra-articular structures is not possible [4].

For imaging rheumatic diseases, both gray-scale (or B-mode) and power Doppler (PD) US are used. Gray-scale US can visualize morphological abnormalities including proliferative synovial tissue, bony erosions, fluid collection in tendon sheaths or within the joints [8]. High frequency (7.5-20 MHz) linear transducers are generally necessary to assess superficial structures like skin, entheses, tendons, ligaments, bursae and small joints, however low frequency transducers (3.5-5 MHz) may be required for deeper structures [4]. Being able to detect low-velocity blood flow, especially the use of power Doppler US (PDUS) is noteworthy for assessing tissue vascularization i.e. mainly inflammation for rheumatic conditions [9, 10].

Overall, some authors even suggest that musculoskeletal US is "a stethoscope for the joints" [11], and the growing interest in this field and its extended use in daily practice promise a bright future for the diagnosis and follow-up of rheumatic diseases. Accordingly, in this chapter, we will discuss the use of US imaging in various rheumatologic conditions, including rheumatoid arthritis, spondyloarthropathies, osteoarthritis, gout, calcium pyrophosphate dihydrate crystal deposition disease, systemic sclerosis, Sjögren's syndrome, and temporal arteritis.

## 13.2 RHEUMATOID ARTHRITIS

Rheumatoid arthritis (RA) is a chronic inflammatory disease characterized by synovial inflammation and pannus formation resulting in progressive joint destruction and deformities. Sensitive and accurate detection of inflammation is crucial for early diagnosis and effective disease activity monitoring. In early inflammatory arthritis, US can detect the early stage of synovial inflammation at different anatomical sites more accurately than clinical examination [12, 13]. In addition, US can also be used to evaluate recent joint damage or progression of pre-existent damage [14].

Gray scale US readily detects structural abnormalities such as synovial hypertrophy, effusion, bone erosions, whereas PDUS shows changes in tissue vascularization [5, 15]. Assessment of the synovial tissue with PDUS is a reliable method to evaluate inflammatory activity within the joint whereby flow signals may be predictive for the development of erosions. It can also be used as a (semi)quantitative indicator of synovial inflammation [16, 17]. Moreover, PD-positive synovial hypertrophy indicates an ongoing inflammation (which might cause joint destruction during clinical remission) predicting short-term relapse [14, 18]. Herewith, the user-dependency disadvantage of US might also pose challenges during PDUS

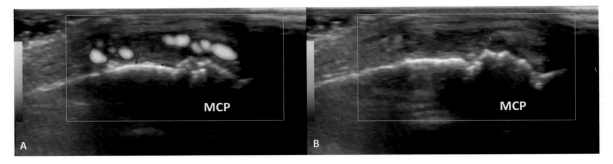

**Figure 13.1**  Longitudinal PDUS imaging of the right 2nd metacarpophalangeal joint (MCP). A - Image shows increased Doppler signal within the MCP joint. Also note the synovial hypertrophy and the cortical irregularity. B - After applying pressure with the probe, the Doppler signal disappeared (the artifacts on the right sides of both images stem from the finger deformity of the patient and inappropriate technical imaging i.e. lack of enough gel application).

imaging. Aside from various technical adjustments one important caution would be not to apply pressure with transducer over the examined tissue. Yet, aberrant pressure may affect the hemodynamics of the visualized tissue resulting in the disappearance of flow signals (Figure 13.1).

Assessment of inflammatory activity in the early period of the disease provides early diagnosis of RA which may further allow early effective treatment. There is still no agreement on which joints are best predictors for assessing disease activity and treatment response; however the wrist (radiocarpal, intercarpal and ulnacarpal joints), metacarpophalangeal (MCP), proximal interphalangeal (PIP), and metatarsophalangeal joints are particularly important in patients with early and established disease [13, 19, 20].

In patients with RA synovitis, synovial hypertrophy, tenosynovitis, and bone erosions are major manifestations which can be assessed/defined by US [4, 15, 21].

### 13.2.1 Synovitis

Synovium is the primary site of the inflammatory process in RA and, if untreated, leads to irreversible damage in the adjacent cartilage and bone [22]. Synovitis is defined as "abnormal hypoechoic, intra-articular tissue that is poorly compressible on gray-scale imaging and can show increased Doppler signals" [15] (Figures 13.2-13.4). Synovitis is observed more frequently on the palmar side of MCP and PIP joints [23]. Further, US can also identify subclinical synovitis, predicting the clinical outcome in early RA [14].

Since it can simultaneously show synovitis and

the related bone lesions, US is superior to conventional radiography in RA. Gray-scale and PDUS findings have also been reported to be highly correlated with those of magnetic resonance imaging (MRI) for the evaluation of synovitis in RA [24,

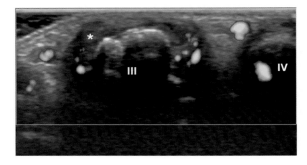

**Figure 13.2**  Transverse PDUS imaging of the 3rd and 4th metacarpal heads. Hypoechoic synovial tissue (*) and increased power Doppler signals are seen. Note the mirror image artifact on the 4th metacarpal.

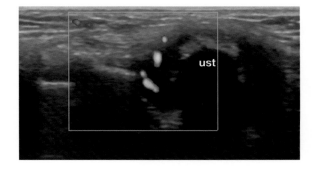

**Figure 13.3**  Longitudinal PDUS imaging shows increased signal within hypoechogenic thickened synovium in the wrist joint. Note the cortical irregularity at the ulnar styloid (ust).

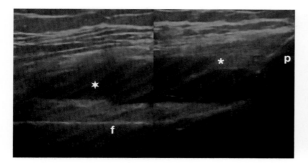

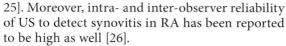

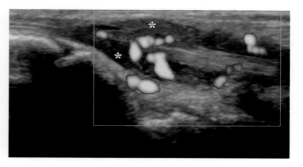

**Figure 13.4**  Knee effusion in a patient with RA. Gray-scale US (longitudinal split screen view) reveals increased hypoechoic fluid within the suprapatellar bursa (star) and synovial hypertrophy (asterisk). f, femur; p, patella.

**Figure 13.5**  PDUS examination (longitudinal view) of the common extensor digitorum tendon in a patient with RA. Tenosynovitis is characterized by heterogeneous synovial hypertrophy (asterisks) with increased power Doppler signals surrounding the tendon.

25]. Moreover, intra- and inter-observer reliability of US to detect synovitis in RA has been reported to be high as well [26].

Several studies have used different quantitative or semi-quantitative scoring systems to grade synovitis. However, as quantitative scoring systems have yet not been standardized or appropriately validated [27], semi-quantitative scoring systems are frequently used in clinical trials and daily practice [21, 23, 28]. Commonly, synovitis is graded as 0 = no effusion/synovial hypertrophy, 1 = mild, 2 = moderate and 3 = extensive [23].

### 13.2.2 Tenosynovitis

Tenosynovitis is also a common feature of RA and may sometimes be the only sign of active dis-

ease. Tendon sheaths of the extensor carpi ulnaris (6th extensor compartment), extensor digitorum, extensor indicis (4th extensor compartment), and the 2nd - 4th flexors appear to be the most commonly affected ones in RA [29].

Sonographic imaging for tenosynovitis (Figure 13.5) is quite sensitive and also very important for assessing disease activity in patients with RA [30]. It is defined as "hypoechoic or anechoic thickened tissue with or without fluid inside the tendon sheath and with positive Doppler signal in two perpendicular planes" [15]. Again, semi-quantitative scoring of tenosynovitis (grading on a 0–3 scale) is noteworthy during the follow-up of these patients [31].

A serious complication of persistent tenosynovitis is tendon rupture which may require surgical reconstruction (Figure 13.6). US may also be used

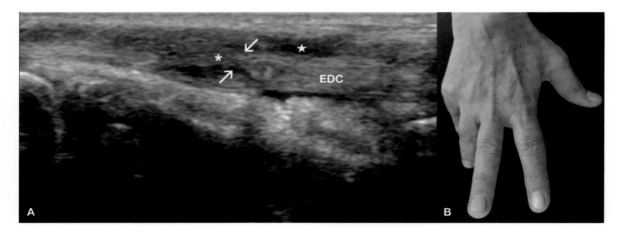

**Figure 13.6**  Extensor tendon rupture in RA. A - Longitudinal gray-scale US of the 4th finger shows irregular hypoechogenic synovium (asterisk) and peritendinous fluid (star). The arrows indicate the ruptured site of the extensor digitorum communis tendon (EDC). B - Photograph of the patient's hand shows the dropped 4th and 5th fingers.

to detect tendon ruptures (full or partial), which are defined as loss of or replacement of the regular hyperechoic fibrillar tendon pattern with irregular intra-tendinous hypoechogenicity (e.g. fluid, blood or fat) [32]. Features like dynamic imaging or testing for tendon compressibility makes US an exclusive diagnostic tool in this regard [33]. Recent classifications for tendon damage in RA also exists in the pertinent literature [34].

### 13.2.3 Bone Erosion

Bone erosions are common findings in RA. Bone erosions (Figures 13.7 and 13.8) are sonographically defined as "intraarticular discontinuity of the bone surface that is visible in two perpendicular planes" [15]. US is more effective than conventional radiographs in detecting early erosions of RA patients and it is comparable with MRI regarding reproducibility [35-37]. US could detect 63% of erosions with 1-10% bone volume loss and 94% of erosions with >10% bone volume loss [38]. In early RA, US is better than MRI for the detection of erosions, however in established RA MRI is superior to US [19, 39-41]. Additionally, since US cannot access some parts of the joints in the wrist and hand, it may have limited value (as compared to MRI) in the detection and follow up of erosive changes over time [19, 30]. In this regard, US scanning protocols usually encompass easily accessible joints (e.g. 2nd and 5th MCP and PIP joints), whereby US becomes advantageous [35, 39]. Several scoring systems, which semi-quantitatively grade erosions (size or extent) and monitor their progression, have been recommended [28, 35, 42-44].

### 13.2.4 Cartilage Damage

In RA, chronic synovitis leads to progressive thinning of the articular cartilage and destruction of the subchondral bone. US can readily be used to monitor changes in the articular cartilage. Sonographic evaluation of the articular cartilage integrity has been shown to be a valid and reliable method particularly in the MCP and PIP joints of RA patients [45].

### 13.2.5 Other Manifestations

*Rheumatoid nodules* are common extra-articular manifestations of RA, usually present on extensor surfaces. They are sonographically described as "oval, generally homogenous, hypoechoic masses that are attached closely to the bone surface with poor internal vascularity" [46]. US can help differentiate these lesions from other subcutaneous nodules.

*Popliteal or Baker's cyst* is the increased production of synovial fluid within the gastrocnemius-semimembranosus bursa, commonplace in RA. The cyst may also rupture and cause sudden swelling/pain in the calf mimicking acute thrombophlebitis, so called as pseudothrombophlebitis [47]. In this sense, either for detecting the simple cyst or its rupture or for the differential diagnosis (e.g. thrombosis of the popliteal vessels) US can be contributory. The presence of anechoic or hypoechoic fluid extending freely between the muscles in the mid-calf or beneath the subcutaneous tissue is a useful and easily detectable sign of pseudothrombophlebitis (Figure 13.9) and PDUS can be used to distinguish vascular pathologies [48].

*Carpal tunnel syndrome* is one of the most common extra-articular features of RA and high

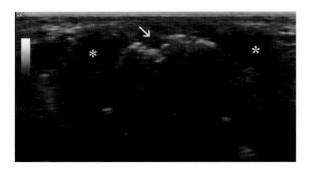

**Figure 13.7** Transverse gray-scale US demonstrating an erosion (arrow) of the 3rd metacarpal head in a patient with RA. Extension of the synovitis is also seen (asterisks).

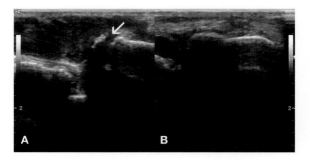

**Figure 13.8** Comparative wrist US imaging (longitudinal view) demonstrates an erosion (arrow) on the right ulnar styloid (A). Normal side (B).

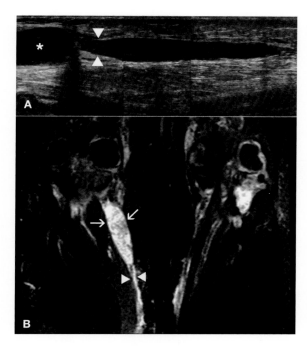

**Figure 13.9** Ruptured Baker's cyst in RA. A - Longitudinal split-screen US image of the posterior calf shows heterogenous Baker's cyst (asterisk) and extension of fluid (arrowheads) distally. B - Bilateral coronal short tau inversion recovery (STIR) sequence reveals hyperintense fluid (arrows) extending inferiorly from the Baker's cyst (arrowheads).

frequency US has been shown to be a sensitive/specific method in its diagnosis (discussed in details in other chapters).

## 13.2.6 Predictive Role of Ultrasound in Rheumatoid Arthritis

Several research groups, which have evaluated the role of US in monitoring response to treatment in RA, showed that there was significant decrease in joint cavity widening, decrease in synovial perfusion and vascularization after intra-articular steroid injections or treatments with biologic agents [49-52]. Additionally, keeping in mind the fact that subclinical inflammation is an important prognostic factor in RA and that US can detect residual disease activity more sensitively than clinical examination both in active disease and in remission, "ultrasonographic remission" may be essential for better RA management [14, 18]. The Targeted Ultrasound Initiative group consists of ultrasonographers and rheumatolo-

gists has devised the Targeted Ultrasound in RA study, where patients with RA in sustained clinical remission are scanned with US in order to determine the presence of PD signals. If there is still evidence of active arthritis on PDUS, the Disease-modifying Antirheumatic Drugs (DMARD) treatment will be increased even if the clinical measures demonstrate remission. Results of the ongoing randomized controlled study will determine significance of subclinical synovitis especially PD and whether suppression of these will have a significant impact on future structural and functional outcomes [53].

## 13.3 SPONDYLOARTHROPATHIES

Spondyloarthropathies (SpA) are a group of inflammatory diseases that comprise ankylosing spondylitis, arthritis/spondylitis associated with psoriasis, reactive arthritis, arthritis/spondylitis associated with inflammatory bowel diseases, and juvenile idiopathic arthritis [54]. The hallmark of SpA is sacroiliitis together with the other main features i.e. spondylitis, arthritis, enthesitis and dactylitis [55]. Early diagnosis gained importance after the invention of new therapeutic agents, including tumor necrosis factor (TNF)-α antagonists which have been shown to be effective not only for patients with established ankylosing spondylitis but also for those with non-radiographic axial SpA [56, 57]. Fortunately, new imaging modalities/techniques are now available for early diagnosis and follow-up [58]. The presence of axial skeletal involvement can be detected early by MRI, even before inflammation becomes evident on radiographs (non-radiographic phase of the disease) [59]. Since entheses, as well as synovia, tendons, ligaments and many other soft tissues can be easily visualized by US, its use in the assessment of SpA is paramount [60]. US is also sensitive for early inflammatory lesions at these sites with the exception of bone marrow edema [61].

### 13.3.1 Enthesitis

An enthesis is a point of union between a tendon, ligament or capsule and the bone. Enthesitis, a characteristic manifestation of SpA, is the inflammation of these sites. Any pathologic process of enthesis whether metabolic, inflammatory,

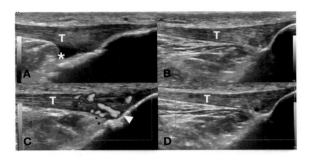

**Figure 13.10** Patellar tendinitis in a 35-year-old man with AS. A - Longitudinal gray-scale US shows decreased echogenicity and thickening of the left patellar tendon (T) at the tibial insertion and infrapatellar bursitis (asterisk). B - Normal side. C - On PDUS, flow signals suggest active inflammation at the attachment site (arrowhead). D - Normal side.

cifications, erosions, tendon tears/thinning may be considered as chronic changes [71] (Figures 13.11 and 13.12). Excellent agreement (>80%) has been reported for hypoechogenicity, calcifications, erosions, thicker tendon insertion, enthesophytes and Doppler activity among experts, with inter-observer reliability being lowest for enthesophytes (0.24) and highest for Doppler activity (0.63) [72].

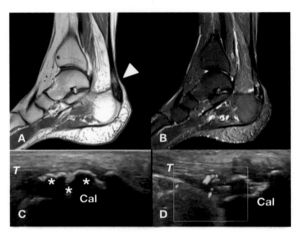

**Figure 13.11** A 37-year-old woman with AS. A - T1-weighted magnetic resonance image (sagittal view) of the left ankle shows irregular and thickened Achilles tendon (arrowhead). B - Short tau inversion recovery image. C - Longitudinal gray-scale US shows calcifications with acustic shadows (asterisks) at the calcaneal (Cal) insertion of the Achilles tendon (T). D - PDUS examination suggests active inflammation.

traumatic or degenerative is referred as enthesopathy, however enthesitis is restricted to inflammatory enthesopathy [62]. It consists of focal, destructive microscopic inflammatory lesions evolving to fibrous scarring and new bone formation [63]. In patients with ankylosing spondylitis, frequency of enthesitis is 25-58% [64, 65]. Entheses are involved in the early stage of SpA, the incidence being higher in men and independent of the SpA subgroup, HLA-B27 status or presentation pattern [66].

Enthesitis usually manifests as swelling, isolated pain or tenderness and plain radiographs have traditionally been used to assess associated bony changes. On the other hand, the accuracy of physical examination or plain radiography is uncertain; yet entheseal bony changes appear late and, with aging the prevalence of asymptomatic enthesopathy increases [67]. As such, US can effectively be used (complimentary/superior to physical examination) for evaluating the structural changes and/or the abnormal vascularization at the enthesal sites in SpA [68, 69] (Figure 13.10).

Despite the wide range of its definitions [70], enthesopathy is usually described as "abnormal hypoechoic (loss of normal fibrillar architecture) and/or thickened tendon or ligament at its bony attachment (may occasionally contain hyperechoic foci consistent with calcification) seen in two perpendicular planes that may exhibit Doppler signal and/or bony changes including enthesophytes, erosions or irregularity" [15]. In addition, changes like hypoechogenicity, thickening, peritendinous fluid and adjacent bursitis may be considered as acute changes of enthesis, whereas cal-

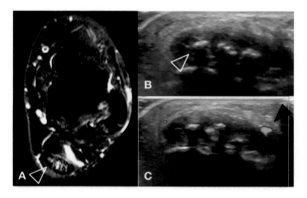

**Figure 13.12** A 37-year-old woman with AS. A - Axial short tau inversion recovery magnetic resonance image shows retrocalcaneal bursitis and thickened Achilles tendon (void arrowhead). B - Transverse gray-scale US shows calcifications (void arrowhead) with acustic shadows inside the Achilles tendon. C - Flow signals suggest active inflammation on PDUS.

Musculoskeletal Ultrasound in Physical and Rehabilitation Medicine

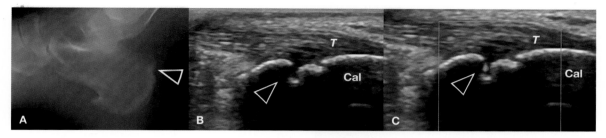

**Figure 13.13** A 35-year-old man with AS. A - Lateral radiograph of the left heel shows an erosion (arrowhead) at the calcaneus. B - Longitudinal gray-scale US shows the same erosion (void arrowhead) on the calcaneus (Cal) and mild thickening in the Achilles tendon (T) as well. C - Flow signal within the erosion is typical for active inflammation on PDUS.

During US examination, a feasible number of entheses should be chosen, preferably from the lower limbs. Yet, a cross-sectional study [63] showed that the most common enthesitic sites of involvement were Achilles tendon and plantar fascia insertions (Figures 13.13 and 13.14). Additionally, if (semi)quantification is necessary, one of the commonly used scales can be included in the examination. For instance, while Glasgow Ultrasound Enthesitis Scoring System evaluates the morphostructural changes of the enthesis at the knees, Achilles tendon and the plantar fascia [68], in Madrid Sonography Enthesitis Index triceps tendon and PDUS assessment are also included [73] and in Sonographic Entheseal Index, the lower extremity enthesopathy is classified as acute (potentially reversible) and chronic (possibly inactive) [74]. It must be kept in the mind that lesions detected by gray-scale US may be observed in both inflammatory and mechanical enthesopathy [75, 76].

When compared to gray-scale US, PDUS may be more informative for enthesitis, because the presence of PD signal indicates entheseal vascularity [63]. It is mainly useful for detecting acute enthesitis in either asymptomatic patients or those with normal radiographs [73, 77]. A recent study showed that PDUS had an excellent sensitivity (but weak specificity) in detecting chronic enthesitis in ankylosing spondylitis patients [78]. PDUS findings of enthesitis has been shown to correlate with clinical measures, pain and tenderness [77]. Of note, PDUS was also reported to be a useful modality for monitoring the therapy [79, 80].

Concerning SpA-associated dactylitis, the clinical scenario may comprise diffuse painful swelling of the digits with findings of enthesitis, synovitis and tenosynovitis altogether [81]. US can depict peritendinous edema, juxta-articular periosteal reactions, pseudotenosynovitis, bony changes and positive Doppler signals [82]. In parallel with the developments in technology (e.g. three-dimensional imaging) assessment for enthesitis seem to improve with better inter-observer reliability [83, 84].

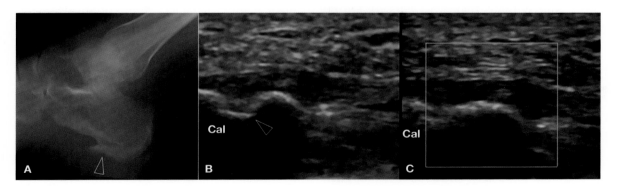

**Figure 13.14** A 35-year-old man with AS. A - Lateral radiograph of the right heel shows a bony erosion and an enthesophyte/spur at the calcaneus. B - Longitudinal gray-scale US shows the same bony erosion (void arrowhead) and thickening of the plantar fascia. C - No flow signal on PDUS. Cal, calcaneus.

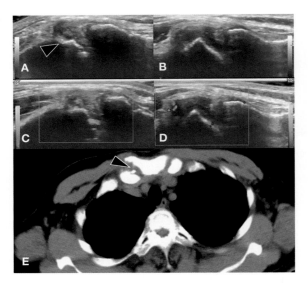

**Figure 13.15** A 35-year-old man with AS. Longitudinal gray-scale US shows a bony erosion (arrowhead) and synovial hypertrophy in the right sternoclavicular joint (A) and synovial hypertrophy on the left side of the patient (B). On PDUS examination, the synovitis is inactive in the right sternoclavicular joint (C) and active on the left side of the patient (D). Axial computed tomography showing the same (aforementioned) bony erosion (arrowhead) (E).

### 13.3.2 Synovitis

Ultrasound examination for synovitis can be performed with the same approach used in RA. US can detect a higher number of inflamed joints and effusion (at knee, hip and fingers) than clinical examination in patients with SpA [85-88] (Figure 13.15). It is a valuable tool in detecting synovial abnormalities of the fingers and toes in patients with suspected psoriatic arthritis [89] and it has been shown that US examination can detect more bone erosions than MRI [90, 91]. On the other hand, the potential of US in the differential diagnosis between RA and psoriatic arthritis has also been investigated but any distinguishing feature could not be determined except peritenon inflammation of the extensor tendons (only found in patients with psoriatic arthritis) [92].

### 13.3.3 Sacroiliitis and Spondylitis

So far, there are few data for US examination of sacroiliac joints (SIJ) and axial skeleton. There is not enough data to derive firm conclusion on the validity of US examination of SIJs. The first study assessing the SIJ of Doppler US suggested that vascularization around the SIJ was more common in patients with sacroiliitis than healthy controls and the mean resistive index (RI, defined as: [Vmax-Vmin/Vmax], where Vmax and Vmin were the maximum and minimum flow rates recorded during one cardiac cycle) value was low in patients with sacroiliitis and increased after the anti-inflammatory therapy [93]. Another study found that color Doppler US might be useful to detect the degree of inflammation by using the same methods in SIJ, lumbar and thoracic vertebral paraspinal areas [94]. A recent study suggest that color Doppler US can be used as a convenient technique in the diagnosis of active sacroiliitis with 92% specificity and 82% sensitivity [95]. Another study showed that color Doppler US detects hypervascularity in SIJ only in 19% of patients with active sacroiliitis [96] and however the same authors demonstrated that contrast-enhanced US can detect active sacroiliitis with 100% sensitivity and 100% specificity [97]. Decrease or disappearance of PD signals and increase in RI values in the sacroiliac joints with infliximab treatment were determined in patients with AS suggesting the use of PDUS in the follow-up of SIJ changes [98]. Actually, intraarticular injections for SIJ are often performed under fluoroscopy or computerized tomography guidance. It should be stated that even peri-articular deposition of steroid appeared sufficient for pain and symptom control in patients with active sacroiliitis [99].

### 13.4 OSTEOARTHRITIS

Osteoarthritis (OA) is the most common rheumatic disease characterized by chronic degenerative changes and loss of cartilage. There is also inflammation in addition to the structural damage in OA [100]. Conventional radiography -still the first-line diagnostic tool in OA- only allows indirect evaluation for the articular cartilage, not being able to show sufficiently the changes in the soft tissues. Herewith, the use of US in the assessment of knee, hip, and hand OA, both for research and clinical practice, continues to evolve. Inflammation (i.e. joint effusion, synovial hypertrophy or vascularization) and structural damage (i.e. osteophytes, cortical bone irregularities, joint cartilage or meniscal abnormalities) can be detected by US [12, 101-104]. Moreover, similar to the aforementioned rheumatic conditions, Doppler imaging can be utilized to distinguish active and inactive lesions [105]. On the other hand, as US waves cannot penetrate through the bone, subchondral sclerosis, cysts or bone marrow lesions can not be evaluated.

### 13.4.1 Synovitis

Synovial pathology is common in the early and late stages of OA and may generate pain [102]. For example, between 47-100% of patients with OA have synovitis and effusion of the symptomatic knee [102]. Ultrasound is more sensitive than clinical examination for detecting synovitis of the knee, small joints of the hands (particularly in erosive hand OA) and feet, also correlating with findings as regards MRI, arthroscopy or histopathology [102, 106, 107]. Further, especially persistent inflammation detected by US has been shown to be independently associated with radiological progression in the following two years in hand OA [108]. As such, US imaging might also play role for the follow-up of particular OA patients. Additionally, US can also demonstrate the presence of accompanying soft tissue pathologies e.g Baker's cysts and pes anserine bursitis in knee OA [109].

Again, similar to the above-quoted disease, synovitis can be semiquantitatively graded on a scale of 0-3 (0: no synovitis; 1: mild synovitis; 2: moderate synovitis; 3: severe synovitis) using B-mode or PDUS [110].

### 13.4.2 Cartilage

Hyaline cartilage is a homogenous low reflective layer parallel to the subchondral bone on US (Figure 13.16) and therefore US imaging has been established as a valid and reliable tool for the as

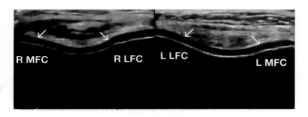

**Figure 13.16** Normal distal femoral cartilage is seen as a regular homogeneous anechoic layer (arrows) on axial view. R; right; L; left; MFC; medial femoral condyle; LFC, lateral femoral condyle.

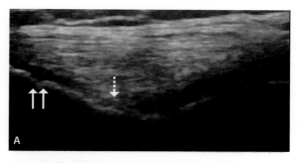

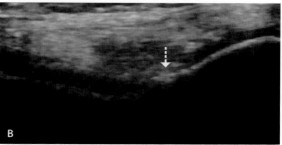

**Figure 13.17** A and B - Comparative gray-scale US imaging (axial view) shows interrupted and thinned femoral cartilage layer (dashed arrows) with a cortical irregularity (double arrow) in a patient with bilateral knee osteoarthritis.

sessment of joint cartilage or for measuring its thickness [111, 112]. In OA, early cartilage abnormalities on US imaging would be blurring of the edges and loss of sharpness on the margins [101, 113, 114]. Thereafter, cartilage loses its homogenity and transparency [112, 113, 115] and finally, thinning of the cartilage and asymmetrical narrowing of the joint space ensues [113] (Figure 13.17). These stages are actually used for sonographic grading of the cartilage in OA as well [116]. In knee OA, protrusion of the medial meniscus can also be visualized, a finding well correlating with clinical and radiological findings of OA [117, 118].

### 13.4.3 Bony Changes

Due to the fact that the US waves do not penetrate through the bones, US is able to show only the periosteum and the cortex (normally a continuous smooth hyperechoic line). On the other hand, especially with the aid of sonopalpation, it is quite sensitive in showing the relevant lesions (erosions, irregularities, and osteophytes) pertaining to the cortex. Osteophytes are frequently seen as irregularities of the bony cortex and cortical protrusions at the joint margins, giving a posterior acoustic shadow [119] and US has been reported to be more effective than radiography in the detection of osteophytes and joint space narrowing in hand OA [119]. Moreover, US has high sensitivity (83%) and specificity (75%) in identifying osteophytes compared with MRI [120]. Osteophytes are evaluated using both dichotomous and semi-quantitative scales (0: no osteopyhtes, 1: mild osteophytes, 2: moderate osteophytes; 3: severe osteophytes) [110].

Bone erosion is defined as "an intra-articular break down of the bone surface, which is visible in two perpendicular planes" [15]. Although erosions are well-known features of RA, they can also be seen in OA, particularly in erosive hand OA [121]. Gray-scale US is a reliable and valid imaging method to assess erosions, when compared to MRI as a reference method in OA [122, 123]. Herewith, in erosive hand OA, erosions characteristically reside at the central aspect of the joint. Therefore, it should be noted that their detection can be more difficult than RA [124]. Lastly, US has again been shown useful in monitoring response to treatment in OA [125, 126].

## 13.5 CRYSTAL ARTHROPATHIES

A group of diseases whereby depositions of crystals are seen in articular and periarticular tissues resulting in inflammation and damage are called as crystal arthropathies. Being capable of depicting those crystals, US has become a useful diagnostic tool in crystal arthropathies. Additionally, US can also demonstrate other pertinent findings e.g. joint effusion, synovitis, bone erosions, cartilage involvement, tendinopathy, bursitis, and precisely guide a likely intervention [127].

### 13.5.1 Gout

Gout is a systemic metabolic inflammatory disease which is characterized by deposition of monosodium urate crystals (MSU) in tissues. The joint cavity may contain "urate milk", tophi and inflamed synovial tissues in gout and demonstration of MSU in the joint fluid is diagnostic. Musculoskeletal US is reliable for detecting MSU deposition in gout and asymptomatic hyperuricemia [128]. Yet, monosodium urate crystals, which re-

flect US waves, can easily be confirmed especially at low gain levels [129]. After sufficient deposition, tophi appear as hyperechoic bands with a posterior acoustic shadow [130].

Specific diagnostic features of gouty arthropathies on US include: a hyperechoic, irregular band over the superficial margin of the articular cartilage, described as a 'double contour sign'; hypoechoic to hyperechoic, inhomogeneous material surrounded by a small anechoic rim (tophus); erosions adjacent to tophaceous material [129]. The sensitivity and specificity for 'double contour sign' are 0.83 and 0.76; and for tophus 0.65 and 0.80, respectively [131]. During urate-lowering treatment, US can also show the disappearance of MSU crystal deposition on hyaline cartilage as uric acid levels return to normal [132]. Follow-up may indisputably include PDUS assessment for synovitis under colchicine therapy [133].

### Synovitis

Acute or chronic synovitis may be present in patients with gout. During acute gout, echogenicity of synovial fluid is variable. Floating of multiple aggregates of MSU crystals may present a snowstorm appearance in the joint cavity. Other sonographic findings would be hyperechoic cloudy areas inside the joint, representing MSU crystal deposits within the thickened synovial membrane. As quoted above, power Doppler signals can be used to differentiate active, inflamed synovium from inactive, non-inflamed synovium and to monitor gouty synovitis [134]. Flow signals may be detected even in asymptomatic joints of patients with gout, corresponding to subclinical chronic inflammation [135].

### Tophus

The tophus represents a chronic inflammatory tissue response to MSU, frequently seen in the advanced stages of the disease [136]. On radiographs, tophi can be visualized as diffuse soft tissue swelling. They appear as nodular deposits almost at any site and can cause erosions to adjacent bone and joint structures.

US is useful to evaluate and differentiate tophi from other subcutaneous nodules e.g. rheumatoid nodules, lipoma and sarcoid nodules [46]. Tophi are generally hyperechoic, heterogeneous,

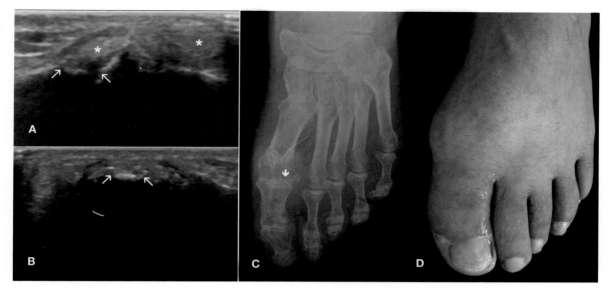

**Figure 13.18** Gout. A - US imaging (longitudinal view) shows cortical erosions (arrows) and an intra-articular tophus -an isoechoic mass (asterisks) with a small anechoic rim in the 1st metatarsophalangeal joint. B - Cortical erosions (arrows) are also seen on the axial view. C - Anteroposterior radiograph shows erosions (arrow) in the 1st and 2nd metatarsal heads. D - Photograph of the patient's foot.

with poorly defined contours, and surrounded by an anechoic halo [137] (Figure 13.18). A soft tophus is visualized as an aggregate of inhomogeneous echogenicity, whereas a hard tophus appears as hyperechoic bands generating posterior acoustic shadowing and mixed tophi show features of both. US findings correlate well with MRI in the detection of tophi [138], its sensitivity being 74% for metatarsophalangeal joints, and specificity being 100% for all sites [139]. During a gout attack, an increased flow signal may reflect active inflammation [140] (Figure 13.19).

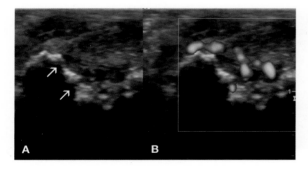

**Figure 13.19** A - Transverse US imaging of the left 1st metatarsal head showing cortical irregularities (arrows). B - Flow signals are seen on PDUS.

## Bone erosion

Bone erosions are manifestations of chronic gout and they have been reported in close association with intra-osseous tophi and synovitis [141, 142]. Concerning imaging, erosions could have been detected three times more frequently by US than radiographs [130]. Likewise, patients who have normal radiographs may have occult destructive arthropathy that can be detected by MRI and US [143]. Further, a sensitive PDUS examination can also document persistent, subclinical inflammation in these erosions. As such, US may assist in the management of gout, by allowing early detection of erosive joint damage and/or tophaceous deposits even in clinically silent joints [130].

## Cartilage involvement

Loss of cartilage and narrowing of the joint space is a late feature of gout. Most commonly seen cartilage abnormality on US is double contour sign (Figure 13.20) which is secondary to deposition of MSU crystals on the superficial surface of hyaline cartilage [128]. It corresponds to a bright hyperechoic irregular band over the superficial margin of the anechoic cartilage over

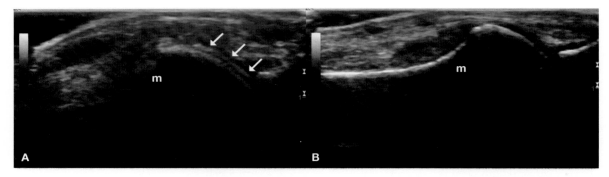

**Figure 13.20**   A - Longitudinal US imaging of the 1st metatarsal head (m) showing the double contour sign (arrows). B - Normal side.

the hyperechoic bone. For metatarsophalangeal joints, the double contour sign is significantly associated with hyperuricemia and disease duration. Although the sensitivity of the double contour sign is variable, its specificity is as high as >98% [130, 139]. On the other hand, the prognostic value of the double contour sign for progression of the cartilage damage is currently unclear.

Of note, two conditions must be considered while promptly distinguishing the double contour sign. First would be the deposition of calcium pyrophosphate dehydrate crystals (CPPD) which tend to aggregate in the middle (not super-

ficial) layer of the hyaline cartilage [144]. Second would be the interface sign in the presence of joint effusion (synovitis). Practically, while the interface sign disappears with a change in the slope of the probe, the double contour sign generally persists.

### Soft tissue involvement

In addition to bone and cartilage involvement, gout may also affect tendons, ligaments and bursae. As described before in this chapter, involvement of the bursae (Figure 13.21) and tendons

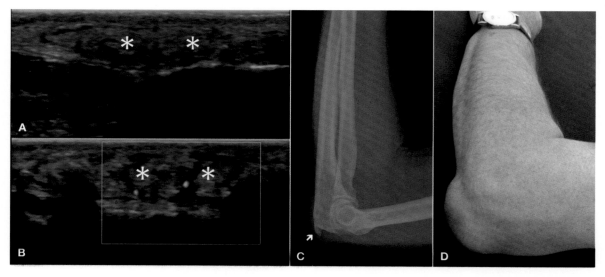

**Figure 13.21**   Tophus at the elbow. A - US imaging (longitudinal view) demonstrates heterogeneous and hyperechoic appearance of the tophus (asterisks) and synovial hypertrophy within the olecranon bursa. B - Tophaceous material (asterisks) with flow signals on PDUS. C - Radiograph of the elbow shows spur formation (arrow) on the olecranon. D - Photograph of the patient's elbow demonstrating soft tissue swelling.

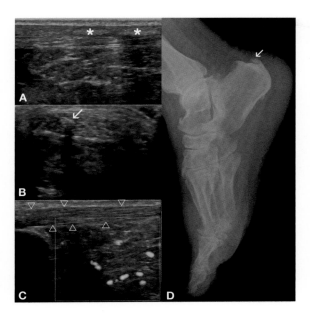

**Figure 13.22** Tophus in the Achilles tendon. A - Longitudinal US imaging shows intratendinous, oval-shaped, heterogeneous and hyperechoic tophi (asterisks). B - Axial view demonstrates the tophus (arrow) giving acoustic shadowing. C - PDUS examination shows also inflammation in the retrocalcaneal fat, Achilles tendon (between arrowheads), calcaneus (Cal). D - Lateral radiograph of the foot showing bony spur formation at the Achilles tendon insertion (arrow).

## 13.5.2 Calcium Pyrophosphate Dihydrate Crystal Deposition Disease

Calcium pyrophosphate dehydrate crystal (CPPD) deposition disease is characterized by the accumulation of pyrophosphate dihydrate crystals in articular and periarticular tissues. Clinical manifestations of CPPD are acute synovitis, chronic arthritis or asymptomatic findings of cartilage calcification. The most commonly involved joints are knee, wrist, symphysis pubis and hip [146]. Demonstration of CPPD crystals in the synovial fluid and plain radiographs is diagnostic for CPPD. Herewith, the sensitivity of US for detection of calcification is higher than radiography in these patients, specificity being 100% for both methods [147, 148].

Sonographic findings of CPPD include a thin hyperechoic band within the cartilage layer, hyperechoic rounded or amorphous shaped areas within the fibrocartilage and homogeneous hyperechoic nodular or oval-shaped deposits in bursae or articular recesses [144, 148]. There is often no acoustic shadowing behind the calcifications [149]. For sure, PDUS can also assess the presence and extent of inflammation.

In CPPD, unlike gout, crystals accumulate within the cartilage layer at different locations including femoral condyle and metacarpal heads. US imaging may show a various types of involvement, ranging from isolated hyperechoic spots to extended large deposits [150, 151]. Hyperechoic regular rounded floating aggregates can even be detected in the synovial fluid. Additionally, CPPD crystals can also be observed in tendons, ligaments, menisci, bursae and articular recesses [144, 148, 152]. Yet, Achilles tendon and plantar fascia

(Figures 13.22 and 13.23) and ligaments can readily be shown by US [135, 145]. Monosodium urate microdeposits may be seen in tendons (with a small hypoechoic halo due to local inflammation) even in asymptomatic subjects. An important late complication of intratendinous tophus would be tendon rupture that can again be visualized substantially using US.

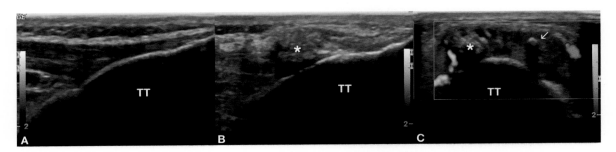

**Figure 13.23** Distal patellar tendon involvement in gout. When compared with the normal side (A), longitudinal US imaging shows a tophus (asterisk) in the distal attachment of the patellar tendon on the tibial tuberosity (TT) (B). PDUS evaluation (axial view) (C) depicts two hyperechoic tophi (asterisk and arrow), the small one giving acustic shadowing (arrow). The flow signals are also seen.

calcifications are commonplace and well identified, used also as an indirect sign of CPPD [153].

## 13.6 OTHER RHEUMATIC DISEASES

### 13.6.1 Systemic Sclerosis

Systemic sclerosis (SSc), also known as scleroderma, is a severe collagen tissue disease characterized by vascular, immune and fibrotic changes in the skin and internal organs [154]. Musculoskeletal involvement is also an important part of the disease and causes significant disability [155]. Further, this type of involvement may be the initial manifestation and early indicator of the disease. It is usually classified as soft tissue, bone, joint and tendon involvement and vascular involvement [156]. Herein, US examination can detect joint and tendon pathologies, subcutaneous calcification and various skin features of SSc patients [157].

Except patients with systemic sclerosis sine scleroderma, skin involvement is the most characteristic finding. It has three phases; an early edematous phase, an indurative phase characterized with collagen deposition and an atrophic phase associated with thinning of the skin [158]. Using high frequency probes, detailed quantitative and qualitative assessment of the skin can be performed different layers of the skin i.e. epidermis, dermis and subcutaneous fat [159, 160]. The echogenicity of the dermis decreases during the initial edematous phase, followed by normal or increased echogenity (reflecting fibrosis) during the disease process [161, 162]. A 17-point dermal US scoring system has already been suggested as a reliable/useful outcome measure for SSc patients [163].

Doppler US can also be used for the evaluation of the localized scleroderma, the most common form of SSc in the pediatric population. Tissue thickness, echogenicity and vascularity can be examined and compared with the contralateral side and this allows not only monitoring the disease activity (i.e. active vs inactive lesions) over time but also evaluating the disease involvement in the deeper tissues [164, 165].

Raynaud's phenomenon is the early manifestation in more than 90% of patients with SSc. It is sometimes difficult to differentiate primary and secondary Raynaud's phenomenon due to underlying connective tissue disease. One study showed that the mean baseline vascularity of the patients with secondary Raynaud's phenomenon was significantly lower than patients with primary Raynaud's phenomenon, and suggested that Doppler US can provide additional information to clinical examination [166].

The earliest manifestations of the SSc are myalgia, fatigue and diffuse swelling of the hands. Furthermore, joint involvement (arthralgia, synovitis and/or tenosynovitis, loss in joint range of motion or flexion contractures) affects 46-97% of SSc patients [167]. However, joint findings are not specific for SSc and have not been included among the preliminary criteria for the very early diagnosis of SSc [168]. There are limited reports on the clinical application of US for SSc patients with joint involvement [169-171]. While radiographs are still being used for the diagnosis and follow-up of SSc, MRI is suggested for detecting bone edema/erosions and US for evaluating synovitis and early calcifications [156, 169, 172]. In a recent study, we have also shown that enthesitis may also be an important musculoskeletal involvement in these patients whereby US imaging would definitely be contributory [173].

Pulmonary involvement, which is one of the main causes of morbidity and mortality, is present approximately in 90% of patients with SSc [174]. Although high-resolution CT is the gold standard method for diagnosis of SSc related interstitial lung disease, transthoracic ultrasound can be used as well to assess pulmonary fibrosis [175]. Its sensitivity and specificity has been reported as 73.58% and 88.23%, respectively [175]. On US, the thickened subpleural interlobar septum causes comet-tail sign, seen as a hyperechoic narrow-based reverberated artifact. Semiquantitative US scoring (normal: 0 - severe: 3) for pulmonary fibrosis has also been defined [175].

In short, still being in its infancy, the use of US imaging in SSC is quite intriguing and definitely requires further studies.

### 13.6.2 Sjögren's Syndrome

Sjögren's syndrome (SS) is a chronic systemic autoimmune disease characterized by lymphocytic infiltration and destruction of the exocrine glands. Its extra-glandular manifestations encompass arthralgia/arthritis, myalgia, neuropathy, vasculitis, pulmonary, renal and gastrointestinal diseases. Salivary dysfunction is the most common manifestation of SS. Although different methods are available for the assessment of salivary glands e.g. minor salivary gland biopsy, salivary flow tests, salivary gland MRI, parotid sialography/sialoscintigraphy; none of them are highly sensitive and specific for the diagnosis of SS [176].

Recently, US of the salivary glands has been introduced as a promising technique in this regard [177, 178]. Since salivary gland US has a diagnostic sensitivity of 82% and specificity of 73%, it can be an alternative imaging technique for the diagnosis of primary SS [179]. Pathological changes of the posterior borders, parenchymal inhomogeneity with hypoechogenic areas and/or hyperechogenic reflections in major salivary glands are the most important US findings [180, 181]. Also, the degree of parenchymal inhomogenicity is positively correlated with disease duration in patients with primary and secondary SS [182]. Several semiquantitative scoring systems are used for grading parenchymal homogeneity, echogenicity, number of hypoechogenic areas, hyperechogenic reflections and clearness of the borders of the salivary glands, [180, 181]. The method proposed by Hocevar et al was suggested to be comparable with scintigraphy and salivary gland biopsy [183].

Additionally, salivary gland US improves the diagnostic performance of the ACR classification criteria for SS [184, 185].

Indisputably, similar to other rheumatic diseases, the aforementioned musculoskeletal manifestations of SS can readily/thoroughly be assessed using US and PDUS [186, 187].

### 13.6.3 Temporal Arteritis

Temporal arteritis is the most common form of systemic vasculitis in adults (commonly aged >50 years) and affects primarily the extracranial branches of the carotid artery. US findings are stenosis of the temporal artery, occlusions, the halo sign which is a hypoechoic edematous wall thickening on Doppler US and compression sign (the arterial wall remained visible upon compression due to vessel wall inflammation). For both the halo and the compression signs, the sensitivity is 79% and specificity is 100% [188]. Diagnostic sensitivity of temporal arteritis may be improved if US and histological examinations are combined [189]. For sure, early detection of large-vessel pathology can help modify treatment and prevent vascular complications in these patients [190].

## REFERENCES

1) Gibbon WW, Wakefield RJ. Ultrasound in inflammatory disease. Radiol Clin North Am. 1999; 37: 633-51.
2) Toprak H, Kilic E, Serter A, Kocakoc E, Ozgocmen S. Ultrasound and Doppler US in evaluation of superficial soft-tissue lesions. J Clin Imaging Sci. 2014; 4: 12.
3) Toprak H, Kilic E, Serter A, Kocakoc E, Ozgocmen S. Doppler US in rheumatic diseases with special emphasis on rheumatoid arthritis and spondyloarthritis. Diagn Interv Radiol. 2014; 20: 72-7.
4) Backhaus M, Burmester GR, Gerber T, Grassi W, Machold KP, Swen WA, et al. Guidelines for musculoskeletal ultrasound in rheumatology. Ann Rheum Dis. 2001; 60: 641-9.
5) Brown AK. Using ultrasonography to facilitate best practice in diagnosis and management of RA. Nat Rev Rheumatol. 2009; 5: 698-706.
6) Hicks A, Adams H, Szczepanski J. Medical imaging and radiographic analysis of the rheumatoid patient. Clin Podiatr Med Surg. 2010; 27: 209-18.
7) Schirmer M, Duftner C, Schmidt WA, Dejaco C. Ultrasonography in inflammatory rheumatic disease: an overview. Nat Rev Rheumatol. 2011; 7: 479-88.
8) Thiele RG. Ultrasonography applications in diagnosis and management of early rheumatoid ar-

thritis. Rheum Dis Clin North Am. 2012; 38: 259-75.

9) Torp-Pedersen ST, Terslev L. Settings and artefacts relevant in colour/power Doppler ultrasound in rheumatology. Ann Rheum Dis. 2008; 67: 143-9.

10) Rubin JM, Bude RO, Carson PL, Bree RL, Adler RS. Power Doppler US: a potentially useful alternative to mean frequency-based color Doppler US. Radiology. 1994; 190: 853-6.

11) Wakefield RJ, Brown A, O'Connor P, Grainger A, Karim Z, McGonagle D, et al. Rheumatological ultrasound. Rheumatology (Oxford). 2003; 42: 1001.

12) Kane D, Balint PV, Sturrock RD. Ultrasonography is superior to clinical examination in the detection and localization of knee joint effusion in rheumatoid arthritis. J Rheumatol. 2003; 30: 966-71.

13) Szkudlarek M, Klarlund M, Narvestad E, Court-Payen M, Strandberg C, Jensen KE, et al. Ultrasonography of the metacarpophalangeal and proximal interphalangeal joints in rheumatoid arthritis: a comparison with magnetic resonance imaging, conventional radiography and clinical examination. Arthritis Res Ther. 2006; 8(2): R52.

14) Scire CA, Montecucco C, Codullo V, Epis O, Todoerti M, Caporali R. Ultrasonographic evaluation of joint involvement in early rheumatoid arthritis in clinical remission: power Doppler signal predicts short-term relapse. Rheumatology (Oxford). 2009; 48: 1092-7.

15) Wakefield RJ, Balint PV, Szkudlarek M, Filippucci E, Backhaus M, D'Agostino MA, et al. Musculoskeletal ultrasound including definitions for ultrasonographic pathology. J Rheumatol. 2005; 32: 2485-7.

16) Kiris A, Ozgocmen S, Kocakoc E, Ardicoglu O. Power Doppler assessment of overall disease activity in patients with rheumatoid arthritis. J Clin Ultrasound. 2006; 34: 5-11.

17) Newman JS, Adler RS, Bude RO, Rubin JM. Detection of soft-tissue hyperemia: value of power Doppler sonography. AJR Am J Roentgenol. 1994; 163: 385-9.

18) Yoshimi R, Hama M, Takase K, Ihata A, Kishimoto D, Terauchi K, et al. Ultrasonography is a potent tool for the prediction of progressive joint destruction during clinical remission of rheumatoid arthritis. Mod Rheumatol. 2013; 23: 456-65.

19) Szkudlarek M, Narvestad E, Klarlund M, Court-Payen M, Thomsen HS, Ostergaard M. Ultrasonography of the metatarsophalangeal joints in rheumatoid arthritis: comparison with magnetic resonance imaging, conventional radiography, and clinical examination. Arthritis Rheum. 2004; 50: 2103-12.

20) Backhaus M, Ohrndorf S, Kellner H, Strunk J, Backhaus TM, Hartung W, et al. Evaluation of a novel 7-joint ultrasound score in daily rheumatologic practice: a pilot project. Arthritis Rheum. 2009; 61: 1194-201.

21) Naredo E, Bonilla G, Gamero F, Uson J, Carmona L, Laffon A. Assessment of inflammatory activity in rheumatoid arthritis: a comparative study of clinical evaluation with grey scale and power Doppler ultrasonography. Ann Rheum Dis. 2005; 64: 375-81.

22) Hitchon CA, El-Gabalawy HS. The synovium in rheumatoid arthritis. Open Rheumatol J. 2011; 5: 107-14.

23) Scheel AK, Hermann KG, Kahler E, Pasewaldt D, Fritz J, Hamm B, et al. A novel ultrasonographic synovitis scoring system suitable for analyzing finger joint inflammation in rheumatoid arthritis. Arthritis Rheum. 2005; 52: 733-43.

24) Taouli B, Guermazi A, Sack KE, Genant HK. Imaging of the hand and wrist in RA. Ann Rheum Dis. 2002; 61: 867-9.

25) Szkudlarek M, Court-Payen M, Strandberg C, Klarlund M, Klausen T, Ostergaard M. Power Doppler ultrasonography for assessment of synovitis in the metacarpophalangeal joints of patients with rheumatoid arthritis: a comparison with dynamic magnetic resonance imaging. Arthritis Rheum. 2001; 44: 2018-23.

26) Cheung PP, Dougados M, Gossec L. Reliability of ultrasonography to detect synovitis in rheumatoid arthritis: a systematic literature review of 35 studies (1,415 patients). Arthritis Care Res (Hoboken). 2010; 62: 323-34.

27) Scheel AK, Backhaus M. Ultrasonographic assessment of finger and toe joint inflammation in rheumatoid arthritis: comment on the article by Szkudlarek et al. Arthritis Rheum. 2004; 50: 1008; author reply -9.

28) Szkudlarek M, Court-Payen M, Jacobsen S, Klarlund M, Thomsen HS, Ostergaard M. Interobserver agreement in ultrasonography of the finger and toe joints in rheumatoid arthritis. Arthritis Rheum. 2003; 48: 955-62.

29) Filippucci E, Gabba A, Di Geso L, Girolimetti R, Salaffi F, Grassi W. Hand tendon involvement in rheumatoid arthritis: an ultrasound study. Semin Arthritis Rheum. 2012; 41: 752-60.

30) Hoving JL, Buchbinder R, Hall S, Lawler G, Coombs P, McNealy S, et al. A comparison of magnetic resonance imaging, sonography, and radiography of the hand in patients with early rheumatoid arthritis. J Rheumatol. 2004; 31: 663-75.

31) Naredo E, D'Agostino MA, Wakefield RJ, Moller I, Balint PV, Filippucci E, et al. Reliability of a consensus-based ultrasound score for tenosyno-

vitis in rheumatoid arthritis. Ann Rheum Dis. 2013; 72: 1328-34.

32) Grassi W, Filippucci E, Farina A, Cervini C. Sonographic imaging of tendons. Arthritis Rheum. 2000; 43: 969-76.

33) Bodor M, Fullerton B. Ultrasonography of the hand, wrist, and elbow. Phys Med Rehabil Clin N Am. 2010; 21: 509-31.

34) Bruyn GA, Hanova P, Iagnocco A, d'Agostino MA, Moller I, Terslev L, et al. Ultrasound definition of tendon damage in patients with rheumatoid arthritis. Results of a OMERACT consensus-based ultrasound score focussing on the diagnostic reliability. Ann Rheum Dis. 2014 Nov; 73(11): 1929-34.

35) Wakefield RJ, Gibbon WW, Conaghan PG, O'Connor P, McGonagle D, Pease C, et al. The value of sonography in the detection of bone erosions in patients with rheumatoid arthritis: a comparison with conventional radiography. Arthritis Rheum. 2000; 43: 2762-70.

36) Scheel AK, Hermann KG, Ohrndorf S, Werner C, Schirmer C, Detert J, et al. Prospective 7 year follow up imaging study comparing radiography, ultrasonography, and magnetic resonance imaging in rheumatoid arthritis finger joints. Ann Rheum Dis. 2006; 65: 595-600.

37) Rowbotham EL, Grainger AJ. Rheumatoid arthritis: ultrasound versus MRI. AJR Am J Roentgenol. 2011; 197: 541-6.

38) Dohn UM, Terslev L, Szkudlarek M, Hansen MS, Hetland ML, Hansen A, et al. Detection, scoring and volume assessment of bone erosions by ultrasonography in rheumatoid arthritis: comparison with CT. Ann Rheum Dis. 2013; 72: 530-4.

39) Dohn UM, Ejbjerg BJ, Court-Payen M, Hasselquist M, Narvestad E, Szkudlarek M, et al. Are bone erosions detected by magnetic resonance imaging and ultrasonography true erosions? A comparison with computed tomography in rheumatoid arthritis metacarpophalangeal joints. Arthritis Res Ther. 2006; 8: R110.

40) Reynolds PP, Heron C, Pilcher J, Kiely PD. Prediction of erosion progression using ultrasound in established rheumatoid arthritis: a 2-year follow-up study. Skeletal Radiol. 2009; 38: 473-8.

41) Baillet A, Gaujoux-Viala C, Mouterde G, Pham T, Tebib J, Saraux A, et al. Comparison of the efficacy of sonography, magnetic resonance imaging and conventional radiography for the detection of bone erosions in rheumatoid arthritis patients: a systematic review and meta-analysis. Rheumatology (Oxford). 2011; 50: 1137-47.

42) Malattia C, Damasio MB, Magnaguagno F, Pistorio A, Valle M, Martinoli C, et al. Magnetic resonance imaging, ultrasonography, and conventional radiography in the assessment of bone erosions in juvenile idiopathic arthritis. Arthritis Rheum. 2008; 59: 1764-72.

43) Gutierrez M, Filippucci E, Ruta S, Salaffi F, Blasetti P, Di Geso L, et al. Inter-observer reliability of high-resolution ultrasonography in the assessment of bone erosions in patients with rheumatoid arthritis: experience of an intensive dedicated training programme. Rheumatology (Oxford). 2011; 50: 373-80.

44) Sommier JP, Michel-Batot C, Sauliere N, Rat AC, Hoenen-Clavert V, Pourel J, et al. Structural lesions in RA: Proposition for a new semiquantitative score (ScuSSEe: Scoring by ultrasound structural erosion). Arthritis Rheum. 2006; 54 Suppl: S140.

45) Moller B, Bonel H, Rotzetter M, Villiger PM, Ziswiler HR. Measuring finger joint cartilage by ultrasound as a promising alternative to conventional radiograph imaging. Arthritis Rheum. 2009; 61: 435-41.

46) Nalbant S, Corominas H, Hsu B, Chen LX, Schumacher HR, Kitumnuaypong T. Ultrasonography for assessment of subcutaneous nodules. J Rheumatol. 2003; 30: 1191-5.

47) Langsfeld M, Matteson B, Johnson W, Wascher D, Goodnough J, Weinstein E. Baker's cysts mimicking the symptoms of deep vein thrombosis: diagnosis with venous duplex scanning. J Vasc Surg. 1997; 25: 658-62.

48) Ward EE, Jacobson JA, Fessell DP, Hayes CW, van Holsbeeck M. Sonographic detection of Baker's cysts: comparison with MR imaging. AJR Am J Roentgenol. 2001; 176: 373-80.

49) Filippucci E, Farina A, Carotti M, Salaffi F, Grassi W. Grey scale and power Doppler sonographic changes induced by intra-articular steroid injection treatment. Ann Rheum Dis. 2004; 63: 740-3.

50) Hau M, Kneitz C, Tony HP, Keberle M, Jahns R, Jenett M. High resolution ultrasound detects a decrease in pannus vascularisation of small finger joints in patients with rheumatoid arthritis receiving treatment with soluble tumour necrosis factor alpha receptor (etanercept). Ann Rheum Dis. 2002; 61: 55-8.

51) Ribbens C, Andre B, Marcelis S, Kaye O, Mathy L, Bonnet V, et al. Rheumatoid hand joint synovitis: gray-scale and power Doppler US quantifications following anti-tumor necrosis factor-alpha treatment: pilot study. Radiology. 2003; 229: 562-9.

52) Terslev L, Torp-Pedersen S, Qvistgaard E, Danneskiold-Samsoe B, Bliddal H. Estimation of inflammation by Doppler ultrasound: quantitative changes after intra-articular treatment in rheumatoid arthritis. Ann Rheum Dis. 2003; 62: 1049-53.

53) Wakefield RJ, D'Agostino MA, Naredo E, Buch

MH, Iagnocco A, Terslev L, et al. After treat-to-target: can a targeted ultrasound initiative improve RA outcomes? Ann Rheum Dis. 2012; 71: 799-803.

54) Khan MA. Update on spondyloarthropathies. Ann Intern Med. 2002; 136: 896-907.

55) Rudwaleit M, van der Heijde D, Landewe R, Akkoc N, Brandt J, Chou CT, et al. The Assessment of SpondyloArthritis International Society classification criteria for peripheral spondyloarthritis and for spondyloarthritis in general. Ann Rheum Dis. 2011; 70: 25-31.

56) Heldmann F, Dybowski F, Saracbasi-Zender E, Fendler C, Braun J. Update on biologic therapy in the management of axial spondyloarthritis. Curr Rheumatol Rep. 2010; 12: 325-31.

57) Rudwaleit M, Khan MA, Sieper J. The challenge of diagnosis and classification in early ankylosing spondylitis: do we need new criteria? Arthritis Rheum. 2005; 52: 1000-8.

58) Rostom S, Dougados M, Gossec L. New tools for diagnosing spondyloarthropathy. Joint Bone Spine. 2010; 77: 108-14.

59) Ozgocmen S, Khan MA. Current concept of spondyloarthritis: special emphasis on early referral and diagnosis. Curr Rheumatol Rep. 2012; 14: 409-14.

60) Riente L, Delle Sedie A, Filippucci E, Iagnocco A, Meenagh G, Grassi W, et al. Ultrasound imaging for the rheumatologist IX. Ultrasound imaging in spondyloarthritis. Clin Exp Rheumatol. 2007; 25: 349-53.

61) D'Agostino MA. Ultrasound imaging in spondyloarthropathies. Best Pract Res Clin Rheumatol. 2010; 24: 693-700.

62) D'Agostino MA, Palazzi C, Olivieri I. Entheseal involvement. Clin Exp Rheumatol. 2009; 27(4 Suppl 55): S50-5.

63) D'Agostino MA, Said-Nahal R, Hacquard-Bouder C, Brasseur JL, Dougados M, Breban M. Assessment of peripheral enthesitis in the spondylarthropathies by ultrasonography combined with power Doppler: a cross-sectional study. Arthritis Rheum. 2003; 48: 523-33.

64) Gerster JC, Vischer TL, Bennani A, Fallet GH. The painful heel. Comparative study in rheumatoid arthritis, ankylosing spondylitis, Reiter's syndrome, and generalized osteoarthrosis. Ann Rheum Dis. 1977; 36: 343-8.

65) Lehtinen A, Taavitsainen M, Leirisalo-Repo M. Sonographic analysis of enthesopathy in the lower extremities of patients with spondylarthropathy. Clin Exp Rheumatol. 1994; 12: 143-8.

66) de Miguel E, Munoz-Fernandez S, Castillo C, Cobo-Ibanez T, Martin-Mola E. Diagnostic accuracy of enthesis ultrasound in the diagnosis of early spondyloarthritis. Ann Rheum Dis. 2011; 70: 434-9.

67) MA DA, Palazzi C, Olivieri I. Entheseal involvement. Clin Exp Rheumatol. 2009; 27(4 Suppl 55): S50-5.

68) Balint PV, Kane D, Wilson H, McInnes IB, Sturrock RD. Ultrasonography of entheseal insertions in the lower limb in spondyloarthropathy. Ann Rheum Dis. 2002; 61: 905-10.

69) Borman P, Koparal S, Babaoglu S, Bodur H. Ultrasound detection of entheseal insertions in the foot of patients with spondyloarthropathy. Clin Rheumatol. 2006; 25: 373-7.

70) Gandjbakhch F, Terslev L, Joshua F, Wakefield RJ, Naredo E, D'Agostino MA. Ultrasound in the evaluation of enthesitis: status and perspectives. Arthritis Res Ther. 2011; 13(6): R188.

71) Kaeley GS. Review of the use of ultrasound for the diagnosis and monitoring of enthesitis in psoriatic arthritis. Curr Rheumatol Rep. 2011; 13: A - 338-45.

72) Terslev L, Naredo E, Iagnocco A, Balint PV, Wakefield RJ, Aegerter P, et al. Defining enthesitis in spondyloarthritis by ultrasound: results of a Delphi process and of a reliability reading exercise. Arthritis Care Res (Hoboken). 2014; 66: 741-8.

73) de Miguel E, Cobo T, Munoz-Fernandez S, Naredo E, Uson J, Acebes JC, et al. Validity of enthesis ultrasound assessment in spondyloarthropathy. Ann Rheum Dis. 2009; 68: 169-74.

74) Alcalde M, Acebes JC, Cruz M, Gonzalez-Hombrado L, Herrero-Beaumont G, Sanchez-Pernaute O. A sonographic enthesitic index of lower limbs is a valuable tool in the assessment of ankylosing spondylitis. Ann Rheum Dis. 2007; 66: 1015-9.

75) Genc H, Cakit BD, Tuncbilek I, Erdem HR. Ultrasonographic evaluation of tendons and enthesal sites in rheumatoid arthritis: comparison with ankylosing spondylitis and healthy subjects. Clin Rheumatol. 2005; 24: 272-7.

76) Falsetti P, Frediani B, Fioravanti A, Acciai C, Baldi F, Filippou G, et al. Sonographic study of calcaneal entheses in erosive osteoarthritis, nodal osteoarthritis, rheumatoid arthritis and psoriatic arthritis. Scand J Rheumatol. 2003; 32: 229-34.

77) Kiris A, Kaya A, Ozgocmen S, Kocakoc E. Assessment of enthesitis in ankylosing spondylitis by power Doppler ultrasonography. Skeletal Radiol. 2006; 35: 522-8.

78) Hamdi W, Bouaziz Chelli M, Ghannouchi MM, Hawel M, Ladeb MF, Kchir MM. Performance of ultrasounds compared with radiographs to detect chronic enthesitis signs in patients with ankylosing spondylitis. Rheumatol Int. 2013; 33: 497-9.

79) Ozgocmen S, Kiris A, Ardicoglu O, Kocakoc E, Kaya A. Glucocorticoid iontophoresis for Achilles tendon enthesitis in ankylosing spondylitis: significant response documented by power Doppler ultrasound. Rheumatol Int. 2005; 25: 158-60.

80) Aydin SZ, Karadag O, Filippucci E, Atagunduz P, Akdogan A, Kalyoncu U, et al. Monitoring Achilles enthesitis in ankylosing spondylitis during TNF-alpha antagonist therapy: an ultrasound study. Rheumatology (Oxford). 2010; 49: 578-82.

81) Healy PJ, Groves C, Chandramohan M, Helliwell PS. MRI changes in psoriatic dactylitis--extent of pathology, relationship to tenderness and correlation with clinical indices. Rheumatology (Oxford). 2008; 47: 92-5.

82) Kelly S, Taylor P, Pitzalis C. Ultrasound imaging in spondyloarthropathies: from imaging to diagnostic intervention. Curr Opin Rheumatol. 2008; 20: 408-15.

83) Iagnocco A, Riente L, Delle Sedie A, Filippucci E, Salaffi F, Meenagh G, et al. Ultrasound imaging for the rheumatologist. XXII. Achilles tendon involvement in spondyloarthritis. A multi-centre study using high frequency volumetric probe. Clin Exp Rheumatol. 2009; 27: 547-51.

84) Naredo E, Moller I, Acebes C, Batlle-Gualda E, Brito E, de Agustin JJ, et al. Three-dimensional volumetric ultrasonography. Does it improve reliabililty of musculoskeletal ultrasound? Clin Exp Rheumatol. 2010; 28: 79-82.

85) Delle Sedie A, Riente L, Filippucci E, Scire CA, Iagnocco A, Meenagh G, et al. Ultrasound imaging for the rheumatologist. XXXII. Sonographic assessment of the foot in patients with psoriatic arthritis. Clin Exp Rheumatol. 2011; 29: 217-22.

86) Riente L, Delle Sedie A, Sakellariou G, Filippucci E, Meenagh G, Iagnocco A, et al. Ultrasound imaging for the rheumatologist XXXVIII. Sonographic assessment of the hip in psoriatic arthritis patients. Clin Exp Rheumatol. 2012; 30: 152-5.

87) Sakellariou G, Iagnocco A, Meenagh G, Riente L, Filippucci E, Delle Sedie A, et al. Ultrasound imaging for the rheumatologist XXXVII. Sonographic assessment of the hip in ankylosing spondylitis patients. Clin Exp Rheumatol. 2012; 30: 1-5.

88) Delle Sedie A, Riente L, Filippucci E, Scire CA, Iagnocco A, Gutierrez M, et al. Ultrasound imaging for the rheumatologist XXVI. Sonographic assessment of the knee in patients with psoriatic arthritis. Clin Exp Rheumatol. 2010; 28: 147-52.

89) De Simone C, Caldarola G, D'Agostino M, Carbone A, Guerriero C, Bonomo L, et al. Usefulness of ultrasound imaging in detecting psoriatic arthritis of fingers and toes in patients with psoriasis. Clin Dev Immunol. 2011; 2011: 390726.

90) Wiell C, Szkudlarek M, Hasselquist M, Moller JM, Vestergaard A, Norregaard J, et al. Ultrasonography, magnetic resonance imaging, radiography, and clinical assessment of inflammatory and destructive changes in fingers and toes of patients with psoriatic arthritis. Arthritis Res Ther. 2007; 9: R119.

91) Weiner SM, Jurenz S, Uhl M, Lange-Nolde A, Warnatz K, Peter HH, et al. Ultrasonography in the assessment of peripheral joint involvement in psoriatic arthritis : a comparison with radiography, MRI and scintigraphy. Clin Rheumatol. 2008; 27: 983-9.

92) Gutierrez M, Filippucci E, Salaffi F, Di Geso L, Grassi W. Differential diagnosis between rheumatoid arthritis and psoriatic arthritis: the value of ultrasound findings at metacarpophalangeal joints level. Ann Rheum Dis. 2011; 70: 1111-4.

93) Arslan H, Sakarya ME, Adak B, Unal O, Sayarlioglu M. Duplex and color Doppler sonographic findings in active sacroiliitis. AJR Am J Roentgenol. 1999; 173: 677-80.

94) Unlu E, Pamuk ON, Cakir N. Color and duplex Doppler sonography to detect sacroiliitis and spinal inflammation in ankylosing spondylitis. Can this method reveal response to anti-tumor necrosis factor therapy? J Rheumatol. 2007; 34: 110-6.

95) Mohammadi A, Ghasemi-Rad M, Aghdashi M, Mladkova N, Baradaransafa P. Evaluation of disease activity in ankylosing spondylitis; diagnostic value of color Doppler ultrasonography. Skeletal Radiol. 2013; 42: 219-24.

96) Klauser AS, Wipfler E, Dejaco C, Moriggl B, Duftner C, Schirmer M. Diagnostic values of history and clinical examination to predict ultrasound signs of chronic and acute enthesitis. Clin Exp Rheumatol. 2008; 26: 548-53.

97) Klauser AS, De Zordo T, Bellmann-Weiler R, Feuchtner GM, Sailer-Hock M, Sogner P, et al. Feasibility of second-generation ultrasound contrast media in the detection of active sacroiliitis. Arthritis Rheum. 2009; 61: 909-16.

98) Hu Y, Zhu J, Xue Q, Wang N, Hu B. Scanning of the sacroiliac joint and entheses by color Doppler ultrasonography in patients with ankylosing spondylitis. J Rheumatol. 2011; 38: 1651-5.

99) Hartung W, Ross CJ, Straub R, Feuerbach S, Scholmerich J, Fleck M, et al. Ultrasound-guided sacroiliac joint injection in patients with established sacroiliitis: precise IA injection verified by MRI scanning does not predict clinical outcome. Rheumatology (Oxford). 2010; 49: 1479-82.

100) Iagnocco A, Meenagh G, Riente L, Filippucci E, Delle Sedie A, Scire CA, et al. Ultrasound imaging for the rheumatologist XXIX. Sonographic assessment of the knee in patients with osteoarthritis. Clin Exp Rheumatol. 2010; 28: 643-6.

101) Moller I, Bong D, Naredo E, Filippucci E, Carrasco I, Moragues C, et al. Ultrasound in the study and monitoring of osteoarthritis. Osteoarthritis Cartilage. 2008; 16 Suppl 3: S4-7.

102) D'Agostino MA, Conaghan P, Le Bars M, Baron G, Grassi W, Martin-Mola E, et al. EULAR report on

the use of ultrasonography in painful knee osteoarthritis. Part 1: prevalence of inflammation in osteoarthritis. Ann Rheum Dis. 2005; 64: 1703-9.

103) Wu PT, Shao CJ, Wu KC, Wu TT, Chern TC, Kuo LC, et al. Pain in patients with equal radiographic grades of osteoarthritis in both knees: the value of gray scale ultrasound. Osteoarthritis Cartilage. 2012; 20: 1507-13.

104) Naredo E, Wakefield RJ, Iagnocco A, Terslev L, Filippucci E, Gandjbakhch F, et al. The OMERACT ultrasound task force--status and perspectives. J Rheumatol. 2011; 38: 2063-7.

105) Iagnocco A, Epis O, Delle Sedie A, Meenagh G, Filippucci E, Riente L, et al. Ultrasound imaging for the rheumatologist. XVII. Role of colour Doppler and power Doppler. Clin Exp Rheumatol. 2008; 26: 759-62.

106) Karim Z, Wakefield RJ, Quinn M, Conaghan PG, Brown AK, Veale DJ, et al. Validation and reproducibility of ultrasonography in the detection of synovitis in the knee: a comparison with arthroscopy and clinical examination. Arthritis Rheum. 2004; 50: 387-94.

107) Guermazi A, Roemer FW, Hayashi D. Imaging of osteoarthritis: update from a radiological perspective. Curr Opin Rheumatol. 2011; 23: 484-91.

108) Kortekaas MC, Kwok WY, Reijnierse M, Kloppenburg M. Inflammatory ultrasound features show independent associations with progression of structural damage after over 2 years of follow-up in patients with hand osteoarthritis. Ann Rheum Dis. 2014 Apr 29. [Epub ahead of print].

109) Acebes JC, Sanchez-Pernaute O, Diaz-Oca A, Herrero-Beaumont G. Ultrasonographic assessment of Baker's cysts after intra-articular corticosteroid injection in knee osteoarthritis. J Clin Ultrasound. 2006; 34: 113-7.

110) Keen HI, Lavie F, Wakefield RJ, D'Agostino MA, Hammer HB, Hensor E, et al. The development of a preliminary ultrasonographic scoring system for features of hand osteoarthritis. Ann Rheum Dis. 2008; 67: 651-5.

111) Myers SL, Dines K, Brandt DA, Brandt KD, Albrecht ME. Experimental assessment by high frequency ultrasound of articular cartilage thickness and osteoarthritic changes. J Rheumatol. 1995; 22: 109-16.

112) Tarhan S, Unlu Z. Magnetic resonance imaging and ultrasonographic evaluation of the patients with knee osteoarthritis: a comparative study. Clin Rheumatol. 2003; 22: 181-8.

113) Grassi W, Filippucci E, Farina A. Ultrasonography in osteoarthritis. Semin Arthritis Rheum. 2005; 34(6 Suppl 2): 19-23.

114) Meenagh G, Filippucci E, Iagnocco A, Delle Sedie A, Riente L, Bombardieri S, et al. Ultrasound im

aging for the rheumatologist VIII. Ultrasound imaging in osteoarthritis. Clin Exp Rheumatol. 2007; 25: 172-5.

115) Spriet MP, Girard CA, Foster SF, Harasiewicz K, Holdsworth DW, Laverty S. Validation of a 40 MHz B-scan ultrasound biomicroscope for the evaluation of osteoarthritis lesions in an animal model. Osteoarthritis Cartilage. 2005; 13: 171-9.

116) Lee CL, Huang MH, Chai CY, Chen CH, Su JY, Tien YC. The validity of in vivo ultrasonographic grading of osteoarthritic femoral condylar cartilage: a comparison with in vitro ultrasonographic and histologic gradings. Osteoarthritis Cartilage. 2008; 16: 352-8.

117) Malas FU, Kara M, Kaymak B, Akinci A, Ozcakar L. Ultrasonographic evaluation in symptomatic knee osteoarthritis: clinical and radiological correlation. Int J Rheum Dis. 2014; 17: 536-40.

118) Carli AB, Akarsu S, Tekin L, Saglam M, Kiralp MZ, Ozcakar L. Ultrasonographic assessment of the femoral cartilage in osteoarthritis patients with and without osteoporosis. Aging Clin Exp Res. 2014; 26: 411-5.

119) Keen HI, Wakefield RJ, Grainger AJ, Hensor EM, Emery P, Conaghan PG. Can ultrasonography improve on radiographic assessment in osteoarthritis of the hands? A comparison between radiographic and ultrasonographic detected pathology. Ann Rheum Dis. 2008; 67: 1116-20.

120) Mathiessen A, Haugen IK, Slatkowsky-Christensen B, Boyesen P, Kvien TK, Hammer HB. Ultrasonographic assessment of osteophytes in 127 patients with hand osteoarthritis: exploring reliability and associations with MRI, radiographs and clinical joint findings. Ann Rheum Dis. 2013; 72: 51-6.

121) Grainger AJ, Farrant JM, O'Connor PJ, Tan AL, Tanner S, Emery P, et al. MR imaging of erosions in interphalangeal joint osteoarthritis: is all osteoarthritis erosive? Skeletal Radiol. 2007; 36: 737-45.

122) Wittoek R, Jans L, Lambrecht V, Carron P, Verstraete K, Verbruggen G. Reliability and construct validity of ultrasonography of soft tissue and destructive changes in erosive osteoarthritis of the interphalangeal finger joints: a comparison with MRI. Ann Rheum Dis. 2011; 70: 278-83.

123) Iagnocco A, Perella C, D'Agostino MA, Sabatini E, Valesini G, Conaghan PG. Magnetic resonance and ultrasonography real-time fusion imaging of the hand and wrist in osteoarthritis and rheumatoid arthritis. Rheumatology (Oxford). 2011; 50: 1409-13.

124) Iagnocco A, Filippucci E, Ossandon A, Ciapetti A, Salaffi F, Basili S, et al. High resolution ultrasonography in detection of bone erosions in pa

tients with hand osteoarthritis. J Rheumatol. 2005; 32: 2381-3.

125) Ceccarelli F, Perricone C, Alessandri C, Modesti M, Iagnocco A, Croia C, et al. Exploratory data analysis on the effects of non pharmacological treatment for knee osteoarthritis. Clin Exp Rheumatol. 2010; 28: 250-3.

126) Salini V, De Amicis D, Abate M, Natale MA, Di Iorio A. Ultrasound-guided hyaluronic acid injection in carpometacarpal osteoarthritis: short-term results. Int J Immunopathol Pharmacol. 2009; 22: 455-60.

127) Filippucci E, Iagnocco A, Meenagh G, Riente L, Delle Sedie A, Bombardieri S, et al. Ultrasound imaging for the rheumatologist. Clin Exp Rheumatol. 2006; 24: 1-5.

128) Howard RG, Pillinger MH, Gyftopoulos S, Thiele RG, Swearingen CJ, Samuels J. Reproducibility of musculoskeletal ultrasound for determining monosodium urate deposition: concordance between readers. Arthritis Care Res (Hoboken). 2011; 63: 1456-62.

129) Thiele RG, Schlesinger N. Diagnosis of gout by ultrasound. Rheumatology (Oxford). 2007; 46: 1116-21.

130) Wright SA, Filippucci E, McVeigh C, Grey A, McCarron M, Grassi W, et al. High-resolution ultrasonography of the first metatarsal phalangeal joint in gout: a controlled study. Ann Rheum Dis. 2007; 66: 859-64.

131) Ogdie A, Taylor WJ, Weatherall M, Fransen J, Jansen TL, Neogi T, et al. Imaging modalities for the classification of gout: systematic literature review and meta-analysis. Ann Rheum Dis. 2014 Jun 10. [Epub ahead of print].

132) Thiele RG, Schlesinger N. Ultrasonography shows disappearance of monosodium urate crystal deposition on hyaline cartilage after sustained normouricemia is achieved. Rheumatol Int. 2010; 30: 495-503.

133) Filippucci E, Ciapetti A, Grassi W. [Sonographic monitoring of gout]. Reumatismo. 2003; 55: 184-6.

134) Schueller-Weidekamm C, Schueller G, Aringer M, Weber M, Kainberger F. Impact of sonography in gouty arthritis: comparison with conventional radiography, clinical examination, and laboratory findings. Eur J Radiol. 2007; 62: 437-43.

135) Pineda C, Amezcua-Guerra LM, Solano C, Rodriguez-Henriquez P, Hernandez-Diaz C, Vargas A, et al. Joint and tendon subclinical involvement suggestive of gouty arthritis in asymptomatic hyperuricemia: an ultrasound controlled study. Arthritis Res Ther. 2011; 13(1): R4.

136) Dalbeth N, Pool B, Gamble GD, Smith T, Callon KE, McQueen FM, et al. Cellular characterization of the gouty tophus: a quantitative analysis. Arthritis Rheum. 2010; 62: 1549-56.

137) de Avila Fernandes E, Kubota ES, Sandim GB, Mitraud SA, Ferrari AJ, Fernandes AR. Ultrasound features of tophi in chronic tophaceous gout. Skeletal Radiol. 2011; 40: 309-15.

138) Perez-Ruiz F, Martin I, Canteli B. Ultrasonographic measurement of tophi as an outcome measure for chronic gout. J Rheumatol. 2007; 34: 1888-93.

139) Ottaviani S, Richette P, Allard A, Ora J, Bardin T. Ultrasonography in gout: a case-control study. Clin Exp Rheumatol. 2012; 30: 499-504.

140) Gerster JC, Landry M, Dufresne L, Meuwly JY. Imaging of tophaceous gout: computed tomography provides specific images compared with magnetic resonance imaging and ultrasonography. Ann Rheum Dis. 2002; 61: 52-4.

141) Dalbeth N, Clark B, Gregory K, Gamble G, Sheehan T, Doyle A, et al. Mechanisms of bone erosion in gout: a quantitative analysis using plain radiography and computed tomography. Ann Rheum Dis. 2009; 68: 1290-5.

142) Thiele RG. Role of ultrasound and other advanced imaging in the diagnosis and management of gout. Curr Rheumatol Rep. 2011; 13: 146-53.

143) Carter JD, Kedar RP, Anderson SR, Osorio AH, Albritton NL, Gnanashanmugam S, et al. An analysis of MRI and ultrasound imaging in patients with gout who have normal plain radiographs. Rheumatology (Oxford). 2009; 48: 1442-6.

144) Grassi W, Meenagh G, Pascual E, Filippucci E. "Crystal clear"-sonographic assessment of gout and calcium pyrophosphate deposition disease. Semin Arthritis Rheum. 2006; 36: 197-202.

145) Filippucci E, Scire CA, Delle Sedie A, Iagnocco A, Riente L, Meenagh G, et al. Ultrasound imaging for the rheumatologist. XXV. Sonographic assessment of the knee in patients with gout and calcium pyrophosphate deposition disease. Clin Exp Rheumatol. 2010; 28: 2-5.

146) Magarelli N, Amelia R, Melillo N, Nasuto M, Cantatore F, Guglielmi G. Imaging of chondrocalcinosis: calcium pyrophosphate dihydrate (CPPD) crystal deposition disease -- imaging of common sites of involvement. Clin Exp Rheumatol. 2012; 30: 118-25.

147) Ellabban AS, Kamel SR, Omar HA, El-Sherif AM, Abdel-Magied RA. Ultrasonographic diagnosis of articular chondrocalcinosis. Rheumatol Int. 2012; 32: 3863-8.

148) Frediani B, Filippou G, Falsetti P, Lorenzini S, Baldi F, Acciai C, et al. Diagnosis of calcium pyrophosphate dihydrate crystal deposition disease: ultrasonographic criteria proposed. Ann Rheum Dis. 2005; 64: 638-40.

149) Guermazi A, Burstein D, Conaghan P, Eckstein F, Hellio Le Graverand-Gastineau MP, Keen H, et al.

Imaging in osteoarthritis. Rheum Dis Clin North Am. 2008; 34: 645-87.

150) Filippucci E, Riveros MG, Georgescu D, Salaffi F, Grassi W. Hyaline cartilage involvement in patients with gout and calcium pyrophosphate deposition disease. An ultrasound study. Osteoarthritis Cartilage. 2009; 17: 178-81.

151) Sofka CM, Adler RS, Cordasco FA. Ultrasound diagnosis of chondrocalcinosis in the knee. Skeletal Radiol. 2002; 31: 43-5.

152) Falsetti P, Frediani B, Acciai C, Baldi F, Filippou G, Prada EP, et al. Ultrasonographic study of Achilles tendon and plantar fascia in chondrocalcinosis. J Rheumatol. 2004; 31: 2242-50.

153) Ellabban AS, Kamel SR, Abo Omar HA, El-Sherif AM, Abdel-Magied RA. Ultrasonographic findings of Achilles tendon and plantar fascia in patients with calcium pyrophosphate deposition disease. Clin Rheumatol. 2012; 31: 697-704.

154) Hinchcliff M, Varga J. Systemic sclerosis/scleroderma: a treatable multisystem disease. Am Fam Physician. 2008; 78: 961-8.

155) Avouac J, Guerini H, Wipff J, Assous N, Chevrot A, Kahan A, et al. Radiological hand involvement in systemic sclerosis. Ann Rheum Dis. 2006; 65: 1088-92.

156) Boutry N, Hachulla E, Zanetti-Musielak C, Morel M, Demondion X, Cotten A. Imaging features of musculoskeletal involvement in systemic sclerosis. Eur Radiol. 2007; 17: 1172-80.

157) Riente L, Delle Sedie A, Filippucci E, Iagnocco A, Meenagh G, Epis O, et al. Ultrasound imaging for the rheumatologist XIV. Ultrasound imaging in connective tissue diseases. Clin Exp Rheumatol. 2008; 26: 230-3.

158) Rodnan GP, Lipinski E, Luksick J. Skin thickness and collagen content in progressive systemic sclerosis and localized scleroderma. Arthritis Rheum. 1979; 22: 130-40.

159) Bendeck SE, Jacobe HT. Ultrasound as an outcome measure to assess disease activity in disorders of skin thickening: an example of the use of radiologic techniques to assess skin disease. Dermatol Ther. 2007; 20: 86-92.

160) Kaloudi O, Bandinelli F, Filippucci E, Conforti ML, Miniati I, Guiducci S, et al. High frequency ultrasound measurement of digital dermal thickness in systemic sclerosis. Ann Rheum Dis. 2010; 69: 1140-3.

161) Akesson A, Hesselstrand R, Scheja A, Wildt M. Longitudinal development of skin involvement and reliability of high frequency ultrasound in systemic sclerosis. Ann Rheum Dis. 2004; 63: 791-6.

162) Hesselstrand R, Scheja A, Wildt M, Akesson A. High-frequency ultrasound of skin involvement in systemic sclerosis reflects oedema, extension and severity in early disease. Rheumatology (Oxford). 2008; 47: 84-7.

163) Moore TL, Lunt M, McManus B, Anderson ME, Herrick AL. Seventeen-point dermal ultrasound scoring system--a reliable measure of skin thickness in patients with systemic sclerosis. Rheumatology (Oxford). 2003; 42: 1559-63.

164) Li SC, Liebling MS. The use of Doppler ultrasound to evaluate lesions of localized scleroderma. Curr Rheumatol Rep. 2009; 11: 205-11.

165) Li SC, Liebling MS, Haines KA, Weiss JE, Prann A. Initial evaluation of an ultrasound measure for assessing the activity of skin lesions in juvenile localized scleroderma. Arthritis Care Res (Hoboken). 2011; 63: 735-42.

166) Keberle M, Tony HP, Jahns R, Hau M, Haerten R, Jenett M. Assessment of microvascular changes in Raynaud's phenomenon and connective tissue disease using colour doppler ultrasound. Rheumatology (Oxford). 2000; 39: 1206-13.

167) Avouac J, Clements PJ, Khanna D, Furst DE, Allanore Y. Articular involvement in systemic sclerosis. Rheumatology (Oxford). 2012; 51: 1347-56.

168) Avouac J, Fransen J, Walker UA, Riccieri V, Smith V, Muller C, et al. Preliminary criteria for the very early diagnosis of systemic sclerosis: results of a Delphi Consensus Study from EULAR Scleroderma Trials and Research Group. Ann Rheum Dis. 2011; 70: 476-81.

169) Cuomo G, Zappia M, Abignano G, Iudici M, Rotondo A, Valentini G. Ultrasonographic features of the hand and wrist in systemic sclerosis. Rheumatology (Oxford). 2009; 48: 1414-7.

170) Iagnocco A, Vavala C, Vasile M, Stefanantoni K, Valesini G, Riccieri V. Power Doppler ultrasound of the hand and wrist joints in systemic sclerosis. Clin Exp Rheumatol. 2013; 31(2 Suppl 76): 89-95.

171) Kilic G, Kilic E, Akgul O, Ozgocmen S. Decreased femoral cartilage thickness in patients with systemic sclerosis. Am J Med Sci. 2014; 347: 382-6.

172) Chitale S, Ciapetti A, Hodgson R, Grainger A, O'Connor P, Goodson NJ, et al. Magnetic resonance imaging and musculoskeletal ultrasonography detect and characterize covert inflammatory arthropathy in systemic sclerosis patients with arthralgia. Rheumatology (Oxford). 2010; 49: 2357-61.

173) Kilic E, Kilic G, Akgul O, Ozgocmen S. High prevalence of enthesitis in patients with systemic sclerosis demonstrated by Doppler ultrasonography. Ann Rheum Dis. 2014; 73(Suppl 2): 465.

174) Shahin AA. Pulmonary involvement in systemic sclerosis. Treatments in respiratory medicine. 2006; 5: 429-36.

175) Mohammadi A, Oshnoei S, Ghasemi-rad M. Com-

parison of a new, modified lung ultrasonography technique with high-resolution CT in the diagnosis of the alveolo-interstitial syndrome of systemic scleroderma. Med Ultrason. 2014; 16: 27-31.

176) Vitali C, Bombardieri S, Jonsson R, Moutsopoulos HM, Alexander EL, Carsons SE, et al. Classification criteria for Sjogren's syndrome: a revised version of the European criteria proposed by the American-European Consensus Group. Ann Rheum Dis. 2002; 61: 554-8.

177) Makula E, Pokorny G, Kiss M, Voros E, Kovacs L, Kovacs A, et al. The place of magnetic resonance and ultrasonographic examinations of the parotid gland in the diagnosis and follow-up of primary Sjogren's syndrome. Rheumatology (Oxford). 2000; 39: 97-104.

178) Salaffi F, Carotti M, Iagnocco A, Luccioli F, Ramonda R, Sabatini E, et al. Ultrasonography of salivary glands in primary Sjogren's syndrome: a comparison with contrast sialography and scintigraphy. Rheumatology (Oxford). 2008; 47: 1244-9.

179) Takagi Y, Kimura Y, Nakamura H, Sasaki M, Eguchi K, Nakamura T. Salivary gland ultrasonography: can it be an alternative to sialography as an imaging modality for Sjogren's syndrome? Ann Rheum Dis. 2010; 69: 1321-4.

180) Salaffi F, Argalia G, Carotti M, Giannini FB, Palombi C. Salivary gland ultrasonography in the evaluation of primary Sjogren's syndrome. Comparison with minor salivary gland biopsy. J Rheumatol. 2000; 27: 1229-36.

181) Hocevar A, Ambrozic A, Rozman B, Kveder T, Tomsic M. Ultrasonographic changes of major salivary glands in primary Sjogren's syndrome. Diagnostic value of a novel scoring system. Rheumatology (Oxford). 2005; 44: 768-72.

182) Wernicke D, Hess H, Gromnica-Ihle E, Krause A, Schmidt WA. Ultrasonography of salivary glands -- a highly specific imaging procedure for diagnosis of Sjogren's syndrome. J Rheumatol. 2008; 35: 285-93.

183) Milic VD, Petrovic RR, Boricic IV, Marinkovic-Eric J, Radunovic GL, Jeremic PD, et al. Diagnostic value of salivary gland ultrasonographic scoring system in primary Sjogren's syndrome: a comparison with scintigraphy and biopsy. J Rheumatol. 2009; 36: 1495-500.

184) Takagi Y, Sumi M, Nakamura H, Iwamoto N, Horai Y, Kawakami A, et al. Ultrasonography as an additional item in the American College of Rheumatology classification of Sjogren's syndrome. Rheumatology (Oxford). 2014; 53(11): 1977-83.

185) Cornec D, Jousse-Joulin S, Marhadour T, Pers JO, Boisrame-Gastrin S, Renaudineau Y, et al. Salivary gland ultrasonography improves the diagnostic performance of the 2012 American College of Rheumatology classification criteria for Sjogren's syndrome. Rheumatology (Oxford). 2014; 53: 1604-7.

186) Iagnocco A, Modesti M, Priori R, Alessandri C, Perella C, Takanen S, et al. Subclinical synovitis in primary Sjogren's syndrome: an ultrasonographic study. Rheumatology (Oxford). 2010; 49: 1153-7.

187) Riente L, Scire CA, Delle Sedie A, Baldini C, Filippucci E, Meenagh G, et al. Ultrasound imaging for the rheumatologist. XXIII. Sonographic evaluation of hand joint involvement in primary Sjogren's syndrome. Clin Exp Rheumatol. 2009; 27: 747-50.

188) Aschwanden M, Daikeler T, Kesten F, Baldi T, Benz D, Tyndall A, et al. Temporal artery compression sign - a novel ultrasound finding for the diagnosis of giant cell arteritis. Ultraschall Med. 2013; 34: 47-50.

189) Schmidt WA, Gromnica-Ihle E. Incidence of temporal arteritis in patients with polymyalgia rheumatica: a prospective study using colour Doppler ultrasonography of the temporal arteries. Rheumatology (Oxford). 2002; 41: 46-52.

190) Ghinoi A, Pipitone N, Nicolini A, Boiardi L, Silingardi M, Germano G, et al. Large-vessel involvement in recent-onset giant cell arteritis: a case-control colour-Doppler sonography study. Rheumatology (Oxford). 2012; 51: 730-4.

# Ultrasound Imaging in Rehabilitation Settings

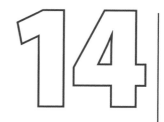

Nuray AKKAYA

Neuromuscular deficits can cause various musculoskeletal changes and disorders. Ultrasound (US), due to its advantages e.g. convenient, high spatial resolution, low cost, acceptance by patients and non-ionizing radiation, has significant clinical relevance on the decisions of clinicians who are interested in rehabilitation medicine. Although US has been used in various musculoskeletal disorders (degenerative/inflammatory joint problems or sport injuries), it is noteworthy that US imaging can also serve as an ideal imaging technique for prompt evaluation of rehabilitation patients [1]. Accordingly, the possible role of US in rehabilitation settings will be summarized in this chapter.

## 14.1 HEMIPLEGIC SHOULDER

Shoulder pain is the most common (5-84%) complication in hemiplegic patients and it delays recovery and lessens the effectiveness of the rehabilitation process [2, 3]. Different mechanisms and factors can contribute to shoulder pain in hemiplegic patients. Shoulder subluxation, soft tissue injuries, impingement syndrome, rotator cuff injuries, adhesive capsulitis, spasticity, and reflex sympathetic dystrophy are the important associated factors [2, 4-7]. Although many physical examination tests are useful in the evaluation of rotator cuff injuries, due to flaccidity and sensory impairment, the diagnosis may not be straightforward in stroke patients [8, 9]. Herein, owing to the aforementioned advantages, US appears to be a convenient imaging method for the evaluation of shoulder and rotator cuff lesions in hemiplegic patients [3, 10]. While the use of standard shoulder US scanning protocol allows for reliable assessment of the hemiplegic shoulder pain [11, 12], due to particular motion restrictions, imaging may become a little challenging. None-theless, the acromion, coracoid, clavicle, lesser and greater tubercles are again the useful bony landmarks for probe positioning [12].

### 14.1.1 Shoulder Subluxation

It is one of the most common causes of hemiplegic shoulder pain [6]. Deterioration of the muscle balance pertaining to the glenohumeral joint in stroke patients, especially in the flaccid period, can result in increased translation of the humeral head from the glenoid fossa due to the effect of gravity - with a palpable gap in between [13, 14]. Since shoulder subluxation significantly impedes the rehabilitation process, its prompt diagnosis and management is paramount [15-17]. Since clinical examination has disadvantages i.e. lack of precision, difficulties in detecting small changes; radiographic comparison (affected vs. unaffected sides) has been used to determine the displacement of the humeral head. However, aside from radiation exposure, radiography has some limitations in detecting hemiplegic shoulder subluxation; anteroposterior radiography are not suitable for detecting subluxations except in the inferior side and its use requires hemiplegic patients to maintain an upright body posture [17-20]. In addition, the tendency for medial displacement of the humeral head can be seen in serious inferior shoulder subluxation, indicating that anterior subluxation can be associated with severe inferior subluxation in hemiplegic patients [19]. Park et al. [21] reported that ultrasonographic subluxation ratios demonstrating both anterior and inferior subluxations correlated more with the clinical situation as compared to the radiographic ratios demonstrating only inferior subluxation. Overall, US seems to be superior in the evaluation of hemiplegic shoulder subluxation [21-23].

Several ultrasonographic measurement techniques with high reproducibility were defined to measure hemiplegic shoulder subluxation [21, 24]. In one method, authors suggested that patients are seated in a standardized position with their hips and knees flexed to 90°, their shoulders in neutral rotation and their elbows unsupported in 90° of flexion - to ensure that there is no elevation of the shoulder and that the forearm is rested on a pillow in the pronation position. Along the longitudinal axis of the humerus, the US transducer is placed over the lateral border of the acromion to image and measure the distance between the lateral border of the acromion and the nearest superior part of the greater tuberosity of the humerus on the frozen US image [21, 24] (Figure 14.1). In lateral longitudinal US imaging of the hemiplegic shoul-der, the distance between the lateral border of the acromion and the humerus can also be measured perpendicular to the medial border of humeral head, and this distance can be used to estimate the subluxation distance by comparison with the un-affected side [25] (Figure 14.2).

## 14.1.2 Soft Tissue Injuries

The decreased strength of the upper limb and muscle imbalance of the shoulder girdle in the hemiplegic shoulder may result in other soft tissue injuries as well. Especially in the flaccid phase of hemiplegia, stretching of the shoulder girdle during transfer activities or the pulling effect of gravity on paralytic upper extremities during rehabilitation tasks (e.g. standing, walking) can cause soft tissue injuries [2]. During US examination of hemiplegic shoulder subluxation, simultaneous imaging can also be performed for tendonitis, effusion, or bursitis which were reported as the other likely reasons for shoulder pain in stroke [4, 5, 11, 26] (Figure 14.3). Huang et al. [4] reported that hemiplegic patients with poor motor function had a higher frequency of soft tissue injuries and subluxation

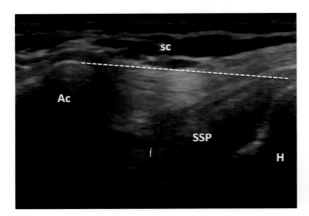

**Figure 14.1** Ultrasound image of the shoulder in a hemiplegic patient (lateral coronal view). The subacromial distance is measured between the lateral border of the acromion and the nearest superior part of the greater tuberosity of the humerus. Ac, acromion; H, humerus; sc, subcutaneous fat tissue; SSP, supraspinatus tendon.

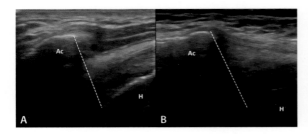

**Figure 14.2** Ultrasound image of the shoulder in a hemiplegic patient (lateral coronal view). The subacromial distance is measured from the lateral border of the acromion (Ac) to the medial border of the humeral head (H) for assessment of shoulder subluxation. A - Normal side. B - Hemiplegic side.

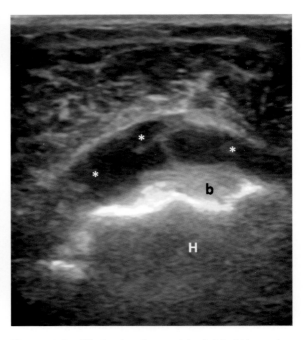

**Figure 14.3** Effusion in subacromial subdeltoid bursa (asterisks) in a hemiplegic patient's shoulder. H, humerus; b, bicipital tendon.

due to the poor protection of an imbalanced shoulder girdle. Further, Lee et al. [23] found no correlation between the severity of US findings and the motor recovery stage and thus concluded that the relevant soft tissue injuries cannot be predicted by Brunnstrom stages and that US is a beneficial method for the imaging hemiplegic shoulder.

The major sites of soft tissue injuries in hemiplegic shoulders were reported as the biceps and supraspinatus tendons (with frequencies of 50% and 47.1%, respectively) in hemiplegic patients with poor motor recovery stage [4]. Transverse, longitudinal, bilateral, and dynamic (with shoulder and elbow motions) scans should be performed. For instance, in addition to the normal shoulder protocol, the integrity of the transverse humeral ligament can be assessed by internal and external rotation of the arm to evaluate the subluxation of the biceps tendon [11, 26].

In brain injury patients, bicipital tendinopathy has been reported as the most common musculoskeletal lesion detected by US [27]. While an anechoic crescent around the extra-articular part of the biceps tendon is commonplace; hypoechoic synovial tissue with or without echotexture changes of the tendon (with or without power Doppler signals) can be observed in different types of tenosynovitis [28] (Figure 14.4). Enlargement of the tendon with heterogeneous echogenicity can be found as a sign of bicipital tendinosis. Partial thickness tears can be seen as hypoechoic areas within the tendon or in case of total rupture, the two separated ends can be observed [11, 26].

### 14.1.3 Impingement Syndrome

For impingement syndrome, dynamic evaluation can be performed while the probe is placed in the coronal oblique position on the lateral edge of the acromion. Normally, the supraspinatus tendon should be observed to disappear smoothly without pain/limitation during shoulder abduction [12].

A wide range of rotator cuff lesions i.e. tendinopathies or partial/full-thickness tears can be seen in the hemiplegic shoulder [3, 4] (Figure 14.5). Ultrasonographic findings are usually similar to those seen in patients without neurological problems, described in Chapter 5 - "Ultrasound Evaluation of the Shoulder".

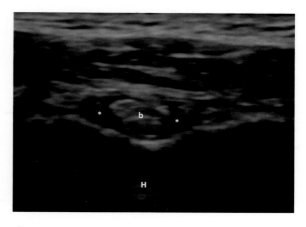

**Figure 14.4** Ultrasound image (axial view) of the biceps tendon (b) in the bicipital groove. Effusion (asterisks) is seen around the tendon which is also inhomogenous as regards echogenicity. H, humeral heal.

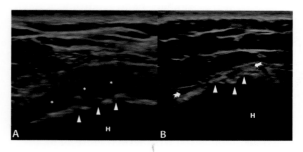

**Figure 14.5** Ultrasound images (axial view) of supraspinatus tendon tears in stroke patients. A - Partial-thickness tear. Multiple hypo-/an-echoic clefts (asterisks) are observed in the tendon overlying the cortical irregularities (white arrowheads). B - Full-thickness tear. The tendon can not be detected (arrows) on the humeral head (H) which is irregular (white arrowheads).

### 14.1.4 Frozen Shoulder

This may be another scenario to be assessed in a hemiplegic shoulder. Falsetti et al. [27] mentioned that they diagnosed frozen shoulder in 8.8% of painful shoulders in their patients with stroke or acquired brain injury. They reported the pertinent US findings as glenohumeral effusion, mild synovitis in the intracapsular tract of the long head of the biceps tendon, no rotator cuff lesions indicating primary capsular inflammation, and an insufficient signal in the rotator cuff outlet using power Doppler US [27].

Of note, the absence of pathognomonic findings may limit the use of US in frozen shoulder.

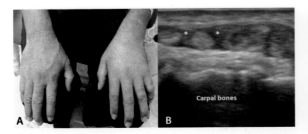

**Figure 14.6** Extensor tenosynovitis. A - Edema is seen on the dorsal side of the patient's left hand. B - Ultrasonographic evaluation (axial view) shows increased fluid (asterisks) in the 4th extensor compartment.

## 14.1.5 Complex Regional Pain Syndrome

Known also as shoulder-hand syndrome, it is one of the common reasons of post-stroke hand edema and pain. In an US study, the frequency of shoulder-hand syndrome was reported as 29.4% in stroke patients [27]. The US findings were reported as moderate effusion in the flexor/extensor tendon sheaths, radiocarpal and midcarpal joints; as well as subcutaneous edema without significant power Doppler signals or with mild synovial inflammatory hypervascularization at the wrist level (Figure 14.6). Presence of the latter can actually be helpful for the management whereby corticosteroid and/or bisphosphonate treatment can be attempted [27, 29].

## 14.2 OVERUSE INJURIES IN WHEELCHAIR USERS

Wheelchair users suffer particular injuries secondary to repetitive incorrect movements or loading of the upper limbs during propulsion, push-up and other daily transfer activities [30]. Tendons and nerves of the upper limbs are commonly affected. Regarding the shoulder girdle; bursitis, impingement syndrome, tendinosis, partial/full thickness tears of the rotator cuff, and tendinitis or tenosynovitis of the biceps have been commonly reported [31-33]. Concerning the elbow, medial and lateral epicondylitis can be observed as edema, increased tendon thickness, loss of fibrillar structure with heterogeneous echotexture, focal hypoechoic areas and bony irregularities of the epicondyles with or without Doppler signals [34, 35] (Figure 14.7). The ulnar nerve can also be

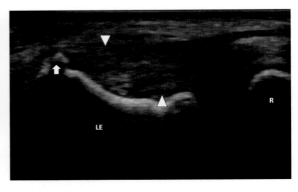

**Figure 14.7** Ultrasonographic evaluation (longitudinal view) of lateral epicondylitis in a patient with elbow pain. There is edema in the superficial and deep fibers of the common extensor tendon (arrowheads) with a small spur (arrow) on the entheseal site. R, radial head; LE, lateral epicondyle.

vulnerable to compression/traction either due to repetitive motions of the elbow or prolonged resting position of the elbow on the wheelchair armrest. The US findings include focal enlargement of the nerve usually proximal to the compression area [36].

Overuse injuries of the wrist in wheelchair users can be caused by inadequate push-up methods which can lead to wrist tendon lesions, especially in quadriparetic patients with no wrist extension. Tenosynovitis of the first extensor compartment is one of the most commonly seen injuries in wheelchair users [25]. The US findings of De Quervain's tenosynovitis comprise distention of the tendon sheath with effusion, heterogeneous hypoechoic swelling of the tendon and positive

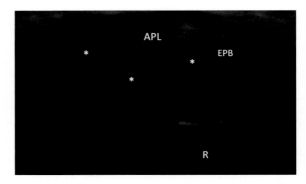

**Figure 14.8** Ultrasound image (axial view) of the 1st extensor compartment in a patient with De Quervain tenosynovitis. Effusion is detected within the tendon sheath (*). Abductor pollicis longus (APL) is enlarged due to edema. EPB, extensor pollicis brevis tendon; R, radius.

Doppler signals in the presence of acute inflammation [1, 37] (Figure 14.8). Repetitive wrist extensions may lead to compressions of the median nerve in the carpal tunnel and the deep branch of the ulnar nerve in Guyon's canal. Aside from prompt diagnosis, subsequent US guided therapeutic interventions can also be applied in these patients [25].

## 14.3 HETEROTOPIC OSSIFICATION

Heterotopic ossification (HO) is defined as the formation of ectopic lamellar bone in soft tissues which can eventually cause pain and limitation in joint motions. In the rehabilitation units, neurogenic HO can generally be detected in association with traumatic brain injury, spinal cord injury, and hemiplegia [38-41]. Hips, knees and elbows are the most commonly affected sites, and HO can begin a few weeks after the onset of a neurogenic disorder and its early inflammatory stage may mimick infection, tumor, acute arthritis, or deep venous thrombosis [39-41]. Firm swelling can be detected in the knee and elbow after a few days, but the detection of a palpable mass around hip may be difficult. The pertinent laboratory findings (i.e. increased serum alkaline phosphatase, C-reactive protein, and erythrocyte sedimentation rate) are of limited help for early diagnosis because of their low specificity [39-41]. In that sense, US can be a convenient bedside imaging tool for early diagnosis. Yet, radiography or computed tomography fail to be contributory especially in the initial 4-8 weeks, and three phase 99m technetium bone scanning and MRI have low sensitivity [39, 42, 43].

B-mode US -as a sensitive method for detection of soft tissue lesions and calcifications- can show the classical "zone phenomenon" of HO, and power Doppler US can be used for semi-quantitative evaluation of the hypervascularization [40, 44, 45]. The zone phenomenon is described as the focal disorganization of the muscle in the affected site with the occurrence of a heterogeneous hypoechoic mass and the absence of longitudinal muscular striation [44, 46]. The appearance of the zone phenomenon in B-mode US is an outer hypoechoic zone next to the normal muscle and an inner hypoechoic core circled by hyperechoic mineralized ring islands. Low compressibility of these early lesions could also be suggestive for HO [38]. A ring-

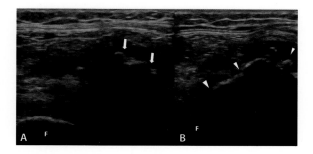

**Figure 14.9** Ultrasound imaging (longitudinal view) of the hip joint in a patient with heterotopic ossification. A - In the early stage (left image), heterotopic ossification (arrows) is detected within the iliopsoas muscle overlying the proximal portion of the femur (F). B - In the late stage (right image), the calcifications (arrowheads) are increased in size.

shaped hyperechoic mineralized tissue thickens with the progression of HO. As a result, US appearance of the zone is lost, representing maturation of the bone formation around 7 weeks after the onset of HO symptoms [44] (Figure 14.9) (see also Chapter 16 - "Ultrasound Imaging in Orthopaedics). Overall, in addition to early diagnosis/treatment, US provides differential diagnosis (e.g. hematoma, deep venous thrombosis, muscle tears) and close follow up with high specificity [44-48].

## 14.4 PRESSURE ULCERS

A pressure ulcer (PU) is a localized lesion of the skin and/or the underlying subcutaneous tissue as a result of pressure or shear over a bony prominence. Early detection and initiation of proper treatment can prevent the progression of the lesion. The prevalence of PU ranges from 0.4-38% for acute care and 2-24% for long-term care [49, 50]. While superficial PUs arise within and/or directly below the epidermis, deep PUs originate in the deeper tissues, and develop in an outward direction [51, 52]. According to a hypothesis on deep tissue injuries, skin signs of a pressure related cutaneous injury can occur after 48 hours to 7 days following the actual event. Initial destruction at the bone-muscle interface and the initial changes of the dermis (e.g. flattening of the collagen fibers) are not visible at first, but they are predictor signs of PU development that appear before visual signs of the epidermis occur. Therefore, it should be kept in mind that severe lesions of the subcuta-

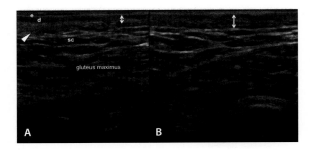

**Figure 14.10** Ultrasound imaging for bilateral pressure ulcers on the gluteal area. A - On the left side, there is edema (arrowhead) on the superficial layer of the subcutaneous fat tissue (sc). B - On the right side, edema is more predominant in the dermis (d). e, epidermis.

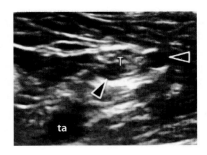

**Figure 14.11** Ultrasound image of a stump neuroma in a transtibial amputee. The tibial nerve (T) is observed to end up with distal anechoic enlargements (arrowheads). ta, posterior tibial artery.

neous tissues may have already ensued while the visible signs are minor on the skin surface. As such, high frequency US (15-20 MHz) has an important/effective role in the assessment of early epidermal and dermal changes over bony prominences [53-55].

The US appearance of a superficial PU is hypoechoic superficial layer representing the subepidermal edema under the intact epidermis [53, 56] (Figure 14.10). US findings of deep tissue injuries include unclear layers (low-contrast foggy appearance with rough resolution), heterogeneous hypoechoic areas (representing hematoma, seroma or necrosis) and discontinuous superficial or deep fascia [56]. The latter two findings have been reported to be more predictive (with high sensitivity and specificity) for future deterioration of a PU [56]. Fluid pockets between the bone and the dermis, and direct extensions of edema into the dermis are also not uncommon in PUs. As a new US technology, elastography can be used to assess PUs as well [57].

## 14.5 AMPUTEE LIMB AND STUMP COMPLICATIONS

Amputees may have associated problems both on the amputated or healthy limbs caused by either the amputation process or overuse of the healthy side. In this regard, US can be used for imaging of various complications such as joint degeneration, soft tissue injuries and neuromas [58-63].

A neuroma related to stump pain is a frequently seen condition in amputees [64]. Assessment of these neuromas with MRI or CT can be challenging; while detection of above-knee neuromas by MRI is available, imaging of below-knee neuromas is limited by muscular fatty atrophy and compact muscles [65]. Similarly, it is difficult to distinguish neuromas from the adjacent soft tissues using CT [66]. On US, neuromas can be observed as hypoechoic, pseudocystic and ovoid mass lesions in which an adjacent nerve enters (Figure 14.11). Further, US guided injections can easily/immediately be performed thereafter [58, 59]. Aside from the neuromas, structural changes of the related peripheral nerves can also be assessed by US quite conveniently [61].

Soft tissue problems in stumps can be imaged by US. The frequency of postoperative fluid collections was reported to be 27% in lower limb amputees. In these patients, US guidance could be used for the drainage of extensive fluid, and this procedure can help to decrease the duration of intravenous antibiotic use [62, 67]. US has a valuable role in the detection of degenerative changes in tendons, muscles, or cartilage after amputation due to the overuse of healthy limbs or the misuse of prosthesis [63, 68, 69]. For instance, thickening of the patellar tendon in below-knee amputees has been previously reported [63]. Muscle atrophy can also be evaluated by US imaging. Significant atrophy in quadriceps and sartorius - but not much in gracilis and hamstring - muscles has been reported in the amputated side of transtibial amputees [69].

Assessment of the bony cortex (for irregularities and spur formation) using sonopalpation is another feasibility of US imaging in amputee patients [1, 60].

## 14.6 SPASTICITY AND ITS MANAGEMENT

Spasticity is one of the main causes of disability in patients with neuromuscular disorders. It is defined as velocity dependent increases in the tonic stretch reflex and causes contractures or joint instability. Spasticity and contractures are reported to be the major problems observed in 18.4% of patients in the rehabilitation process [27]. For localized spasticity, botulinum toxin A (BonT-A) injection is a preferred treatment. Electromyography (EMG) or US can be used for needle guidance during BonT-A injections and correct placement of the needle in the muscle is important to obtain more functional improvements and to ensure fewer side effects [70-75]. EMG can identify muscle contractions, but it does not differentiate individual muscles, particularly co-contracting adjacent muscles. EMG and electrical stimulation are painful procedures, especially for children. Moreover, they require the patient's cooperation as well as expensive disposable monopolar Teflon coated needle electrodes [76, 77]. On the other hand, advantages of US-guided BonT-A injections are precise needle placement, avoidance of injuries in the adjacent tissues (e.g. vessels and nerves) and unnecessity for expensive needles. For sure, US provides information about the muscle architecture (fibroadipose degeneration, changes in thickness, fascicle length, and pennation angle) as well [72-75, 78, 79] (Figure 14.12).

The US-guided injections can be performed using an indirect or direct method. In the former method, the muscle is scanned, the injection place and depth are determined and then the injection is performed without real-time imaging. The disadvantages would be the changes in muscle depth according to probe compression and the difficulty in estimating the exact length of the inserted needle due to absence of markers on the needles. With the direct method, placement of the needle in the target muscle and distribution of the solution can be seen (as an echogenic cloud) with real-time imaging [78].

Peripheral nerve blocks (PNBs) also can be performed for treating spasticity or other painful situations. Compared to palpation of anatomic landmarks or nerve stimulation techniques, US guided PNBs have several advantages as regards precision, real-time imaging and decreased side effects [80,

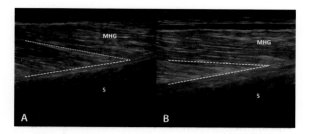

**Figure 14.12** Ultrasound image (longitudinal view) demonstrating the pennate angle measurements from the medial head of the gastrocnemius muscle (MHG) in a stroke patient with spasticity. A - Normal side. B - Hemiplegic side. S, soleus.

81]. The latter includes avoidance of nearby vessels and also the use of smaller amounts of local anesthetics. In the treatment of painful conditions, diagnostic PNBs with local anesthetics can first be performed and then, if necessary, followed with other injections (e.g. corticosteroids) [82]. In rehabilitation practice, a suprascapular nerve block (SSNB) with local anesthetics or in combination with corticosteroids or phenol can be performed for shoulder pain in patients with stroke or traumatic brain injury [83]. Thereby, blockage of 70% of the joint, capsule, subacromial space, acromioclavicular joint and coracoacromial ligament facilitates the rehabilitation process due to the shoulder pain relief and also the risk of pneumothorax and nerve injury is decreased [84, 85].

Phenol injections for perineural blocks have been used to treat spasticity for many years, with the reported failure rates of blind injections being up to 20% [86]. Adverse effects include dysesthesia, numbness and hematoma [87]. Median, ulnar, or musculocutaneous nerves for the upper extremities and obturator or tibial nerves for the lower extremities are the common targets [88]. US guided PNB was reported with a success rate of 100% for spasticity without any adverse effects [89]. Although US guided PNB provides visualization of the distribution of the injected material around the nerve, intensive training is required for this injection technique [90].

## 14.7 IMAGING OF THE DIAPHRAGM

Diaphragm paralysis can be caused by several etiologies e.g. central nervous system disorders, motor neuron diseases, phrenic nerve injuries and direct traumatic injury. Dysfunction of the diaphragm, which is the major respiratory muscle of quiet breathing, is usually underdiagnosed because of its nonspecific findings such as unexplained respiratory distress, dyspnea, asymmetric breathing pattern, paradoxical movement of the epigastrium and recurrent pneumonia [91, 92]. Therefore, early assessment of the diaphragm functions is important in the management of various rehabilitation patients.

Diaphragm elevation may be detected on the weak side of the diaphragm on chest radiographs which have relatively low sensitivity and a poor prediction rate for normal motion [93, 94]. In the case of unilateral paralysis, the paradoxical movement of the diaphragm is detected by fluoroscopy. However, because of the compensatory respiratory mechanisms, normal descent of both sides may be seen in bilateral paralysis [95-96]. Moreover, fluoroscopic imaging causes a significant amount of radiation exposure and it also requires spontaneous breathing of the patient [97]. While CT has a limited role in the dynamic evaluation of diaphragm motion, new dynamic MRI techniques - with the drawbacks of limited availability, operator dependency and high costs - can evaluate the quantitative excursion and velocity of the diaphragm motion [98, 99].

Phrenic nerve conduction studies and EMG are the nonimaging techniques for assessment of diaphragmatic neural continuity [100]. Diaphragm EMG can detect the presence (and the reason) of denervation with high sensitivity and specificity, even in patients on full ventilator support. In addition, EMG provides information about the severity/chronicity of the disorder and its recovery pattern. However, the clinical use of diaphragm EMG is limited by drawbacks such as pneumothorax risk, liver bleeding and discomfort for patients [94, 101, 102]. US guidance for EMG needle localization improves the precision of the process with real-time imaging. Under direct US imaging, the insertion of the needle between the midclavicular and anterior axillary lines can be performed with an in-plane technique, via placing the probe parallel to the ribs at the 7th or 8th intercostal space or with an out-plane technique with the probe perpendicular to the ribs [103-105]. However, the out-plane technique is not preferred because of the risk of puncturing vital structures during inspiration.

Diaphragm US has several advantages, such as bedside real-time imaging, availability of both structure and motion evaluation, no exposure to ionizing radiation and similar accuracy rate with other imaging techniques [92, 101, 104, 106-108]. The lateral and posterior parts of the diaphragm are the most commonly evaluated structures containing muscular components, which are innervated by the phrenic nerve [96]. The echotexture of the diaphragm can also be evaluated by US. In longitudinal view, the appearance of the diaphragm is seen as the hypoechoic muscle fibers separated by the hyperechoic perimysium. In transverse view, a starry night appearance of muscles is observed [103]. The normal diaphragm thickens during inspiration; however, the thickness of the diaphragm and changes in its thickness during inspiration decrease in case of diaphragm paralysis [104]. In severe cases, an atrophic diaphragm may not move with inspiration and will appear as a very thin strip deep to the intercostal muscles [97, 104, 109].

The motion and position of the diaphragm is affected by the patient's position; therefore, supine position, which has less overall variability and has greater reproducibility, is the preferred examination position [92, 99]. Moreover, any compensatory active expiration masking the paralysis by the anterior abdominal wall is limited, and caudal expansion of the lungs provides additional safety in this position [96]. Patients are scanned during spontaneous respiration and deep breaths are avoided. Different frequency probes can be used depending on the imaged part of the diaphragm and the body features of the patient [103]. A high frequency linear-array transducer (7-18 MHz) can be used perpendicu-

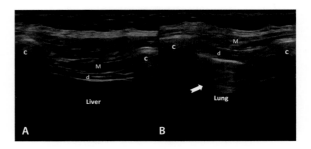

**Figure 14.13** Ultrasound imaging of the diaphragm. The probe is positioned perpendicular to the long axes of the 7th and 8th costae (C). A - The diaphragm (d) can be visualized between the intercostal muscle (M) and liver at rest. B - With inspiration, the lung shadow (arrow) can also be seen.

lar to the ribs at the anterior axillary line (Figure 14.13). On the other hand, the preferred view for the evaluation of diaphragm excursion would be the anterior subcostal placement of the transducer which requires a lower frequency curvilinear transducer (2-6 MHz). In this view, the B-mode is first used to visualize the diaphragm moving away from the transducer, and then M-mode is used to measure the excursion and velocity of the diaphragm [93, 98, 110, 111]. Similar to the anterior subcostal view, the posterior subcostal view is also performed by placement of the probe in the posterior subcostal area in the sagittal planes, enabling the measurement of the excursion [94]. Since the posterior subcostal view requires the patient to be seated, it could not be performed in mechanically ventilated patients. Another position for evaluating the diaphragm excursion is the subxiphoid view which requires the placement of a low frequency curvilinear transducer (2-6 MHz) below the xiphoid in the transverse position [98, 112, 113].

# REFERENCES

1) Özçakar L, Tok F, De Muynck M, Vanderstraeten G. Musculoskeletal ultrasonography in physical and rehabilitation medicine. J Rehabil Med. 2012; 44: 310-8.

2) Turner-Stokes L, Jackson D. Shoulder pain after stroke: a review of the evidence base to inform the development of an integrated care pathway. Clin Rehabil. 2002; 16: 276-98.

3) Pong YP, Wang LY, Huang YC, Leong CP, Liaw MY, Chen HY. Sonography and physical findings in stroke patients with hemiplegic shoulders: a longitudinal study. J Rehabil Med. 2012; 44: 553-7.

4) Huang YC, Liang PJ, Pong YP, Leong CP, Tseng CH. Physical findings and sonography of hemiplegic shoulder in patients after acute stroke during rehabilitation. J Rehabil Med. 2010; 42: 21-6.

5) Van Ouwenaller C, Laplace PM, Chantraine A. Painful shoulder in hemiplegia. Arch Phys Med Rehabil. 1986; 67: 23-6.

6) Lo SF, Chen SY, Lin HC, Jim YF, Meng NH, Kao MJ. Arthrographic and clinical findings in patients with hemiplegic shoulder pain. Arch Phys Med Rehabil. 2003; 84: 1786-91.

7) Tepperman PS, Greyson ND, Hilbert L, Jimenez J, Williams JI. Reflex sympathetic dystrophy in hemiplegia. Arch Phys Med Rehabil. 1984; 65: 442-7.

8) Park HB, Yokota A, Gill HS, El Rassi G, McFarland EG. Diagnostic accuracy of clinical tests for the different degrees of subacromial impingement syndrome. J Bone Joint Surg Am. 2005; 87: 1446-55.

9) Beaudreuil J, Nizard R, Thomas T, Peyre M, Liotard JP, Boileau P, et al. Contribution of clinical tests to the diagnosis of rotator cuff disease: a systematic literature review. Joint Bone Spine. 2009; 76: 15-9.

10) Waldt S, Bruegel M, Mueller D, Holzapfel K, Imhoff AB, Rummeny EJ, et al. Rotator cuff tears: assessment with MR arthrography in 275 patients with arthroscopic correlation. Eur Radiol. 2007; 17: 491-8.

11) Naredo E, Iagnocco A, Valesini G, Uson J, Beneyto P, Crespo M. Ultrasonographic study of painful shoulder. Ann Rheum Dis. 2003; 62: 1026-7.

12) Petranova T, Vlad V, Porta F, Radunovic G, Micu MC, Nestorova R, et al. Ultrasound of the shoulder. Med Ultrason. 2012; 14: 133-40.

13) Huang SW, Liu SY, Tang HW, Wei TS, Wang WT, Yang CP. Relationship between severity of shoulder subluxation and soft tissue injury in hemiplegic stroke patients. J Rehabil Med. 2012; 44: 733-9.

14) Murie-Fernández M, Carmona Iragui M, Gnanakumar V, Meyer M, Foley N, Teasell R. Painful hemiplegic shoulder in stroke patients: causes and management. Neurologia. 2012; 27: 234-44.

15) Najenson T, Yacubovich E, Pikielni SS. Rotator cuff injury in shoulder joints of hemiplegic patients. Scand J Rehabil Med. 1971; 3: 131-7.

16) Roy CW, Sands MR, Hill LD. Shoulder pain in acutely admitted hemiplegics. Clin Rehabil. 1994; 8: 334-40.

17) Zorowitz RD, Hughes MB, Idank D, Ikai R, Johnston MV. Shoulder subluxation after stroke: a comparison of four supports. Arch Phys Med Rehabil. 1995; 76: 763-71.

18) Boyd EA, Goudreau L, O'Riain MD, Grinnell DM, Torrance GM, Gaylard A. A radiological

measure of shoulder subluxation in hemiplegia: its reliability and validity. Arch Phys Med Rehabil. 1993; 74: 188-93.

19) Prevost R, Arsenault AB, Dutil E, Drouin G. Shoulder subluxation in hemiplegia: a radiologic correlational study. Arch Phys Med Rehabil. 1987; 68: 782-5.

20) Van Langenberghe HV, Hogan BM. Degree of pain and grade of subluxation in the painful hemiplegic shoulder. Scand J Rehabil Med. 1988; 20: 161-6.

21) Park GY, Kim JM, Sohn SI, Shin IH, Lee MY. Ultrasonographic measurement of shoulder subluxation in patients with post-stroke hemiplegia. J Rehabil Med. 2007; 39: 526-30.

22) Pong YP, Wang LY, Wang L, Leong CP, Huang YC, Chen YK. Sonography of the shoulder in hemiplegic patients undergoing rehabilitation after a recent stroke. J Clin Ultrasound. 2009; 37: 199-205.

23) Lee IS, Shin YB, Moon TY, Jeong YJ, Song JW, Kim DH. Sonography of patients with hemiplegic shoulder pain after stroke: correlation with motor recovery stage. Am J Roentgenol. 2009; 192: 40-4.

24) Kumar P, Bradley M, Gray S, Swinkels A. Reliability and validity of ultrasonographic measurements of acromion-greater tuberosity distance in poststroke hemiplegia. Arch Phys Med Rehabil. 2011; 92: 731-6.

25) Ozçakar L, Carli AB, Tok F, Tekin L, Akkaya N, Kara M. The utility of musculoskeletal ultrasound in rehabilitation settings. Am J Phys Med Rehabil. 2013; 92: 805-17.

26) Backhaus M, Burmester GR, Gerber T, Rassi W, Machold KP, Swen WA, et al.; Working Group for Musculoskeletal Ultrasound in the EULAR Standing Committee on International Clinical Studies including Therapeutic Trials. Guidelines for musculoskeletal ultrasound in rheumatology. Ann Rheum Dis. 2001; 60: 641-9.

27) Falsetti P, Acciai C, Carpinteri F, Palilla R, Lenzi L. Bedside ultrasonography of musculoskeletal complications in brain injured patients. J Ultrasound. 2010; 13: 134-41.

28) Middleton WD. Ultrasonography of the shoulder. Radiol Clin North Am. 1992; 30: 927-40.

29) Kondo I, Hosokawa K, Soma M, Iwata M, Maltais D. Protocol to prevent shoulder-hand syndrome after stroke. Arch Phys Med Rehabil. 2001; 82: 1619-23.

30) Dyson-Hudson TA, Kirshblum SC. Shoulder pain in chronic spinal cord injury, Part I: Epidemiology, etiology, and pathomechanics. J Spinal Cord Med. 2004; 27: 4-17.

31) Ballinger DA, Rintala DH, Hart KA. The relation of shoulder pain and range-of-motion problems

to functional limitations, disability, and perceived health of men with spinal cord injury: a multifaceted longitudinal study. Arch Phys Med Rehabil. 2000; 81: 1575-81.

32) Mercer JL, Boninger M, Koontz A, Ren D, Dyson-Hudson T, Cooper R. Shoulder joint kinetics and pathology in manual wheelchair users. Clin Biomech (Bristol, Avon). 2006; 21: 781-9.

33) van Drongelen S, Boninger ML, Impink BG, Khalaf T. Ultrasound imaging of acute biceps tendon changes after wheelchair sports. Arch Phys Med Rehabil. 2007; 88: 381-5.

34) Kijowski R, De Smet AA. The role of ultrasound in the evaluation of sports medicine injuries of the upper extremity. Clin Sports Med. 2006; 25: 569-90.

35) Miller TT, Shapiro MA, Schultz E, Kalish PE. Comparison of sonography and MRI for diagnosing epicondylitis. J Clin Ultrasound. 2002; 30: 193-202.

36) Kara M, Özçakar L, De Muynck M, Tok F, Vanderstraeten G. Musculoskeletal ultrasound for peripheral nerve lesions. Eur J Phys Rehabil Med. 2012; 48: 665-74.

37) Tok F, Özçakar L, De Muynck M, Kara M, Vanderstraeten G. Musculoskeletal ultrasound for sports injuries. Eur J Phys Rehabil Med. 2012; 48: 651-63.

38) Falsetti P, Acciai C, Palilla R, Carpinteri F, Patrizio C, Lenzi L. Bedside ultrasound in early diagnosis of neurogenic heterotopic ossification in patients with acquired brain injury. Clin Neurol Neurosurg. 2011; 113: 22-7.

39) van Kuijk AA, Geurts ACH, van Kuppevelt HJM. Neurogenic heterotopic ossification in spinal cord injury. Spinal Cord. 2002; 40: 313-26.

40) Youssefian T, Sapena R, Carlier R, Bos C, Denormandie A, Denys P, et al. Nodular osteochondrogenic activity in soft tissue surrounding osteoma in neurogenic para osteo-arthropathy: morphological and immunohistochemical study. BMC Musculoskelet Disord. 2004; 5: 46.

41) Taly AB, Nair KP, Jayakumar PN, Ravishankar D, Kalaivani PL, Indiradevi B, et al. Neurogenic heterotopic ossification: a diagnostic and therapeutic challenge in neurorehabilitation. Neurol India. 2001; 49: 37-40.

42) May DA, Disler DG, Joner EA, Balkissoon AA, Manaster BJ. Abnormal signal intensity in skeletal muscle at MR imaging: patterns, pearls and pitfalls. Radiographics. 2000; 20: 295-315.

43) Wick L, Berger M, Knecht H, Gluker T, Ledermann HP. Magnetic resonance signal alterations in the acute onset of heterotopic ossification in patients with spinal cord injury. Eur Radiol. 2005; 15: 1867-75.

# Ultrasound Imaging in Pediatric Conditions

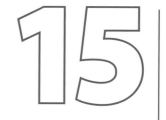

Martine DE MUYNCK, Erkan DEMİRKAYA,
Willem GOETHALS, Mileen DE VLEESCHHOUWER

Owing to the lack of radiation and capability of dynamic imaging, ultrasound (US) assessment is well tolerated in babies and children, and also well accepted by their parents. The immature skeleton allows an excellent visualization, with information on bone and cartilage as well as on soft tissues [1].

## 15.1 NORMAL IMAGING

Imaging of joint pathology in children is unique and differs from that in adults in several aspects. In terms of development, the articular cartilage derives from the immature articular epiphyseal

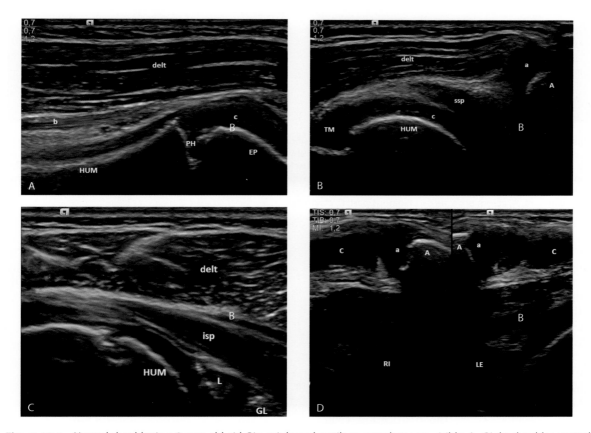

**Figure 15.1**  Normal shoulder in a 8-year-old girl. Big epiphyseal cartilage complexes are visible. A - Right shoulder, ventral vertical view. EP, epiphysis; HUM, humerus; PH, physis; b, tendon of the long head of the biceps; c, cartilage of the humeral head; delt, deltoid muscle. B - Right shoulder, coronal view. A, bony acromion; HUM, humerus; TM, tuberculum majus (greater tubercle); a, cartilaginous acromion; c, cartilage of the humeral head; delt, deltoid muscle; ssp, supraspinatus tendon. C - Right shoulder, dorsal horizontal view. Humerus (HUM) covered by cartilage, bony glenoid (GL), fibrocartilaginous hyperechoic labrum (L), deltoid muscle (delt), infraspinatus (isp). D - Right (RI) and left (LE) shoulder, acromio-clavicular joint. A, acromion; a, its cartilaginous part; C, cartilaginous clavicula.

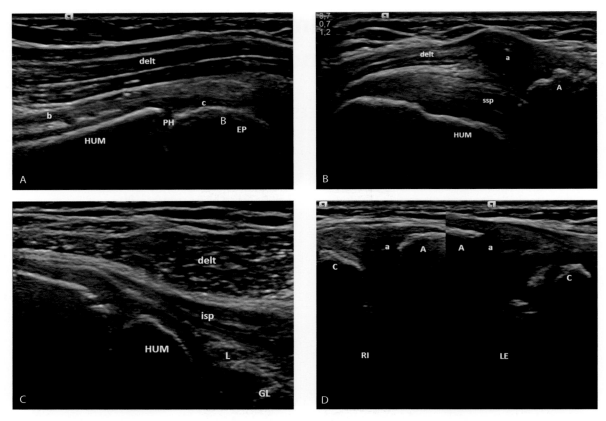

**Figure 15.2** Normal shoulder in a 14-year-old boy. More ossification centres are apparent and epiphyseal cartilage progressively ossified. A - Right shoulder, ventral vertical view. EP, epiphysis; HUM, humerus; PH, physis; b, tendon of the long head of the biceps; c, cartilage of the humeral head; delt, deltoid muscle. B - Right shoulder, coronal view. A, bony acromion; HUM, humerus; a, cartilaginous acromion; delt, deltoid muscle; ssp, supraspinatus tendon. C - Right shoulder, dorsal horizontal view. HUM, humerus; GL, glenoid; L, labrum; delt, deltoid muscle; isp, infraspinatus. D - Right (RI) and left (LE) shoulder, acromioclavicular joint. A, acromion; a, its cartilaginous part; C, clavicula.

cartilage complex, so that the cartilage of the epiphysis and the articular cartilage are initially continuous with each other. During growth, the epiphyseal cartilage progressively ossifies, leaving only the covering layer of the articular cartilage at the end of maturation [2] (Figures 15.1 and 15.2). On US examination, since the epiphyseal cartilage of the unossified skeleton is formed by hyaline cartilage, it appears hypo-/an-echoic with evenly spread brighter foci probably reflecting vessels, whereas the overlying articular cartilage is completely anechoic. Later, the ossification centers become visible as highly reflective surfaces [3].

Comparing symptomatic/asymptomatic sides is even more important than in adults. As illustrated in figures 15.1 and 15.2, it is more difficult to recognize the bone shapes and the hypo-/anechoic cartilage can easily be mistaken for a fluid collection. Comparing both sides and exerting slight compression can help to differentiate. The thickness of the overlying soft tissue layers will depend on the age of the child and also here, looking for right/left difference is advocated.

## 15.2 IMAGING FOR PATHOLOGIES

### 15.2.1 Congenital Pathologies

*Developmental dysplasia of the hip*

Where available, US is now the preferred method for diagnostic imaging of the immature hip [4]. It allows direct visualization of the cartilaginous components of the hip joint. When the femoral head becomes ossified, the acetabulum can be in-

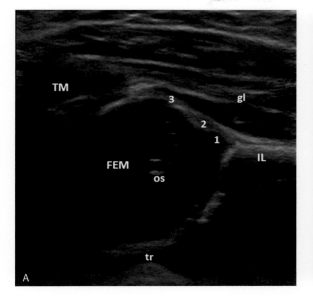
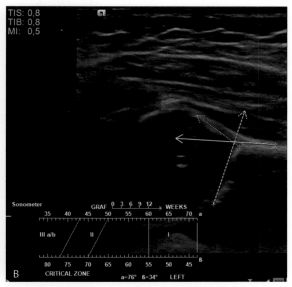

**Figure 15.3**  A 2-month-old baby boy. Standard coronal view. A - Normal left hip. More than half of the femoral head (FEM) is covered by bone, the ossification centre (os) in the head is becoming visible. The bony promontory of the ilium (IL) is slightly rounded. TM, greater trochanter; gl, gluteal muscles; tr, triradiate fibrocartilage; 1, hyaline part of the labrum; 2, fibro-cartilaginous labrum; 3, capsule. B - Baseline (solid line), bony roof line (interrupted line), and cartilaginous roof line (dotted line) are drawn. Alpha (76°) and beta (34°) angles are thus defined and shown in the "sonometer" of Graf: Ib type hip, mature hip.

adequately visualized and the value of US diminishes (certainly above the age of 12 months).

In 1978, the Austrian orthopaedic surgeon Graf started to investigate infant hips by US. He introduced an exact, reproducible procedure to evaluate congenital hip dysplasia and dislocation [5-7].

Besides this morphological examination method, there is a dynamic method of Harcke, and other modified/combined methods as well [8]. Graf uses a single-view (coronal) and looks for morphological characteristics with quantification (mainly used in Europe) [5-7]. The Harcke method is multiplanar, dynamic and semi-quantitative (more used in the USA) [8]. For the American Institute of Ultrasound in Medicine, the diagnostic examination for developmental dysplasia of the hip (DDH) incorporates two orthogonal planes: a coronal view in the standard plane at rest and a transverse view of the flexed hip with and without stress [4]. The Barlow stress maneuver is performed to evaluate for hip instability with the hip and knee flexed and the thigh adducted. If the femoral head is subluxated or dislocated, reducibility can be assessed by the Ortolani maneuver (abducting and externally rotating the hip).

The standard coronal plane is defined by iden-

tifying a straight iliac line, the transition from the os ilium to the triradiate cartilage (lower rim of the ilium) and the tip of the acetabular labrum. Alpha (bony covering) and beta (cartilaginous covering) angles must be measured. The base line is parallel with the ilium. The bony roof line starts from the lower limb of os ilium and is tangent with the bony roof. The alpha angle is defined by the base line and the bony roof line. For the beta angle, the cartilage roof line is needed, from the crossing point of the bony roof (concave to convex) through the middle of the labrum. Ideally the alpha angle is >60°. In younger babies (<3 months), it can be smaller, conforming to age (immature hip IIa) (Figure 15.3).

Graf [5-7] discriminates different sonographic hip types (I: mature, IIa: immature <3 months, IIb: immature >3 months, IIc: critical zone hip, IId: decentering hip, III: eccentric, IV: eccentric head luxated), and proposes appropriate treatment for each type (Figure 15.4). Ultrasound can be used for baseline evaluation and for serial assessment during treatment (IIb, c hips need maturation and thus Pavlik harness; unstable IIc, d hips need retention and thus plaster; III, IV need repositioning or surgery).

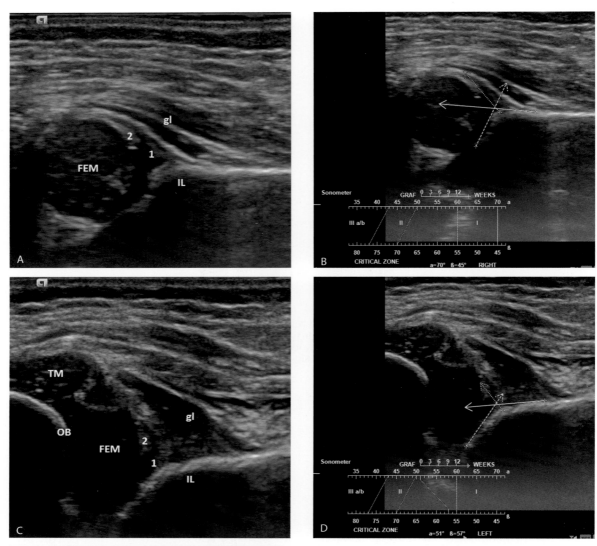

**Figure 15.4** A 6-week-old baby girl. Standard coronal view. A - Normal right hip. The ossification centre in the femoral head (FEM) is not yet visible. IL, ilium; gl, gluteal muscles; 1, hyaline part of the labrum; 2, fibrocartilaginous labrum. B - Baseline (solid line), bony roof line (interrupted line) and cartilaginous roof line (dotted line) are drawn. Alpha (70°) and beta (45°) angles are thus defined and shown in the "sonometer" of Graf: Ib type hip, mature hip. C - Pathological left hip: highly deficient bony modeling of the bony roof; cartilaginous roof still covering the femoral head. TM, greater trochanter; FEM, femoral head; IL, ilium; OB, osseous boundary of the femur; gl, gluteal muscles; 1, hyaline part of the labrum; 2, fibrocartilaginous labrum. D - Baseline (solid line), bony roof line (interrupted line) and cartilaginous roof line (dotted line) are drawn. Alpha (51°) and beta (57°) angles are thus defined and shown in the "sonometer" of Graf: IIa (-) type hip, immature hip with maturational deficit. E - Serial exam 6 weeks later. No positive evolution at all: the bony modeling remains highly insufficient. FEM, femoral head; IL, ilium; OB, osseous boundary between head and diaphysis of the femur, TM, greater trochanter; gl, gluteal muscles.

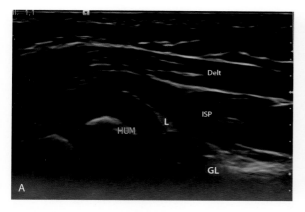 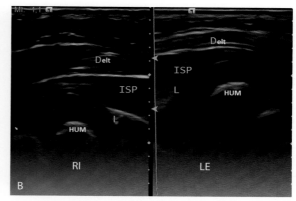

**Figure 15.5** A 5-month-old baby girl with Erb's palsy on the left side. A - Right shoulder, dorsal horizontal view. HUM, ossification centre of humeral head; GL, glenoid. B - Right (RI) and left (LE) shoulder, dorsal horizontal view. There is muscular atrophy, mainly of the deltoid muscle, but the position of the humeral head in relation to the glenoid is normal. HUM, humerus; L, labrum; Delt, deltoid muscle; ISP, infraspinatus.

There are limitations with regard to accuracy: US is able to detect abnormality not apparent on clinical examination, therefore it is inherently a more sensitive test. Intra- and inter-observer agreement in reproducing scans are less than in interpreting the images. Substantial training and attention to technical details and evaluation of results are necessary to obtain reliable results [9]. The dynamic technique is more prone to subjectivity and standardization is more difficult to establish. A few studies reported an adequate repeatability for the static and the combined static/dynamic methods, while no such reports exist for the dynamic US techniques [10].

Besides, questions remain about whom (all newborns? Those at risk? At risk according to the history and/or physical examination?) and when to screen (better not at the time of birth, but later at 4 weeks or 6 weeks?). Used selectively, hip US is clearly indicated for all infants with abnormal findings on clinical examination and for those with risk factors for DDH.

Ultrasound screening may lead to overdiagnosis and overtreatment; costs and benefits are debated. Overtreatment and delayed treatment rates of DDH are believed to be minimized by the use of both morphological and dynamic US methods in the evaluation of the newborn hip [11]. There is still insufficient evidence to give clear recommendations for practice. There is inconsistent evidence that universal US results in a significant increase in treatment compared to the use of targeted US or clinical examination alone. Neither of

the US strategies has been demonstrated to improve clinical outcomes including late diagnosed DDH and surgery [12].

### Brachial plexus injuries

In experienced hands, US can be helpful in demonstrating nerve lesions outside the spinal canal [1]. Two findings can be identified: traumatic neuroma, and pseudomeningocele. Neuromas are fusiform hypoechoic masses, in continuity with the nerve or on a retracted stump. Pseudomeningoceles are collections near the intervertebral foramina [1]. Assessment of the position of the humeral head in relation to the acromion and the glenoid is also possible, looking for secondary (sub)luxation (Figure 15.5).

Other conditions like congenital clubfoot and tarsal coalition can also be evaluated in babies and children [1]. In babies with inability to move the interphalangeal joint of the thumb, congenital tenosynovitis of flexor pollicis longus can be looked for [1].

### 15.2.2 Hereditary Diseases

#### Hemophylia

With US, acute or subclinical bleeding in a joint can be detected; the regression and organisation of hemarthrosis can be followed as well [1] (Figure 15.6). Bleeding occurring repeatedly can cause early osteoarthritis [1]. The following pa-

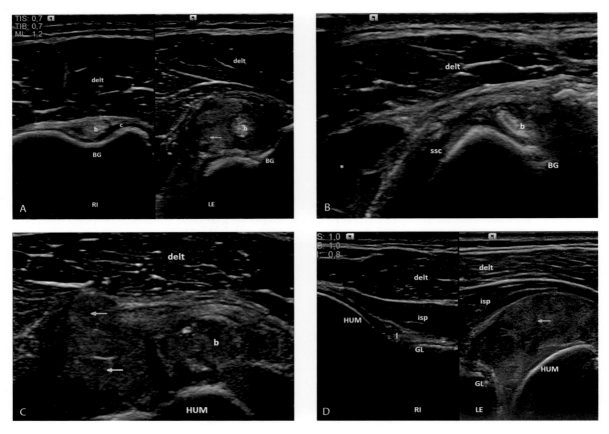

**Figure 15.6** A 15-year-old boy with hemophilia, and recent bleeding in the left shoulder. A - Right (RI) and left (LE) shoulder, ventral horizontal view. Big amount of blood (arrow) surrounding the biceps tendon (b). The fluid is compressible, rather hyperechoic. BG, bicipital groove; c, cartilage of the physis; delt, deltoid muscle. B - Left shoulder, ventral horizontal view. There is also fluid in the subacromio-subdeltoid bursa (*), fluid in 2 compartments being suggestive of a full thickness rotator cuff rupture. BG, bicipital groove; b, biceps tendon; delt, deltoid muscle; ssc, subscapularis tendon. C - Left shoulder, coraco-acromial view. Blood (arrows) is filling the space medially from the biceps (b) (which cannot clearly be differentiated from surrounding blood), the image is suggestive of subscapularis rupture. HUM, humerus; delt, deltoid muscle. D - Right (RI) and left (LE) shoulder, dorsal horizontal view. A big amount of intra-articular blood (arrow) is covering the humeral head (HUM). GL, glenoid; delt, deltoid muscle; isp, infraspinatus; l, labrum.

rameters can be evaluated using US: synovial hypertrophy, synovial hyperaemia, cartilage loss, and bone surface erosion [13]. The first stage of degenerative cartilage in hemophilic arthropathy is characterised by loss of the anechoic appearance, reduction of sharpness and cartilage thinning. This is followed by moderate or severe cartilage loss. Ultrasound has proven to be an excellent modality for detection of early bone erosions with a sensitivity superior to plain films. The use of US might allow frequent monitoring of patients with hemophilia and early detection of arthropathy [13]. A simplified US scanning procedure and scoring method, named "Haemophilia Early Arthropathy Detection with US" [HEAD-US], was

developed to evaluate joints of patients with hemophilic arthropathy [14]. Three comprehensive and evidence-based US scanning procedures to image the elbow, knee and ankle were established, in order to increase sensitivity in detection of early signs of joint involvement. Each procedure includes systematic evaluation of synovial recesses and selection of a single osteochondral surface for damage analysis. A simplified scoring system based on an additive scale was created, to define the joint status and to evaluate disease progression [14].

Bleeding may also occur in muscles. US allows the visualization and follow-up of the hematoma. Eventual complications such as an encapsulated

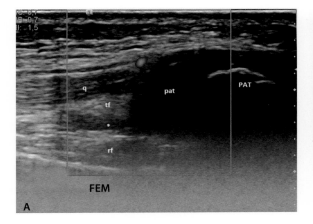

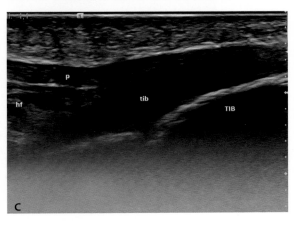

**Figure 15.7** Normal knee of a 5-year-old girl. A - Suprapatellar vertical view. Insertion of the quadriceps tendon (q) with Doppler signal in the distal part of the tendon. FEM, femur; PAT, ossification centre of the patella; pat, cartilaginous part of the patella; rf, rectangular fat body; tf, triangular fat body; *, suprapatellar recess. B - Infrapatellar vertical view. PAT, ossification centre of the patella; hf, Hoffa fat; p, insertion of the patellar tendon; pat, cartilaginous part of the patella; TIB, tibia; tib, cartilaginous apophysis of the tibia. C - Infrapatellar vertical view. Distal insertion of the patellar tendon (p), maturation Ducher stage 1 or cartilage attachment. TIB, tibia; hf, Hoffa fat; tib, cartilaginous apophysis of the tibia.

collection or non-contractile scar tissue can be diagnosed as well [1].

### Neuromuscular disorders

Ultrasound could become an additional tool to electromyography in the diagnosis and follow-up of peripheral nerve and muscle disorders. Yet, US is more sensitive to detect fasciculations, and it has also been demonstrated that even the smaller fibrillations can be visualized [15]. Measuring muscle thickness or other architectural parameters (i.e. pennation angle, fascicle length) and determining muscle echo intensity with computer-assisted gray-scale analysis could be helpful for the detection and differentiation of neuromuscular disorders [16, 17].

### 15.2.3 Apophyseal Injuries

Between the ages of 10 and 16 years, the ossification centers of most apophyses are still imma-

ture and the cartilage cannot give firm stability to the osteotendinous junction [1] (Figure 15.7). Acute apophyseal injury is caused by a single indirect major trauma. The apophyses of the pelvis (the anterior superior and inferior iliac spine, the pubis and ischial tuberosity) and the elbow (medial and lateral epicondyle) are most commonly affected [1]. There can be partial or complete detachment of the apophysis onto which the tendon is attached [1].

Chronic apophyseal lesions, with a sequence of overlapping damage-repair processes, are common at the knee (Osgood-Schlatter disease (OSD), and Sinding-Larsen-Johansson disease) and ankle (Sever disease) [1, 18] (Figures 15.8 and 15.9).

Ultrasound is able to depict cartilage swelling, fragmentation of the apophyseal ossification centre, insertional tendon swelling and infrapatellar bursitis. Already in 1989, De Flaviis et al. [19] proposed a classification for OSD, based on the involvement of both apophysis and soft tissues. Type 1 shows a hypoechoic zone superficial

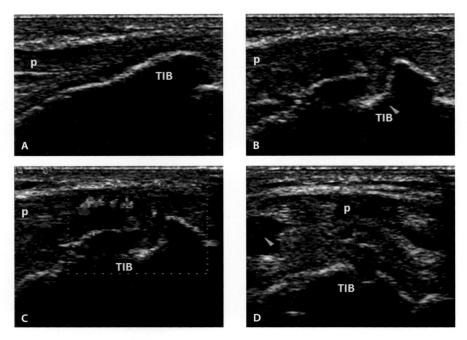

**Figure 15.8** Osgood-Schlatter disease, De Flaviis type 4. A - Infrapatellar vertical view. Asymptomatic side, maturation Ducher stage 2 or insertional cartilage. TIB, tibia; p, patellar tendon. B - Infrapatellar vertical view. Symptomatic side. Fragmented (arrowhead) ossification centre of the tibia (TIB) and swollen patellar tendon (p). C - Infrapatellar vertical view, symptomatic side. Doppler signal in the swollen, patellar tendon (p). TIB, tibia. D - Infrapatellar horizontal view. Symptomatic side. Fluid collection in the retrotendinous bursa (arrowhead). TIB, tibia; p, patellar tendon.

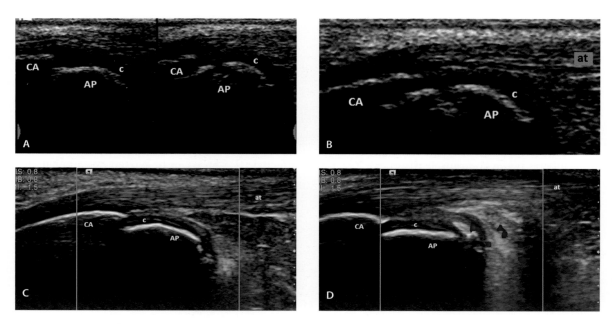

**Figure 15.9** Sever disease. A - Older machine and probe. Right asymptomatic and left symptomatic heel, showing asymmetrical ossification centres, with fragmentation on the left side. B - Older machine and probe, showing mainly the fragmented ossification centre. C - High end machine and probe, showing more details of cartilage and soft tissues at the asymptomatic side of a 12-year old boy. D - High end machine and probe. Swollen, inhomogenous, blurred cartilage and Doppler signal in the cartilage and the overlying soft tissues. CA, calcaneus; AP, apophysis; c, cartilage; at, Achilles tendon.

Musculoskeletal Ultrasound in Physical and Rehabilitation Medicine

to the apophysis (cartilaginous swelling); type 2 shows a fragmented and hypoechoic ossification centre as well; in type 3 there is swelling of the insertion of the patellar tendon; in type 4 there is a fluid collection in the retrotendinous bursa (see figure 15.8). It should be noted that the sonographic appearance of tibial tuberosity depends on the age of the child. Ducher et al. [20, 21] showed that irregularity of the apophysis and presence of different ossicles are part of normal development. They staged the maturation process of the patellar tendon attachment: stage 1 or cartilage attachment is characterized by a large amount of apophyseal cartilage, with or without interspersed ossicles; in stage 2 or insertional cartilage, a thin layer of cartilage is still visible and the apophyseal surface appears smoother; stage 3 represents a mature enthesis and the attachment of the collagen fibers on the bone is complete and no apophyseal cartilage remains (see figures 15.7 and 15.8). Sailly et al. [22] also used color Doppler and described that neo-vessels started from the prepatellar bursa and extended into the distal end of the patellar tendon. Positive Doppler signal was associated with higher pain on palpation and resisted static contraction. They also found that the stage of cartilage attachment with visible ossicles (late stage 1

of Ducher) could be the critical stage of development of symptomatic OSD [22].

The normal pediatric enthesis can nevertheless exhibit Doppler signals and this might be especially relevant during periods of rapid growth with increased mechanical strain [23]. No Doppler signals were seen directly at the bone/cartilage surface in the enthesis, but Doppler signals were seen at 2 mm of the tibial tuberosity and certainly at 10 mm distance (30% in flexed vs. 20% in neutral position) in asymptomatic children [23].

### 15.2.4 The "Irritable Hip"

The "irritable" hip is common in children: it refers to an acute painful hip with limping or refusal to walk. Ultrasound can help to differentiate between possible causes, such as transient synovitis, septic arthritis, Leg-Calvé-Perthes disease, and slipped capital femoral epiphysis [24] (Figure 15.10).

*Transient synovitis*

Transient synovitis of the hip typically occurs in 3 to 8-year-old children. Etiology is still unknown. The hip is often held in an antalgic posi-

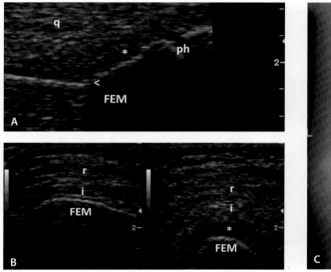
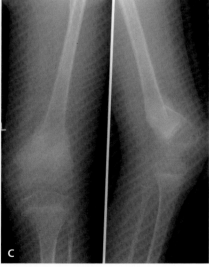

**Figure 15.10**  A 8-year-old girl with cerebral palsy, refusing to walk (irritable hip?). Normal US exam of the hips. Much pain when moving and touching the thigh more distally during the exam. A - The cortex of the femur (FEM) is showing an angulation (<) and overlying swelling of the periosteum (*), suggestive of fracture. ph, physis; q, quadriceps muscle. B - Transverse view, confirming the soft tissue swelling (*). FEM, femur; vastus intermedius (i) and rectus (r) parts of the quadriceps muscle. C - Corresponding radiographic follow-up, showing formation of callus at the fracture site.

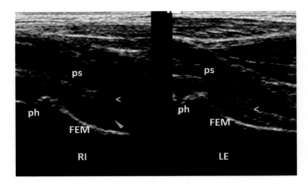

**Figure 15.11** Irritable hip, transient synovitis. Ventral vertical view of right (RI) and left (LE) hip. Convex aspect of the capsule (<) in the right hip, with anechoic fluid (arrowhead). FEM, femur neck; ph, physis; ps, psoas muscle.

tion of flexion/abduction/external rotation. The hip is examined in an anterior approach, in a parasagittal plane parallel with the femoral neck. US image is characterized by widening of the joint space - the distance between the femoral neck and the ventral margin of the joint capsule becoming more than 5 mm [25] (Figure 15.11). Futami et al. [25] attributed the widening to effusion in transient synovitis and to synovial thickening in Leg-Calvé-Perthes disease. Robben et al. [26] illustrated that the anterior joint capsule of the hip comprises an anterior and posterior layer, mainly composed of fibrous tissue, lined by only a minute synovial membrane. Both fibrous layers were identified separately at US in 84% of normal hips

and in all hips with transient synovitis [26] (Figures 15.12 and 15.13). Normally the capsule follows the curve of the femur and is concave. In case of effusion, it becomes convex. One should be very meticulous in positioning the patient: in extension/internal rotation the capsule can become a little convex in normal hips - in flexion/abduction/external rotation less fluid will be seen under the capsule. In case of transient synovitis, pain lasts for a mean of five days and fluid remains for a mean of nine days [27]. If fluid is visible for a longer time, close follow-up is necessary; certainly if longer than 24 days, Leg-Calvé-Perthes should be suspected [27].

### Septic arthritis

Typically occurs earlier (<3 years-old) than transient synovitis. The appearance of synovitis is non-specific. Turbid fluid, debris, synovial thickening and hyperaemia may also be found in non-infected joints [24]. Kocher et al. [28] described four independent multivariate predictors for septic arthritis: non-weight bearing, fever, sedimentation rate of >40 mm/hour and serum white blood count of >12000/mm³. Predicted probability of 93.1% for three predictors and 99.6% for 4 predictors was found. If septic arthritis is suspected and US is negative, it is advised to repeat the exam after 24 hours, because there can be a delay between the appearance of the symptoms and fluid becoming visible. If septic arthritis is suspected,

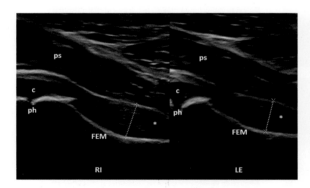

**Figure 15.12** Irritable right hip in a 7-year-old boy. Ventral vertical view of right (RI) and left (LE) hip. Rather convex aspect of the capsule on both sides, with distance between femoral neck (FEM) and ventral margin of the capsule of 7.1 and 6.7 mm. A small fluid layer (*) is visible between posterior and anterior tissue layer. Physis (ph), cartilage (c) on the femoral head; ps, psoas muscle.

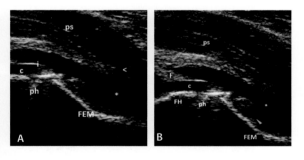

**Figure 15.13** Irritable hip and transient synovitis in a 6-year-old boy. A - Ventral vertical view. Convex aspect of the capsule (<), with anechoic fluid (*) and interface sign (i) between it and the cartilage (c) on the femoral head. FEM, femur neck; ph, physis; ps, psoas muscle. B - Ventral vertical view. Detail: anechoic fluid (*) and swelling of the deep soft issue layer (arrowhead). FEM, femur neck; FH, femoral head; c, cartilage covering it; l, labrum; ph, physis; ps, psoas muscle.

needle aspiration of hip effusion is necessary for confirming the diagnosis (Figure 15.14).

Pressure exerted on feeding vessels by the effusion in transient synovitis, might be a predisposition for ischemia of the femoral head [24]. Long-standing hip joint effusion (lasting at least 3 weeks) needs close follow-up. Thickening of the cartilage covering the femoral head may help to distinguish *Leg-Calvé-Perthes disease*. An irregularly fragmented and flattened appearance of the femoral epiphysis as well as wasting of the ipsilateral quadriceps muscle can also be present [24].

## Epiphysiolysis

Slipped upper femoral epiphysis or epiphysiolysis is a Salter-Harris type-1 injury of the hip in adolescents. Predisposing factors include increased body weight and the status of intrinsic weakness of the cartilaginous growth plate at the end of puberty, combined with mechanical stress [24, 29]. In the acute phase, US can assess the epiphyseal slipping by measuring the width of the physeal step using an anterior approach [24, 29].

## 15.2.5 Rheumatic Diseases

Juvenile Idiopathic Arthritis (JIA), a condition which is also referred to as juvenile rheumatoid arthritis or juvenile chronic arthritis, is the most common chronic inflammatory arthropathy in childhood, accounting for approximately 6-19 cases per $10^6$ children per year [30]. It is a heterogeneous group of disorders, the majority of which are different from adult seropositive rheumatoid arthritis [31]. It is characterized by articular and periarticular tissue inflammation that persists for a minimum of 6 consecutive weeks in one or more joints, starting before the age of 16 years (Figure 15.15). The extent of this inflammation may cause cartilage and bone damage and lead to permanent alterations in joint structures [32, 33]. The main goal in the management of JIA is getting an early and extensive diagnosis of inflammatory activity in order to avoid physical disability in adult age.

Traditionally, the gold standard for detecting joint inflammation has been the clinical assessment of affected joints and laboratory analyses. However, clinical assessment of joint swelling and pain in children has proven to be difficult and not entirely reliable, both in diagnosis and follow-up [34]. Laboratory measures have the limitation of

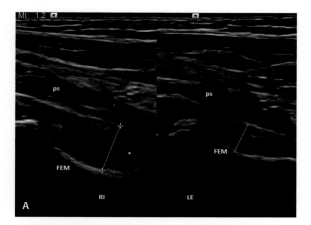

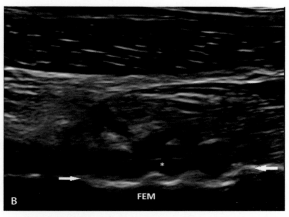

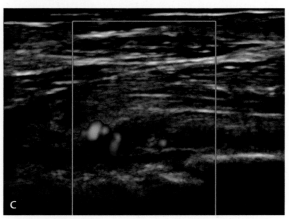

**Figure 15.14** A 5-year-old boy, in therapy for neuroblastoma, with fever and refusal to walk (septic arthritis of hip? other?). No response to antibiotics, US and MRI inconclusive, biopsy showed metastasis. A - Right (RI) and left (LE) hip, ventral vertical view, with fluid (*) in the right hip (distance between neck and capsule 9.3 mm on the right side, 5.9 mm on the left). FEM, femur; ps, psoas muscle. B - More distally, area with irregular cortex of the femur (FEM). Small fluid layer (*) covering the area. C - More distally, along the femur (FEM), positive Doppler signal in the soft tissues over this area.

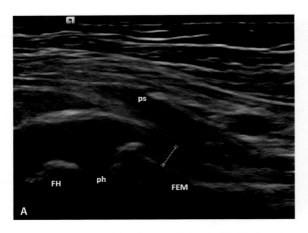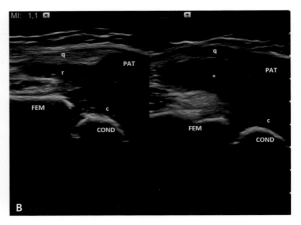

**Figure 15.15** Possible relapse of irritable left hip in a 2-year-old boy. A - Ventral vertical view showing no fluid in the hip joint (distance between femoral neck (FEM) and capsule only 2.9 mm). FH, femoral head; ph, physis; ps, psoas muscle. B - On the contrary, there is intra-articular fluid (*) in the left knee joint. The right condylar cartilage (c) seems to be irregular and swollen. COND, condyle; FEM, femur; PAT, cartilaginous patella; q, quadriceps tendon; r, suprapatellar recess. Finally diagnosed as juvenile idiopathic arthritis.

not directly measuring inflammation at the primary site of pathology and may be subject to confounding influences [35]. Therefore, it is necessary to perform imaging to better understand and to monitor processes in the joint [36, 37]. Magnetic resonance imaging and US have come to the forefront. Both are capable of directly visualizing and quantifying synovial inflammation and also enable better and earlier detection of cartilage and bone changes in children with JIA [38]. Ultrasound is the best available imaging tool to guide aspirations and injections [39].

Pathological findings include the following:

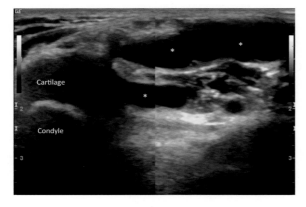

**Figure 15.16** Ultrasound imaging for Baker cyst in a child. Axial (split-screen) image shows the large anechoic cartilage layer overlying the medial femoral condyle next to the cystic lesion (asterisks).

non-compressible hypoechoic synovial hypertrophy, compressible hypoechoic/anechoic joint effusion, hypoechoic/anechoic tissue within the tendon sheath, hypoechoic and/or thickened tendons, ligaments, capsules or fasciae on bony insertions, enthesitis, cartilage thickening or thinning and bone erosions seen as localized cortical defects [38]. Additionally, Power Doppler US (PDUS) allows the evaluation of synovial/tissue hyperemia and discrimination between active and inactive joint disease [40]. Apart from the articular cartilage, the epiphyseal cartilage and the shape/contour of the epiphysis and growth plate is almost invariably involved in JIA, possibly leading to important and lasting consequences on maturation and growth.

Herewith, US assessment in growing children is challenging, as physiologic findings may be misinterpreted as pathologic (Figure 15.16). As such, experience and a thorough knowledge of the age-related changes of normal anatomy are essential for precise identification of JIA related pathologies in children [3].

### Synovitis

The synovial membrane is an important connective tissue lining the inner surface of the joint capsule, tendon sheath and bursa and the place where inflammation usually originates. US is well suited to understand and assess the pathological changes seen in the synovium [34]. Similar to

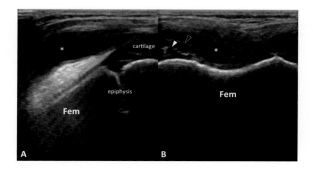

**Figure 15.17** Knee effusion in a child with juvenile idiopathic arthritis. Anechoic fluid in the suprapatellar bursa (asterisks) is seen in the longitudinal (A) and axial (B) views. The distal femoral cartilage and the ossification areas (white arrowhead) are observed during maximum knee flexion (B). Note the interface sign (black arrowhead) between fluid and cartilage.

adult rheumatoid arthritis, US has proven to be more sensitive and specific than radiographs or clinical examination in detection of synovial activity [2, 41-43]. Identification of subclinical synovitis is relevant for patient classification in the different JIA categories and taking decisions in patient treatment as well [44]. The presence of active disease in at least five joints is necessary for the diagnosis of polyarticular JIA, as well as being a prerequisite for patient inclusion in clinical trials of second-line or biologic agents [45-47].

In JIA, as in any other inflammatory arthritis, the synovium undergoes changes leading to the formation of a mass of synovial tissue. The presence of joint, bursal or tendon sheath effusion is used as an excellent, indirect correlate of synovial inflammation (Figure 15.17). Further, its presence (as an anechoic structure) technically enables a better visualization of the synovial thickening [37, 48]. The characteristics of synovial inflammation include hypertrophy and edema caused by proliferation of the capillaries and postcapillary venules. US is a sensitive method for detecting synovial thickening and synovial cysts [38, 49]. Synovial hypertrophy is seen as a solid, non-compressible, abnormally thickened hypoechoic tissue associated with joint lines or surrounding tendons [50, 51]. In the absence of an effusion, synovitis is diagnosed by the presence of an abnormally thickened hypoechoic region, usually measured in a standard plane with reference to an established normal range or to the contralateral normal joint.

PDUS assessment of synovial vascularization

has been shown to be more sensitive than serum markers of inflammation and in the identification of active disease in JIA [52, 53].

Lastly, serial examinations may significantly contribute to monitoring disease activity and in evaluating response to therapy [54]. Of note, it is more challenging to assess synovial hypertrophy in younger children than in adolescents and adults even though image quality is actually better in children.

## Effusion

Effusion is an indirect sign of synovitis in rheumatic diseases. Morever, effusion may allow a better monitoring of disease course than synovial proliferation. Sureda et al. [55] reported no significant differences in synovial thickness between patients with clinically active disease and those in clinical remission. Changes in the amount of fluid after clinical improvement seemed to occur faster than changes in synovial thickness [55].

However, there is no consensus concerning the amount of intra-articular fluid in healthy individuals in pediatric ages. Muller et al. [56] reported that relatively large amounts of fluid that had previously been considered to be pathological in adults may be seen in some joints of healthy children. Graded compression or sonopalpation may be useful in distinguishing isolated effusion from synovial proliferation.

Effusions as small as 1 ml can be detected with an interobserver agreement of 79% in hand and foot joints [57]; US has been found superior to clinical examination in the detection of effusion, even in a large and relatively easily palpable joint such as the knee joint [58]. The presence of knee effusion in JIA was also highly correlated with disease activity [59].

Moreover, US cannot accurately differentiate whether a fluid collection is inflammatory, infectious or hematogenous, but it provides precise guidance for aspiration (and laboratory analysis) [60].

## Enthesitis

Enthesitis, inflammation at the insertions of tendons, ligaments and capsules or fascia into the bone, is a distinctive feature of enthesitis-related arthritis that constitutes 20% of all JIA categories [32]. The entheses commonly involved in children are the calcaneal attachment sites of the plantar

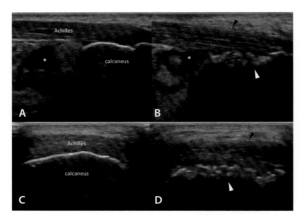

**Figure 15.18** Bilateral imaging for enthesopathy in a child with enthesis related arthritis; longitudinal (A, B) and axial (C, D) views. While there is only retrocalcaneal bursitis (asterisk) on one side (A, C); on the other side (B, D), there is also edema in the Achilles tendon (black arrowheads) and enthesitis (white arrowheads) at its insertion on the calcaneus.

fascia and the Achilles' tendon and the insertions of the patellar tendon [34].

The soft tissue components of an enthesis have traditionally been evaluated by clinical examination based on the presence of tenderness and/or swelling while conventional radiography has been used to assess associated bony changes (i.e. calcifications, enthesophytes and bony erosions) which usually reveal the late stages of the disease [61].

Grey-scale US can detect abnormal enthesis with changed echogenicity, increased thickness, focal or diffuse loss of normal tendon or ligament fibrillar structure, intratendinous or intraligamentous calcification, enthesophytes, bone erosions and bursitis (Figure 15.18). Again, PDUS examination may give additional information as regards inflammation/vascularization.

Although the US appearance of enthesitis is generally the same irrespective of age, especially in young children the presence of higher amount of cartilage, physiological vascularization areas inside it and irregular ossification centers should be kept in mind [62-64].

## Tenosynovitis

Ultrasound imaging is particularly useful in the study of tendon involvement, which often accompanies and sometimes precedes arthritis. The range of tendon pathologies in JIA is wide and includes distension of tendon sheath, loss of fibril-

lar echotexture, loss of definition of tendon margins and partial or complete loss of tendon continuity [65].

Tendon sheath widening is generally the hallmark of early tendon involvement in JIA. The appearance of sheath content is characteristically anechoic in patients with acute tenosynovitis. On the contrary, if synovial fluid is rich in proteinaceous material or has an elevated cellular content, a variable degree of echoes can be detected, which indicate chronic tenosynovitis. Synovial hypertrophy, which appears as an irregular thickening of the synovial layer and/or villous vegetations, can also be seen. In addition, the amount of synovial fluid within a widened tendon sheath may vary considerably, ranging from minimal homogeneous widening (difficult to detect if the pressure with the transducer is high) to balloon-like distension [35, 65].

Assessment of tendon echotexture or loss of its substance is crucial for a complete US exam [37, 65]. PDUS evaluation can help to better understand the inflammatory process involving the tendons [37, 38].

Overall, the use of US imaging seems to provide a platform for a better anatomical classification of JIA as well [66, 67].

## Cartilage damage

Sonographically detected cartilage loss may be an early marker of joint damage in JIA. Radiographs do not directly visualize cartilage, and joint space narrowing is a relatively late finding [35]. Ultrasound can well be used for evaluation of the integrity of cartilage in the immature skeleton and has been shown to be a sensitive modality to detect alterations in the articular cartilage in patients with JIA [41]. Articular cartilage is normally seen as an anechoic structure with a smooth outline over the bone surfaces. Although US is a valid tool for assessing cartilage in JIA patients, it should be taken into account that cartilage thickness is affected by several non-disease-related factors, including maturation, pubertal stage, height, weight and BMI [68, 69]. Further, owing to different aforementioned factors, either the B-mode or PDUS evaluation of cartilage should be carefully performed in children [70-72].

Cartilage edema in early stages of JIA can be detected sonographically as thickening of the articular cartilage. Chronic inflammation of the cartilage results in permanent damage to the articular surface, observed as blurring of the articular surface. Continued destruction of the cartilage is seen as pitting of the articular surface and thinning of the cartilage [37].

The reliability of the assessment of cartilage thickness with US has been demonstrated [73, 74].

## Bone erosions

Studies evaluating long-term outcome of JIA have shown that a relevant proportion of patients may develop progressive joint destruction and serious physical disability [75]. The development of erosions early in the disease course has been associated with a higher risk of progressive disease and has been included among the poor prognostic indicators of long-term outcome [76, 77]. With the advent of new disease-modifying therapy for JIA, early detection of damage and aggressive disease control can decrease the chance of further disability.

In this sense, conventional radiography is quite insensitive as it usually shows late and often irreversible signs of bone erosion [78]. Over the last few years, several studies in JIA have confirmed that US is more sensitive than radiographs for detection of bone erosions [68, 75-77]. This higher sensitivity in detection of erosions depends both on the high resolution and on the possibility of carrying out multiplanar examination.

In adults, the joint cartilage surface is not vascularised, protecting the underlying cortex from inflammation-driven destructive processes [40]. Accordingly, bone erosions in adults are typically marginal. However, in children the epiphyses are vascularised, and metaphyseal and epiphyseal vessels anastomose through the growth plate. Consequently, inflammation affecting the epiphyseal cartilage can readily spread to the ossification center, causing excessive growth, deformities or destruction with epiphyseal erosions, rather than marginal erosions [79].

On US, bone erosions can sensitively be visualized as interruption of the smooth, continuous hyperechogenic line corresponding to the bony cortex [75]. For sure, US can not detect erosions whereby sound waves fail to have access to certain areas/joints or intramedullary lesions [75, 80]. Again, the unique anatomy of growing children makes assessment of erosive changes challenging, since the presence of physiological bone irregularities in recently ossified bones can be misinterpreted as cortical erosions.

## Local injections

Aspiration and steroid injection are frequently used in the treatment of JIA [81]. To improve accuracy, image-guided interventions are required and, especially for pediatric patients (with small joint size and subcutaneous fat masking the bone landmarks), US is the best available technique.

## REFERENCES

1) Martinoli C, Valle M, Mallatia C, Damasio MB, Tagliafico A. Paediatric musculoskeletal US beyond the hip joint. Pediatr Radiol. 2011; 41: 113-24.
2) Lamer S, Sebag GH. MRI and ultrasound in children with juvenile chronic arthritis. Eur J Radiol. 2000; 33: 85-93.
3) Martinoli C, Valle M. Pediatric musculoskeletal ultrasound. In: Bianchi S, Martinoli C, editors. Ultrasound of the musculoskeletal system. 1st ed. Berlin: Springer; 2007.
4) American Institute of Ultrasound in Medicine. AIUM practice guideline for the performance of an ultrasound examination for detection and assessment of developmental dysplasia of the hip. J Ultrasound Med. 2013; 32: 1307-17.

5) Graf R. The diagnosis of congenital hip-joint dislocation by the ultrasonic Combound treatment. Arch Orthop Trauma Surg. 1980; 97: 117-33.
6) Graf R. Fundamentals of sonographic diagnosis of infant hip dysplasia. J Pediatr Orthop. 1984; 4: 735-40.
7) Graf R. Guide to sonography of the infant hip. Stuttgart: Thieme; 1987.
8) Harcke HT, Grissom LE. Performing dynamic sonography of the infant hip. AJR Am J Roentgenol. 1990; 155: 837-44.
9) Graf R, Mohajer M, Plattner F. Hip sonography update. Quality-management, catastrophes - tips and tricks. Med Ultrason. 2013; 15: 299-303.
10) Rosendahl K, Toma P. Ultrasound in the diagnosis

of developmental dysplasia of the hip in newborns. The European approach. A review of methods, accuracy and clinical validity. Eur Radiol. 2007; 17: 1960-7.

11) Koşar P, Ergun E, Unlübay D, Koşar U. Comparison of morphologic and dynamic US methods in examination of the newborn hip. Diagn Interv Radiol. 2009; 15: 284-9.

12) Shorter D, Hong T, Osborn DA. Screening programmes for developmental dysplasia of the hip in newborn infants. Cochrane Database Syst Rev. 2011; 9: CD004595.

13) Muça-Perja M, Riva S, Grochowska B, Mangiafico L, Mago D, Gringeri A. Musculoskeletal ultrasonography of haemophilic arthropathy. Haemophilia. 2012; 18: 364-8.

14) Martinoli C, Della Casa Alberighi O, Di Minno G, Graziano E, Molinari AC, Pasta G, et al. Development and definition of a simplified scanning procedure and scoring method for Haemophilia Early Arthropathy Detection with Ultrasound (HEAD-US). Thromb Haemost. 2013; 109: 1170-9.

15) Pillen S, van Alfen N. Skeletal muscle ultrasound. Neurol Res. 2011; 33: 1016-24.

16) Pillen S, Scholten RR, Zwarts MJ, Verrips A. Quantitative skeletal muscle ultrasonography in children with suspected neuromuscular disease. Muscle Nerve. 2003; 27: 699-705.

17) Pillen S, Arts IM, Zwarts MJ: Muscle ultrasound in neuromuscular disorders. Muscle Nerve. 2008; 37: 679-93.

18) Draghi F, Danesino GM, Coscia D, Precerutti M, Pagani C. Overload syndromes of the knee in adolescents: sonographic findings. J Ultrasound. 2008; 11: 151-7.

19) De Flaviis L, Nessi R, Scaglione P, Balconi G, Albisetti W, Derchi LE. Ultrasonic diagnosis of Osgood-Schlatter and Sinding-Larsen-Johansson diseases of the knee. Skelet Radiol. 1989; 18: 193-7.

20) Ducher G, Cook J, Spurrier D, Coombs P, Ptasznik R, Black J, et al. Ultrasound imaging of the patellar tendon attachment to the tibia during puberty, a 12-month follow-up in tennis players. Scand J Med Sci Sports. 2010; 20: 35-40.

21) Ducher G, Cook J, Lammers G, Coombs P, Ptasznik R, Black J, et al. The ultrasound appearance of the patellar tendon attachment to the tibia in young athletes is conditional on gender and pubertal stage. J Sci Med Sport. 2010; 13: 20-3.

22) Sailly M, Whiteley R, Johnson A. Doppler ultrasound and tibial tuberosity maturation status predicts pain in adolescent male athletes with Osgood-Schlatter's disease: a case series with comparison group and clinical interpretation. Br J Sports Med. 2013; 47: 93-7.

23) Roth J, diGeso L. Power and colour Doppler findings in lower extremity entheses of healthy children - effect of measurement distance from insertion and joint position. Arthritis Rheumatol. 2014; 66 Suppl S3: S45.

24) Martinoli C, Garello I, Marchetti A, Palmieri F, Altafini L, Valle M, et al. Hip ultrasound. Eur J Radiol. 2012; 81: 3824-31.

25) Futami T, Kasahara Y, Suzuki S, Ushikubo S, Tsuchiya T. Ultrasonography in transient synovitis and early Perthes' disease. J Bone Joint Surg Br. 1991; 73: 635-9.

26) Robben SG, Lequin MH, Diepstraten AF, den Hollander JC, Entius CA, Meradji M. Anterior joint capsule of the normal hip and in children with transient synovitis: US study with anatomic and histologic correlation. Radiology. 1999; 210: 499-507.

27) Bickerstaff DR, Neal LM, Booth AJ, Brennan PO, Bell MJ. Ultrasound examination of the irritable hip. J Bone Joint Surg Br. 1990; 72: 549-53.

28) Kocher MS, Zurakowki D, Kasser JR. Differentiating between septic arthritis and transient synovitis of the hip in children: An evidence-based clinical prediction algorithm. J Bone Joint Surg Am. 1999; 81: 1662-70.

29) Gill K. Pediatric hip: Pearls and pitfalls. Semin Musculoskelet Radiol. 2013; 17: 328-38.

30) Buchmann RF, Jaramillo D. Imaging of articular disorders in children. Radiol Clin North Am. 2004; 42: 151-68.

31) Martini A. Systemic juvenile idiopathic arthritis. Autoimmun Rev. 2012; 12: 56-9.

32) Petty RE, Southwood TR, Manners P, Baum J, Glass DN, Goldenberg J, et al. International League of Associations for Rheumatology classification of juvenile idiopathic arthritis: second revision, Edmonton, 2001. J Rheumatol. 2004; 31: 390-2.

33) Collado P, Jousse-Joulin S, Alcalde M, Naredo E, D'Agostino MA. Is ultrasound a validated imaging tool for the diagnosis and management of synovitis in juvenile idiopathic arthritis? A systematic literature review. Arthritis Care Res. 2012; 64: 1011-9.

34) Ramos PC, Ceccarelli F, Jousse-Joulin S. Role of ultrasound in the assessment of juvenile idiopathic arthritis. Rheumatology. 2012; 51 Suppl 7: vii10-2.

35) Lanni S, Wood M, Ravelli A, Magni Manzoni S, Emery P, Wakefield RJ. Towards a role of ultrasound in children with juvenile idiopathic arthritis. Rheumatology. 2013; 52: 413-20.

36) Ozçakar L, Tok F, De Muynck M, Vanderstraeten G. Musculoskeletal ultrasonography in physical and rehabilitation medicine. J Rehabil Med. 2012; 44: 310-8.

37) Tok F, Demirkaya E, Ozçakar L. Musculoskeletal ultrasound in pediatric rheumatology. Pediatr Rheumatol Online J. 2011; 9: 25.

38) Laurell L, Court-Payen M, Boesen M, Fasth A. Imaging in juvenile idiopathic arthritis with a focus on ultrasonography. Clin Exp Rheumatol. 2013; 31: 135-48.

39) De Muynck M, Parlevliet T, De Cock K, Vanden Bossche L, Vanderstraeten G, Özçakar L. Musculoskeletal ultrasound for interventional physiatry. Eur J Phys Rehabil Med. 2012; 48: 675-87.

40) Breton S, Jousse-Joulin S, Finel E, Marhadour T, Colin D, de Parscau L, et al. Imaging approaches for evaluating peripheral joint abnormalities in juvenile idiopathic arthritis. Semin Arthritis Rheum. 2012; 41: 698-711.

41) Damasio MB, Malattia C, Martini A, Tomà P. Synovial and inflammatory diseases in childhood: role of new imaging modalities in the assessment of patients with juvenile idiopathic arthritis. Pediatr Radiol. 2010; 40: 985-98.

42) Magni-Manzoni S, Epis O, Ravelli A, Klersy C, Veisconti C, Lanni S, et al. Comparison of clinical versus ultrasound-determined synovitis in juvenile idiopathic arthritis. Arthritis Rheum. 2009; 61: 1497-504.

43) Haslam KE, McCann LJ, Wyatt S, Wakefield RJ. The detection of subclinical synovitis by ultrasound in oligoarticular juvenile idiopathic arthritis: a pilot study. Rheumatology. 2010; 49: 123-7.

44) Rebollo-Polo M, Koujok K, Weisser C, Jurencak R, Bruns A, Roth J. Ultrasound findings on patients with juvenile idiophatic arthritis in clinical remission. Arthritis Care Res. 2011; 63: 1013-9.

45) Lovell DJ, Giannini EH, Reiff A, Cawkwell GD, Silverman ED, Nocton JJ, et al. Etanercept in children with polyarticular juvenile rheumatoid arthritis. Pediatric Rheumatology Collaborative Study Group. N Engl J Med. 2000; 342: 763-9.

46) Giannini EH, Brewer EJ, Kuzmina N, Shaikov A, Maximov A, Vorontsov I, et al. Methotrexate in resistant juvenile rheumatoid arthritis. Results of the USA-USSR double-blind, placebo-controlled trial. The Pediatric Rheumatology Collaborative Study Group and the Cooperative Children's Study Group. N Engl J Med. 1992; 326: 1043-9.

47) Ruperto N, Murray KJ, Gerloni V, Wulffraat N, de Oliveira SK, Falcini F, et al. Pediatric Rheumatology International Trials Organization. A randomized trial of parenteral methotrexate comparing an intermediate dose with a higher dose in children with juvenile idiopathic arthritis who failed to respond to standard doses of methotrexate. Arthritis Rheum. 2004; 50: 2191-201.

48) Kane D, Grassi W, Sturrock R, Balint PV. Musculoskeletal ultrasound - a state of the art review in rheumatology. Part 2: Clinical indications for musculoskeletal ultrasound in rheumatology. Rheumatology. 2004; 43: 829-38.

49) El-Miedany YM, Housny IH, Mansour HM, Mourad HG, Mehanna AM, Megeed MA. Ultrasound versus MRI in the evaluation of juvenile idiopathic arthritis of the knee. Joint Bone Spine. 2001; 68: 222-30.

50) Wakefield RJ, Balint PV, Szkudlarek M, Filippucci E, Backhaus M, D'Agostino MA, et al. OMERACT 7 Special Interest Group. Musculoskeletal ultrasound including definitions for ultrasonographic pathology. J Rheumatol. 2005; 32: 2485-7.

51) Backhaus M, Burmester GR, Gerber T, Grassi W, Machold KP, Swen WA, et al. Working Group for Musculoskeletal Ultrasound in the EULAR Standing Committee on International Clinical Studies including Therapeutic Trials. Guidelines for musculoskeletal ultrasound in rheumatology. Ann Rheum Dis. 2001; 60: 641-9.

52) Sparchez M, Fodor D, Miu N. The role of power Doppler ultrasonography in comparison with biological markers in the evaluation of disease activity in juvenile idiopathic arthritis. Med Ultrason. 2010; 12: 97-103.

53) Shahin AA, Shaker OG, Kamal N, Hafez HA, Gaber W, Shahin HA. Circulating interleukin-6, soluble interleukin-2 receptors, tumor necrosis factor alpha, and interleukin-10 levels in juvenile chronic arthritis: correlations with soft tissue vascularity assessed by power Doppler sonography. Rheumatol Int. 2002; 22: 84-8.

54) Eich GF, Hallé F, Hodler J, Seger R, Willi UV. Juvenile chronic arthritis: imaging of the knees and hips before and after intra-articular steroid injection. Pediatr Radiol. 1994; 24: 558-63.

55) Sureda D, Quiroga S, Arnal C, Boronat M, Andreu J, Casas L. Juvenile rheumatoid arthritis of the knee. Evaluation with US. Radiology. 1994; 190: 403-6.

56) Müller LS, Avenarius D, Damasio B, Eldevik OP, Malattia C, Lambot-Juhan K, et al. The paediatric wrist revisited: redefining MR findings in healthy children. Ann Rheum Dis. 2011; 70: 605-10.

57) Szkudlarek M, Court-Payen M, Jacobsen S, Klarlund M, Thomsen HS, Ostergaard M. Interobserver agreement in ultrasonography of the finger and toe joints in rheumatoid arthritis. Arthritis Rheum. 2003; 48: 955-62.

58) Kane D, Balint PV, Sturrock RD. Ultrasonography is superior to clinical examination in the detection and localization of knee joint effusion in rheumatoid arthritis. J Rheumatol. 2003; 30: 966-71.

59) Frosch M, Foell D, Ganser G, Roth J. Arthrosonography of hip and knee joints in the follow up of juvenile rheumatoid arthritis. Ann Rheum Dis. 2003; 62: 242-4.

60) Raza K, Lee CY, Pilling D, Heaton S, Situnayake RD, Carruthers DM, et al. Ultrasound guidance allows accurate needle placement and aspiration

from small joints in patients with early inflammatory arthritis. Rheumatology. 2003; 2: 976-9.

61) Resnick D, Niwayama G. Entheses and enthesopathy. Anatomical, pathological, and radiological correlation. Radiology. 1983; 146: 1-9.

62) Jousse-Joulin S, Breton S, Cangemi C, Fenoll B, Bressolette L, de Parscau L, et al. Ultrasonography for detecting enthesitis in juvenile idiopathic arthritis. Arthritis Care Res. 2011; 63: 849-55.

63) D'agostino MA, Aegerter P, Jousse-Joulin S, Chary-Valckenaere I, Lecoq B, Gaudin P, et al. How to evaluate and improve the reliability of power Doppler ultrasonography for assessing enthesitis in spondylarthritis. Arthritis Rheum. 2009; 61: 61-9.

64) Balint PV, Kane D, Wilson H, McInnes IB, Sturrock RD. Ultrasonography of entheseal insertions in the lower limb in spondyloarthropathy. Ann Rheum Dis. 2002; 61: 905-10.

65) Martino F, Silvestri E, Grassi W, Garlaschi G, Filippucci E, Martinolli C, et al. Pathological findings in rheumatic diseases. In: Martino F, Silvestri E, Grassi W, Garlaschi G, editors. Musculoskeletal sonography. 1st ed. Milano: Springer; 2007.

66) Rooney ME, McAllister C, Burns JF. Ankle disease in juvenile idiopathic arthritis: ultrasound findings in clinically swollen ankles. J Rheumatol. 2009; 36: 1725-9.

67) McGonagle D, Benjamin M. Towards a new clinico-immunopathological classification of juvenile inflammatory arthritis. J Rheumatol. 2009; 36: 1573-4.

68) Ravelli A, Martini A. Early predictors of outcome in juvenile idiopathic arthritis. Clin Exp Rheumatol. 2003; 21: 89-93.

69) Larché MJ, Roth J. Toward standardized ultrasound measurements of cartilage thickness in children. J Rheumatol. 2010; 37: 2445-7.

70) Laurell L, Court-Payen M, Nielsen S, Zak M, Boesen M, Fasth A. Ultrasonography and color Doppler in juvenile idiopathic arthritis: diagnosis and follow-up of ultrasound-guided steroid injection in the ankle region. A descriptive interventional study. Pediatr Rheumatol Online J. 2011; 9: 4.

71) Karmazyn B. Ultrasound of pediatric musculoskeletal disease: from head to toe. Semin Ultrasound CT MR. 2011; 32: 142-50.

72) Shahin AA, el-Mofty SA, el-Sheikh EA, Hafez HA, Ragab OM. Power Doppler sonography in the evaluation and follow-up of knee involvement in patients with juvenile idiopathic arthritis. Z Rheumatol. 2001; 60: 148-155.

73) Spannow AH, Stenboeg E, Pfeiffer-Jensen M, Herlin T. Ultrasound measurement of joint cartilage thickness in large and small joints in healthy children: a clinical pilot study assessing observer variability. Pediatr Rheumatol Online J. 2007; 2: 5-3.

74) Möller B, Bonel H, Rotzetter M, Villiger PM, Ziswiler HR. Measuring finger joint cartilage by ultrasound as a promising alternative to conventional radiograph imaging. Arthritis Rheum. 2009; 61: 435-41.

75) Malattia C, Damasio MB, Magnaguagno F, Pistorio A, Valle M, Martinoli C, et al. Magnetic resonance imaging, ultrasonography, and conventional radiography in the assessment of bone erosions in juvenile idiopathic arthritis. Arthritis Rheum. 2008; 59: 1764-72.

76) Magni-Manzoni S, Rossi F, Pistorio A, Temporini F, Viola S, Beluffi G, et al. Prognostic factors for radiographic progression, radiographic damage, and disability in juvenile idiopathic arthritis. Arthritis Rheum. 2003; 48: 3509-17.

77) Ravelli A, Martini A. Early predictors of outcome in juvenile idiopathic arthritis. Clin Exp Rheumatol. 2003; 21: 89-93.

78) Doria AS, Babyn PS, Feldman B. A critical appraisal of radiographic scoring systems for assessment of juvenile idiopathic arthritis. Pediatr Radiol. 2006; 36: 759-72.

79) Karmazyn B, Bowyer SL, Schmidt KM, Ballinger SH, Buckwalter K, Beam TT. US findings of metacarpophalangeal joints in children with idiopathic juvenile arthritis. Pediatr Radiol. 2007; 37: 475-82.

80) Buchmann RF, Jaramillo D. Imaging of articular disorders in children. Radiol Clin North Am. 2004; 42: 151-68.

81) Bloom BJ, Alario AJ, Miller LC. Intra-articular corticosteroid therapy for juvenile idiopathic arthritis: report of an experiential cohort and literature review. Rheumatol Int. 2011; 31: 749-56.

# Ultrasound Imaging in Orthopaedics

Thierry PARLEVLIET, Luc VANDEN BOSSCHE

**16**

## 16.1 INTRODUCTION

Ultrasound (US) can offer valuable information in the diagnosis and follow-up of various orthopaedic conditions. Further, especially in PRM practice, when rehabilitation after surgery is not progressing as expected, or when prosperous rehabilitation starts to "go wrong", US can really be helpful in the immediate setting. Yet, imaging for such patients may otherwise pose great challenges as regards contrast use for computed tomography (in elderly patients), or magnetic resonance imaging compatibility of the prosthesis.

## 16.2 HETEROTOPIC OSSIFICATION AND MYOSITIS OSSIFICANS

Heterotopic ossification is defined as the formation of lamellar bone in soft tissues outside the skeleton. It most often occurs around joints, as referred to in the old term "periarticular ossification" (Figures 16.1 and 16. 2). Heterotopic ossification is a frequent complication following central nervous system disorders (brain injuries, tumours, encephalitis, spinal cord lesions), multiple injuries, hip surgery, and burns. In addition to this acquired form, hereditary causes also exist (e.g. fibrodysplasia ossificans progressiva).

Heterotopic ossification (HO) has to be distinguished from metastatic calcifications, which mainly occur in hypercalcemia, and dystrophic calcifications in tumors. Moreover, HO must not be confused with traumatic myositis ossificans (MO), a condition in which -after direct injury- ectopic bone is formed within muscles and soft tissues.

Ectopic calcification is characterised by calci-

um deposits rather than new bone formation inside soft tissue structures, usually in response to chemical or physical trauma as in tendinitis calcarea [1]. A limitation of the range of joint motion has serious consequences for the daily functioning of patients. Therefore, prompt diagnosis is mandatory.

Ultrasound detects HO or MO sooner than conventional radiography [2,3]. Moreover, it is the best modality not only for the early identification but also for the follow-up of HO. It has high sensitivity and specificity for the early diagnosis of HO one week after total hip arthroplasty [2-7].

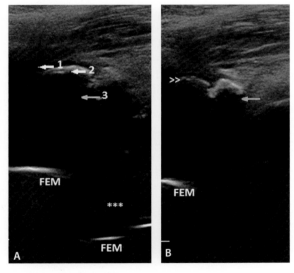

**Figure 16.1**   A - Hip, ventral vertical view. Hypo-hyper-hypo-echoic zone phenomenon (arrows 1, 2, 3) above the femoral head. Heterotopic ossification, onset. Femur prosthesis (FEM) covered by fluid collection (***). B - Hip, slightly more lateral view. Hyperechoic zone (>>) without shadow, leaving the underlying femur (FEM) visible, next to hyperechoic zone (arrow) with shadow. Heterotopic ossification, onset.

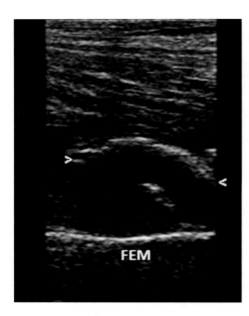

**Figure 16.2** Hip, adductor region, longitudinal view. Hyperechoic zone (> <) without shadow. Heterotopic ossification, onset. FEM, femur.

## 16.2.1 Clinical Diagnosis and Pathology

The initial clinical features of HO are increased joint stiffness, limited range of motion, warmness, swelling and erythema in the affected region. Differentiation between HO and deep venous thrombosis may also be difficult; actually, HO and DVT can often be associated as well. Because of their mass effect and local inflammatory reaction and,

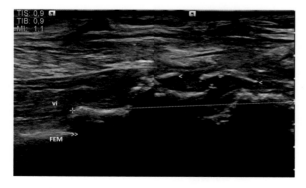

**Figure 16.3** Femur longitudinal view (split image). A 5 cm long (between + +) very irregular hyperechoic zone in vastus intermedius (vi), with complete shadow ( >>) on the femur cortex (FEM). Myositis ossificans. There are also some hyperechoic zones (<) without shadow.

due to swelling and venous compression, HO may give rise to phlebitis [8].

On the other hand, MO often occurs after muscular or soft tissue trauma, usually in sports. It has the highest rate of incidence among adolescents and young adults. The large muscle groups of the thigh and upper arms are areas with increased susceptibility for developing MO. The clinical signs and symptoms associated with MO include tenderness, swelling, muscle hardening within 2-8 weeks after the injury [9-12].

Concerning pathogenesis, HO and MO are fundamentally different. In HO, mature lamellar bone is observed, surrounded by a capsule of compressed muscle fibers and connective tissue. It is suggested that bone forms in connective tissue between muscle planes and not in the muscle itself. Mature HO shows cancellous bone and mature lamellar bone with blood vessels and bone marrow with only a small amount of hematopoiesis [1].

Herewith, MO is a pseudo-inflammatory tumor in the skeletal muscle and corresponds to a heterotopic, metaplastic, non-malignant bone tumor [13, 14] (Figure 16.3). MO develops secondary to a muscular trauma whereby the presentation is mostly an inflammatory, rapidly growing painful muscular mass [13, 15]. These ossifications are similar to HO but should be distinguished from soft tissue ossifications by other causes, e.g. periarticular ossifications (paraosteoarthropathies) that usually occur in a context of central neurologic pathologies, burns, total hip arthroplasty, and long term mechanical ventilation.

Heterotopic ossification and myositis ossificans develop in three characteristic phases the "zone phenomenon". The acute phase lasts one week. The proliferation is composed of mesenchymal cells secreting a myxoid matrix as well as fibroblasts exhibiting numerous mitoses, which gives it a pseudo-fibrosarcomatous appearance [16]. The subacute phase takes about 10 days, with differentiation of the fibroblasts into osteoblasts and secretion of an osteoid matrix at the periphery of the initial myxoid zone (pseudo-osteosarcomatous appearance) [16]. The last phase (maturation phase) starts between the second and fifth weeks of evolution. Bone production can be observed at the periphery of the lesion. Later on fatty metaplastic evolution can also appear at the lesion centre [16].

## 16.2.2 Ultrasound Diagnosis

Ultrasound is the most sensitive imaging tool to depict the early zone phenomenon in bone formation. Often fluid can be detected in the joint as well. US demonstrates the characteristic findings before de novo ossifications can be reported by other diagnostic modalities [17]. Thomas et al. described three concentric zones, corresponding to the described MO zones. The first more peripheral is hypoechoic and encircles the lesion with contiguous hyperemia. The second, thinner zone is hyperechoic and corresponds to the ossifications. The third and central zone is hypoechoic and corresponds to the central stromal fibroblastic component [17]. Due to this bone formation, MO and HO show a hyperechoic area with acoustic shadowing and the bony margins of the underlying skeletal structures become irregular or even undetectable.

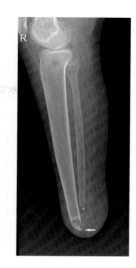

**Figure 16.4** X-Ray of amputation stump in a 17-year old girl. Orthotopic bony overgrowth (arrow) distally on the tibia. Several surgical clips are present.

## 16.3 ORTHOTOPIC OSSIFICATION OR ORTHOTOPIC BONY OVERGROWTH

In rehabilitation medicine, physicians are frequently confronted with amputee patients complaining of stump pain, the causes of which can be widely divergent. The diagnosis is not always straightforward and the treatment is still controversial.

Bony overgrowth of the residual limb after an amputation is a well-documented complication in the pediatric amputee population (Figures 16.4 and 16.5). It can cause pain, problems with skin breakdown and poor prosthetic fit [18]. Also in adult amputees, bony overgrowth is reported more and more frequently; however its prevalence may well be underestimated because symptoms arise more slowly. Because of the high prevalence of bony overgrowth in juvenile amputees, a prophylactic capping procedure during primary construction of the stump is justified. Simple resection is only indicated in adults and in adolescents having almost skeletal maturity, or in case of an infected primary amputation.

The clinical findings are usually non-specific (redness, swelling, pain). Imaging is thus essential in the diagnosis of amputation stump pain. The causes of stump pain can be due to extrinsic and intrinsic causes. The former (prosthesis-induced

pain) comprises improper prosthetic fit or uneven loading leading to bursitis, soft-tissue inflamma-

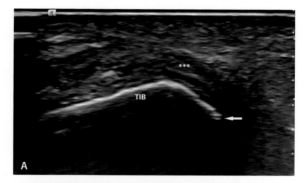

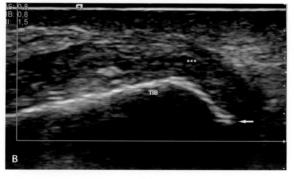

**Figure 16.5** A - Ultrasound image of same patient. Remark the sharp bony ending (arrow) which suggests bony overgrowth. TIB, tibia; ***, overlying muscle. B - This is often associated with neovascularization, but not in this patient.

tion, stress fractures, bruising and skin breakdown. The second group includes intrinsic causes of stump pain, i.e. primarily originating in the stump itself, e.g. osteomyelitis, neuroma, aggressive bone edges, heterotopic ossifications and bony overgrowth (orthotopic ossification).

Radiography with the prosthesis in a weight-bearing position allows to functionally assess the relation between the soft tissues, bone and prosthesis. Complementary US will demonstrate soft-tissue complications such as abscesses and fluid collections, inflammatory changes, tumors, neuroma and beginning of bony overgrowth.

Clinically the overgrowth phenomenon can be observed as a disproportionate growth between the bony stump end and the soft tissue covering. The distal end of bone elongates with gradual stretching of the distal skin, which becomes reddened, irritated and secondarily infected. The sharp bone end does not push the distal skin ahead of it, but rather becomes fixed to the distal soft tissues, eventually protrudes through them, and a chronic infection results [19].

## 16.4 TRAUMATIC NEUROMA

Neuromas are common causes of residual limb pain in amputees. They cause pain and altered sensation along the course of the affected nerve. As such, an amputee can have pain during prosthetic design, fitting and gait rehabilitation or standing. Neuromas are formed after trauma (major trauma or repetitive microtrauma) and they are often connected to bony spurs or are terminating in scar tissue (Figures 16.6 and 16.7).

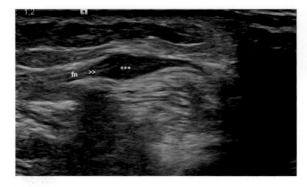

**Figure 16.6** Same patient, longitudinal view of fibular nerve (fn) ending. Remark the swollen, hypoechoic nerve ending (***), with a "rat tale" (>>) going in.

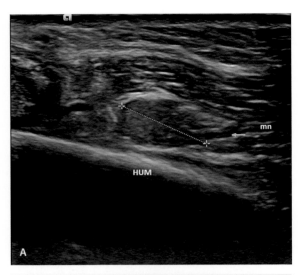

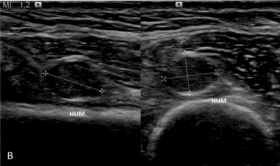

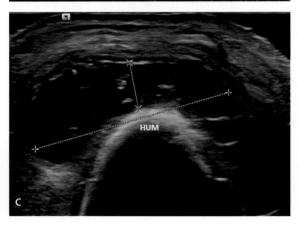

**Figure 16.7** A - Upper arm amputation, longitudinal view of the stump. Hypoechoic bulbous nerve ending (between + +), with the "rat tale" (arrow) of the median nerve (mn) going in. HUM, humerus. B - Same patient, longitudinal and axial view of amputation stump. Remark the hypoechoic bulbous nerve ending (between + +) surrounded by a hyperechoic layer of connective tissue. HUM, humerus. C - Same patient, distal axial view of the amputation stump. There is a big anechoic fluid collection (between + +), with multiple inclusions, covering the humerus (HUM).

Neuromas can present in different ways; mushroom form, lobulated, radiating network of tiny nerves etc. Typical for traumatic neuromas are the non-organised neural bundles that grow from the end of the injured nerve.

On US, the nerve fascicles are seen as hypoechoic bands in longitudinal view. In axial or transverse scan, hypoechoic dots surrounded by hyperechoic connective tissue are observed.

In case of a neuroma, swollen and hypoechoic nerve ending is seen, the bulbous end often arising from the nerve sheath.

## 16.5 ULTRASOUND EVALUATION AFTER HIP REPLACEMENT/ RESURFACING

The most common application for US after arthroplasty is the detection of effusion. In addition, establishing the cause of pain in patients with hip arthroplasty can be challenging: there are numerous possible causes of pain including both intrinsic (e.g. infection, wear debris synovitis, loosening) and extrinsic reasons (e.g. iliopsoas tendinosis, gluteus tendon abnormality, trochanteric pain). Computed tomography and magnetic resonance imaging can cause artefacts due to the prosthetic components which may limit image interpretation [20]. As such, US is an excellent technique to evaluate the soft tissues around the hip. It has the additional advantage of dynamic examination and Doppler imaging for neovascularity. Moreover, US is not affected by metallic artefacts as much as the aforementioned techniques, and lesions lying close to metals can be assessed.

### 16.5.1 Effusion

Ultrasound is a sensitive imaging technique for evaluating hip joint effusion, with sensitivities reported up to 92% [21, 22]. Hip effusions on US are seen as hypoechoic or anechoic fluid that anteriorly displaces the joint capsule or pseudocapsule from the cortex of the femoral neck [23] (Figure 16.8). Van Holsbeeck et al. [23] found that the distance between the anterior pseudocapsule and the anterior cortex of the femur is normally less than 3.2 mm and that patients with infected hip replacements had large joint effusions with a mean capsule-to-bone distance of 10.2 mm. These are not absolute quantifiable criteria for diagnosing the effusion be-

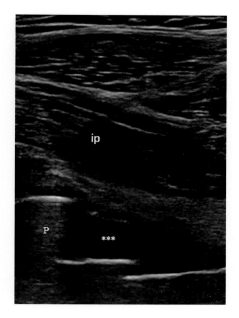

**Figure 16.8** Hip, ventral vertical view. Hypoechoic appearance of fluid (***) within the hip joint. P, hip prosthetic material; ip, iliopsoas muscle.

cause others found no difference in size of the distension of the anterior recess of the joint capsule [24]. While differentiation between septic and aseptic effusions is not always easy, US guided aspirations can relieve pain and also be used for further laboratory analysis. Lastly, checking for fluid at the region of the surgical scar is also noteworthy.

### 16.5.2 Solid and Cystic Periprosthetic Masses

Solid and cystic periprosthetic masses can be seen following hip replacements [25]. The exact cause still remains uncertain but is believed to be related to elevated wear of the material. That is also why they are called reactive masses or pseudotumors. The symptoms usually range from minor discomfort to disabling pain, sometimes they may be asymptomatic as well [26]. These masses appear either as solid structures anterior to the joint or as cystic lesions arising from the posterior joint space. US shows a hypoechoic lesion with little or no internal vascularity on Doppler imaging (Figure 16.9). When deeply localized, it may be difficult to differentiate between solid and cystic lesions. A practical tip would be to palpate with the probe, trying to displace fluid from one part of the lesion to another, proving its

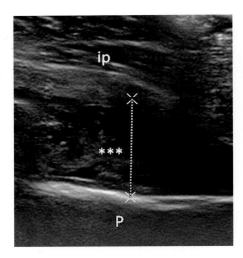

**Figure 16.9** Hip, ventral vertical view. Hyperechoic structure within the hip joint (***). The complete proximal joint space is filled (dotted line). P, hip prosthetic material; ip, iliopsoas muscle.

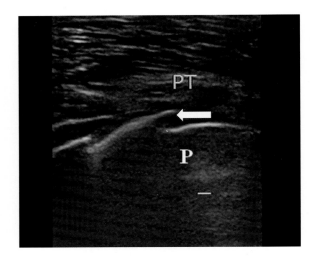

**Figure 16.10** Hip, ventral vertical view. Psoas tendon friction against hip prosthetic material (arrow). PT, psoas tendon; P, prosthetic material.

cystic nature. This may not be possible if the fluid is under pressure though.

### 16.5.3 Iliopsoas Tendon Pathology

Iliopsoas tendon pathology is a known extrinsic cause of hip pain after hip replacement. It is usually caused by impingement or friction of the posterior aspect of the tendon on the anterior aspect of the acetabular or femoral head component of the prosthetic material, but has also been reported in patients without definite contact of the tendon with the component [27]. On US, the symptomatic tendon appears as thickened with or without hypoechogenicity. A possible scanning plane to demonstrate such impingement is the long-axis along the iliopsoas tendon, although the short-axis view is also used (Figure 16.10). As a result of local repetitive friction an inflammatory reaction and effusion in the bursa can occur. In long lasting conditions, attritional wear can lead to tendon thinning and even full thickness tear.

### 16.6 ABSCESS

A likely complication in the immediate postoperative period is abscess formation. Its appearance on US is quite variable in echotexture, ranging from an anechoic to irregularly hyperechoic structure with or without hyperechoic sediment, septae or even gas (Figure 16.11). The shape may be round and generally well-defined to irregularly lobulated. In most cases, an abscess is seen as a fluid-filled hypoechoic structure with posterior acoustic enhancement. In the centre, there may be variable amounts of echogenic debris. A slight pressure may help to confirm the liquid nature of the mass. Doppler imaging is helpful in identifying hyperemia at the abscess wall, internal septa and surrounding tissues [28].

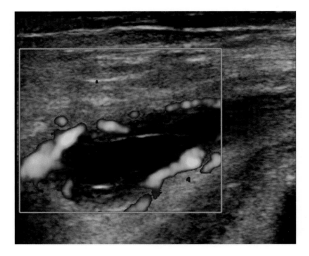

**Figure 16.11** Abscess: hypoechoic mass with irregular margins. Marked peripheral hypervascularity on power Doppler.

## 16.7 FOREIGN BODIES

Foreign bodies are common problems in musculoskeletal practice. Mostly found are wood, glass or metallic objects. They can be found in the soft tissue after a penetrating skin or traumatic injury (or postoperatively metal components). It is important not to overlook foreign bodies because they can otherwise trigger a granulomatous reaction, secondary soft-tissue infection or an eventual abscess. Therefore, an early diagnosis and removal of the foreign body is necessary to prevent these complications. It is also necessary to examine a wide area around the wound as foreign bodies may migrate away from the penetration site.

In this sense, US is an excellent imaging modality for detecting foreign bodies of the musculoskeletal system [29]. The appearance on US varies greatly depending on its nature (metal, glass, wood, etc.), shape and size [30]. The echogenicity of a foreign body is mostly hyperechogenic and the body produces a posterior acoustic shadowing (in case of wood) or reverberations and comet tail artifacts (in case of glass or metal) (Figure 16.12).

These findings are not specific, but can help to identify even small fragments that would otherwise be missed. When an inflammatory reaction occurs around the foreign body (i.e. granulation tissue), a hypoechoic halo surrounding the body can be found, also showing hypervascularity on Doppler imaging. Once the foreign body is detected, the relationship with adjacent tendons, nerves and vessels can necessarily be defined as well. Measuring the depth of the foreign body and marking the skin overlying the fragment would be helpful for navigating the surgeon.

## 16.8 ULTRASOUND AFTER TENDON REPAIR

Ultrasound of a repaired tendon can show variable echogenicity varying from hypo- to hyperechoic. Mostly a persistent swelling of the sutured

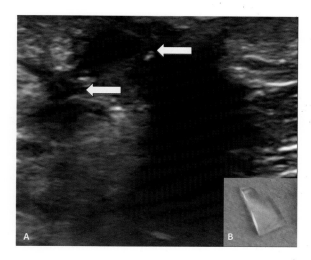

**Figure 16.12**    A - Foreign body (glass) in the subcutaneous tissues is located between the two arrows and surrounded by a hypoechoic halo. B - Glass fragment after removal.

tendon will be found even years after the tendon repair. It is important to distinguish a postoperative tendon from recurrent tendon tear. US can show an obvious gap or disruption whereby suture materials can exhibit acoustic shadowing. Additionally, dynamic US imaging can be effectively used to differentiate between tendon rupture or sticking when there is lack of gliding in the early postoperative period.

The postoperative rotator cuff is abnormally echogenic and can be very similar in appearance to a small rotator cuff tear in non-operated patients [31]. Sonographic evaluation of repaired rotator cuff at or near the 3rd post-operative month may be as important as the clinical examination due to limited motions and pain. The majority of recurrent rotator cuff tears occur within the first 3 months of surgical repair [32]. Although it tends to decrease over time, increased thickness of repaired supraspinatus tendon may persist even 9 months after surgery [33, 34]. The suture material(s), although absorbable, can be visible even after long periods.

# REFERENCES

1) Vanden Bossche L, Vanderstraeten G. Heterotopic ossification: a review. J Rehabil Med. 2005; 37: 129-36.

2) Pistarini C, Carlevati S, Contardi A. The echographic diagnosis of neurogenic paraosteoarthropathies in myelosis patients. G Ital Med Lav. 1993; 15: 159-3.

3) Snoecx M, De Muynck M, Van Laere M. Association between muscle trauma and heterotopic ossification in spinal cord injured patients: reflections on their causal relationship and the diagnostic value of ultrasonography. Paraplegia. 1995; 33: 464-8.

4) Pistarini C, Carlevati S, Contardi A, Cannizzaro G. Use of ultrasonography methods in the diagnosis of neurogenic paraosteoarthropathy in spinal cord injury. Recenti Prog Med. 1995; 86: 483-8.

5) Cassar-Pullicino VN, McClelland M, Badwan DA, McCall IW, Pringle RG, el Masry W. Sonographic diagnosis of heterotopic bone formation in spinal injury patients. Paraplegia. 1993; 31: 40-50.

6) Thomas EA, Cassar-Pullicino VN, Mc Call IW. The role of ultrasound in the early diagnosis and management of heterotopic bone formation. Clin Radiol. 1991; 43: 190-6.

7) Popken F, Konig DP, Tantow M, Rutt J, Kausch T, Peters KM. Possibility of sonographic early diagnosis of heterotopic ossification after total hip replacement. Unfallchirurg. 2003; 106: 28-31.

8) Colachis SC, Clinchot DM, Venesy D. Neurovascular complications of heterotopic ossification following spinal cord injury. Paraplegia. 1993; 31: 51-7.

9) Massey GV, Kuhn JG, Nog J, Spmottswood SE, Narla LD, Russel EC. Case report: the spectrum of myositis ossificans in haemophilia. Haemophilia. 2004; 10: 189-3.

10) Beiner JM, Joki P. Muscle contusion injury and myositis ossificans traumatica. Clin Orthop Relat Res. 2002; 403: 110-9.

11) Wieder DL. Treatment of traumatic myositis ossificans with acetic acid iontophoresis. Phys Ther. 1992; 72: 133-7.

12) Smith TO, Hunt NJ, Wood SJ. The physiotherapy management of muscle haematomas. Phys Ther Sport. 2006; 7: 201-9.

13) Kransdorf MJ, Meis JM. From the archives of the AFIP. Extraskeletal osseous and cartilaginous tumors of the extremities. Radiographics. 1993; 13: 853-84.

14) Olsen KM, Chew FS. Tumoral calcinosis: Pearls, polemics, and alternative possibilities. Radiographics. 2006; 26: 871-85.

15) Spencer JD, Missen GA. Pseudomalignant heterotopic ossification ("myositis ossificans"). Recurrence after excision with subsequent resorption. J Bone Joint Surg Br. 1989; 71: 317-9.

16) Mirra JM. Osseous soft tumors. In: Mirra JM, Picci P, Gold RH. Bone tumors: Clinical, radiologic and pathologic correlations. London: Lea & Febiger; 1989; p. 1549-86.

17) Thomas EA, Cassar-Pullicino VN, McCall IW. The role of ultrasound in the early diagnosis and management of heterotopic bone formation. Clin Radiol. 1991; 43: 190-6.

18) Dudek NL, DeHaan MN, Marks MB. Bone overgrowth in the adult traumatic amputee. Am J Phys Med Rehabil. 2003; 82: 897-900.

19) Swanson AB. Phocomelia and Congenital Limb Malformations - Surgical Reconstruction and Prosthetic Replacement. Am J Surg. 1965; 109: 294-9.

20) Long SS, Surrey D, Nazarian LN. Common sonographic findings in the painful hip after hip arthroplasty. J Ultrasound Med. 2012; 31: 301-12.

21) Bureau NJ, Chhem RK, Cardinal E. Musculoskeletal infections: US manifestations. Radiographics. 1999; 19: 1585-92.

22) Foldes K, Balint P, Balint G, Buchanan WW. Ultrasound-guided aspiration in suspected sepsis of resection arthroplasty of the hip joint. Clin Rheumatol. 1995; 14: 327-9.

23) Van Holsbeeck MT, Eyler WR, Sherman LS, et al. Detection of infection in loosened hip prostheses: efficacy of sonography. AJR Am J Roentgenol. 1994; 163: 381-4.

24) Weybright PN, Jacobson JA, Murry KH, et al. Limited effectiveness of sonography in revealing hip joint effusion: preliminary results in 21 adult patients, with native and postoperative hip. AJR Am J Roentgenol. 2003; 181: 215-8.

25) Boardmann DR, Middleton FR, Kavanagh TJ. A benign psoas mass following metal on metal resurfacing of the hip. J Bone Joint Surg Br. 2006; 88: 402-4.

26) Kwon YM, Ostlere SJ, McLardy-Smith P, et al. "Asymptomatic" pseudotumors after metal-on-metal hip resurfacing arthroplasty: prevalence and metal ion study. J Arthroplasty. 2010; 26: 511-8.

27) Hanssen AD. Revision total hip arthroplasty: the painful hip. J Bone Joint Surg Am. 2009; 91: 22.

28) Arslan H, Sakarya ME, Bozkurt M, et al. The role of power Doppler sonography in the evaluation of superficial soft tissue abscesses. Eur J Ultrasound. 1998; 8: 101-6.

29) Dean AJ, Gronczewski CA, Costantino TG. Technique for emergency medicine bedside ultrasound identification of a radiolucent foreign body. J Emerg Med. 2003; 24: 303-8.

30) Horton LK, Jacobson JA, Powell A, et al. Sonography and radiography of soft-tissue foreign bodies. AJR Am J Roentgenol. 2001; 176: 1155-9.

31) Crass JR, Craig EV, Feinberg SB. Sonography of the postoperative rotator cuff. AJR Am J Roentgenol. 1986; 146: 561-4.

32) Kluger R, Bock P, Mittlbock M, et al. Longterm survivorship of rotator cuff repairs using ultrasound and magnetic resonance imaging analysis. Am J Sports Med. 2011; 39: 2071-81.

33) Lasbleiz J, Benkalfate T, Morelli JN, Jan J. Sonographic evaluation of the post-operative rotator cuff: Does tendon thickness matter? Open J Clin Diagn. 2013; 3: 78-84.

34) Mafulli N, Dymond NP, Regine R. Surgical repair of ruptured Achilles tendon in sportsmen and sedentary patients: a longitudinal ultrasound assessment. Int J Sports Med. 1990; 11: 78-84.

# Ultrasound Imaging for Tumors

Martine DE MUYNCK, Anne OOMEN

## 17.1 INTRODUCTION

Already in the eighties, ultrasound (US) was used for the initial evaluation and follow-up of soft tissue lesions in the extremities, because of its unique possibility of imaging in various planes, providing a better definition of a lesion [1]. Differentiating cystic structures from solid masses was then described to be an important first step in the working-out. In observing a soft tissue mass, the parameters size, border, topography (depth), and echogenicity have to be studied [1]. Doppler US can be helpful in assessing the vascularity of soft tissue masses, which may be important for diagnosis or presurgical planning [2]. In the follow-up, US may be useful for detecting suspected tumor recurrence, especially in patients who have implanted hardware, and artifact precludes other means of imaging [2]. Ultrasound has also earned a role during rehabilitation and follow-up of these (often young) patients.

## 17.2 ULTRASOUND IN DIAGNOSIS

In the diagnosis of soft tissue masses, first orientation is given by anamnesis and clinical exam.

Anamnesis: age and sex of the patient? How long does the swelling exist? How did it occur: spontaneous appearance or post-trauma? Is it painful? If yes, is there pain during the night? Is the swelling increasing or does it remain *statu quo*? Are there complaints due to compression by the mass? Are there general complaints: fever, loss of weight? Is there a history of former surgery for masses at the same site or at another site? Is there a family history of masses?

Clinical exam: where is the swelling situated? Is it a deep or superficial mass? Is it adherent to the skin? Is there a change in colour of the skin? Is

there pain during palpation? Are there signs of neurovascular compression?

US can be used as the first choice technique for an initial evaluation of a soft tissue swelling. Two important questions to be answered are: "is there a lesion (yes/no)?" and "is it a cyst or a soft tissue mass?". If it is a cyst (see later), examination can often be terminated.

### 17.2.1 Differential Diagnosis between Cystic Lesions and Soft Tissue Masses

A synovial cyst has synovial lining and communicates with a joint cavity (for example at the wrist or at the knee - popliteal cyst) or a tendon sheath, though it can be difficult to visualize this "stem". A ganglion cyst is not a true cyst, since it lacks an epithelial wall. It arises from a joint capsule, a tendon sheath, a ligament or pulley, also often at wrist and hand. Labral and meniscal cysts are also ganglionic.

Cysts contain fluid and are homogeneous, hypo- or an-echoic and have sharp borders (Figure 17.1). Solid structures on the contrary are not

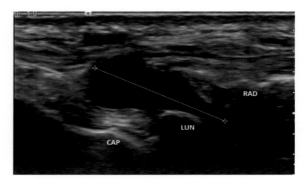

**Figure 17.1** Wrist, dorsal longitudinal view: 13 mm long anechoic cyst between radius (RAD) and lunate (LUN). CAP, capitate.

acoustically homogeneous. There is minimal attenuation of sound waves within a cyst; the area behind the cyst thus will appear bright (posterior enhancement). There is also no internal vascularisation within a cyst (no Doppler signal) (there can be some around it, certainly in ruptured cysts) [3]. However, not all cystic masses can be identified using these criteria and some of these findings can be present in solid soft tissue tumors as well [4]. In a series by Lee et al. [4], the incidence of solid tumors demonstrating cystic appearances on gray scale US was found to be 5.3%. Those tumors were often schwannomas or masses with a fibrous component such as giant cell tumors of tendon sheath. Any solid tumor with a high cell-to-matrix ratio and a homogeneous cellular composition can appear to be well-defined, homogeneous, and hypoechoic with posterior acoustic enhancement [4].

Internal vascularity is not always identified in all soft tissue tumors, certainly not in the small ones (1-2 cm). Appropriate technique and optimization of Doppler parameters are definitely essential. Further, it is important to use a lot of gel and give little transducer pressure so as not to compress the small vessels [4].

Compressibility is another parameter to examine. Non-compressibility is one of the US features of ganglion cysts of the wrist [4]. Compression by the transducer can make internal debris moving, helping to differentiate complex cystic masses such as ruptured cysts, abscesses and bursitis.

## 17.2.2 Differential Diagnosis between Pseudotumors and Tumors

The ratio of malignant/benign soft tissue lesions is about 1/100 [3, 5]. There are more than 80 possible histopathological diagnoses [5]. Giving a complete pictorial essay of tumors is beyond the scope of this chapter. Making a specific diagnosis of a type of soft tissue tumor with US is often impossible, because of the lack of specificity of the exam. However, it is important to be able to differentiate between cyst/tumor and to decide whether a tumor is suspicious and the patient needs to be referred for further assessment/imaging.

Anamnesis, clinical exam, and US are frequently sufficient to differentiate tumor-like lesions or pseudotumors, such as cysts, epidermal inclusion cysts, hematoma, hygroma, abscess, Morton's neuroma (a mechanically induced degenerative neuropathy) [3, 5].

For soft tissue tumors, in 2002 a World Health Organization Classification of Tumors was established [3, 5]. It includes ten groups:
- adipocytic tumors (e.g. lipoma, liposarcoma);
- fibroblastic/myofibroblastic tumors (e. g. nodular fasciitis, myositis ossificans, elastofibroma, musculoskeletal fibromatosis, fibrosarcoma);
- ibrohistiocytic tumors (e.g. giant cell tumour of the tendon sheath, benign fibrous histiocytoma);
- smooth muscle tumors (e.g. leiomyosarcoma);
- pericytic (perivascular) tumors (e.g. glomus tumour);
- skeletal muscle tumors (e.g. rhabdomyosarcoma);
- vascular tumors (e.g. hemangioma);
- chondro-osseous tumors (e.g. extraskeletal osteosarcoma);
- neurogenic tumors (e. g. schwannoma, neurofibroma, malignant peripheral nerve sheath tumor);
- tumors of uncertain differentiation (e.g. synovial sarcoma).

Most *lipomas* are situated in the subcutaneous fat tissue. They are often poorly marginated, and echogenicity can be variable (iso-, hypo-, hyperechogenic in comparison with the surrounding normal fat) (Figure 17.2). They are generally not detectably vascularised. All deep lesions (intra- or inter-muscular) have a chance to be a liposarcoma- the deeper and larger a lesion, the more it is suspicious. Hypervascularity, irregular and thick septations, calcifications and areas of pseudocystic necrosis are also indicative of malignancy [3].

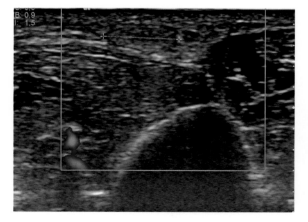

**Figure 17.2**  Same patient as in figures 17.7. Because of history of malignancy, she is worried about a small soft nodule on the forearm. Isoechoic mass compared with the surrounding subcutis, relatively sharp borders and not markedly vascularised: 7 mm long lipoma.

*Elastofibroma dorsi* is located between the chest wall and the inferior scapular angle, underneath the latissimus dorsi muscle. It is thought to be a reaction to repeated mechanical irritation (e.g. using crutches for a long time). On US, it has an ovoid appearance, with alternating hyper-/hypo-echoic layers [5] (Figures 17.3). *Musculoskeletal fibromatosis* is divided into superficial lesions (palmar fibromatosis or Dupuytren disease and plantar fibromatosis or Ledderhose disease) and deep lesions (e.g. fibromatosis colli) [3]. The former ones are seen as hypoechoic nodules with respect to the aponeurosis and they do not infiltrate muscles/subcutaneous fat.

*Giant cell tumor of the tendon sheath* is a common tumor in the hand, in contact with a tendon sheath (so not gliding with the tendon during dynamic evaluation). It is most often homogeneous, hypoechoic and vascularized. There can be cortical erosions underneath [3].

*Glomus tumors* are usually found on the dorsal side of the fingers, under the nail. US can show a sub-ungual hypoechoic mass with hypervascularisation [5].

*Rhabdomyosarcoma* is the most frequent soft tissue tumor in children. It is hypoechoic and will show the characteristics of malignant masses described below [5]. Pathognomonic characteristic of peripheral nerve sheath tumors is their connection with a nerve, with a "rat tail" going in/out of the lesion.

*Schwannomas* lie eccentrically in the nerve; uninvolved fascicles can be found passing the mass. They have sharp borders and are usually hypoechoic, sometimes with a vacuolar (honey-

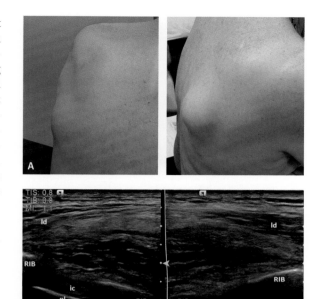

**Figure 17.3** A - Two clinical presentations of elastofibroma dorsi, on the left a more laterally located example than on the right. B - Elastofibroma dorsi, left clinical case. Split image with vertical reconstruction: large oval mass with lamellar hyper-/hypo-echoic aspect, between latissimus dorsi muscle (ld) and ribs (RIB). ic, intercostal muscles; pl, pleura.

comb) aspect. There can be posterior enhancement. Schwannomas are usually vascularized on Doppler US [3] (Figure 17.4). *Neurofibromas*, on

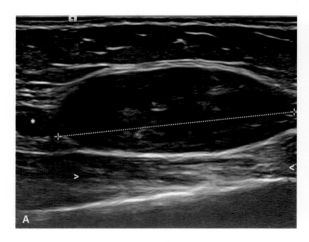
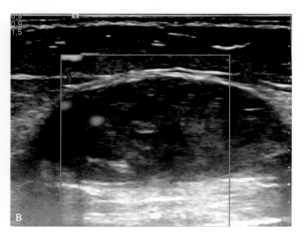

**Figure 17.4** A - A 59-year-old female with known schwannoma in the subcutis of the upper arm: 31 mm long hypoechoic oval mass with vacuolar aspect, in continuity with a nerve (*). There is acoustic enhancement behind it (> <). B - Same mass, with power Doppler signal.

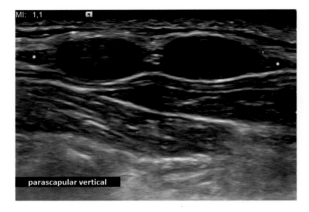

**Figure 17.5** String of pearls: neurofibromata in the subcutis of the parascapular region, in a 16 year old girl with known neurofibromatosis. Two hypoechoic masses, in continuity with a nerve (*).

the contrary, lie concentrically and are less vascularized (Figure 17.5). Multifocal neurofibromas (multiple hypoechoic nodules as well in superficial locations as deeper, in the muscles) and plexiform variants can be present in neurofibromatosis syndromes [3]. *Malignant peripheral nerve sheath tumor* (MPNST) will infiltrate the nerves and thus cause more pain and neurological symptoms.

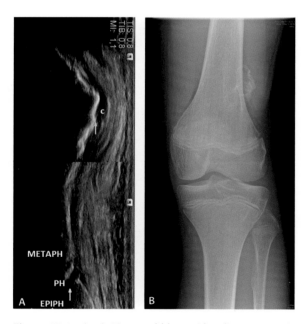

**Figure 17.6** A - A 13-year-old boy with solitary exostosis (arrow) near the physis (PH) of the femur, split image with vertical reconstruction. EPIPH, epiphysis; METAPH, metaphysis; c, small cartilage cap. B - Corresponding radiograph.

In neurofibromatosis, there should be close follow-up mainly in proximal (plexus) lesions that can deteriorate and become MPNST [5].

*Synovial sarcoma* is one of the most common types of soft tissue sarcoma. The name seems misleading, because most of the times it occurs in para-articular tissues (mainly in the lower limbs of young patients). It often is lobulated, inhomogeneous and hypoechoic and vascularized.

Metastases of carcinomas (e. g. hypernephroma, thyroid carcinoma), sarcomas and melanomas usually have unsharp borders, are inhomogeneous and hypoechoic and hypervascularized. Calcifications and pseudocystic necrosis can occur [3, 5].

Bone tumors are classified according to their type of matrix (osteoid, chondroid, fibrous, fatty, or other cell types, like in Ewing sarcoma and metastases).

*Osteochondroma* is the most common of benign bone tumors. It is a cartilage-capped tumor that often appears as a stalk on the surface of the bone [2]. It is probably a developmental malformation rather than a true neoplasm and is usually found in the metaphysis of the distal femur, proximal tibia or proximal humerus (Figure 17.6).

*Multiple hereditary exostoses* is a hereditary disorder characterized by multiple exostoses (multiple osteochondromas). The genetic abnormality results in a defect in the osteoclastic activity at the metaphyseal ends of the bone during the remodeling process in childhood or early adolescence. The metaphyses develop benign bony outgrowths, often capped by cartilage. A small number undergo neoplastic transformation. US can be used for follow-up of the thickness of the cartilage cap (often <1 cm, >2 cm being suspicious for deterioration) and to evaluate complications (e.g. nerve compression) [2].

For malignant bone tumors and metastases, a cortical "break down" with very irregular, interrupted bony edges and sometimes large soft tissue mass with hypervascularization can be visualized with US. Of course, a mass staying well within the boundaries of bone cortex will be out of reach for detection with US.

## 17.2.3 Differential Diagnosis between Benign/Malignant Masses

Malignant tumors are usually inhomogeneous/hypoechoic and often hypervascular. Doppler US imaging allows visualization of flow in small vessels within a mass, but also does not allow to differentiate definitely between benign vs. malignant. Furthermore, US can be used to monitor response of tumor vascularity during therapy.

The center of malignant soft tissue masses often has an increased interstitial pressure with a decrease towards the periphery. Only 1-10% of a tumor's volume is occupied by blood vessels; the rest is filled by connective tissue, separating cancer cells from feeding vessels. This interstitial matrix is generally more extensive in malignant than in benign masses. In this sense, a central region with reduced vascularization and eventual necrosis and a highly vascularized outer rim are characteristic for malignant masses (with malignant anarchic vascular architecture such as trifurcations, loops, corkscrew vessels, stenoses and occlusion) [3, 6] (Figure 17.7). Internal irregular septations, calcifications, pseudocystic necrosis areas also are suspicious. Benign lesions on the contrary have well-arranged and perfused inner areas, and do not exhibit vascularity with an irregular angiogenesis pattern [3, 6].

Most soft tissue tumors are benign, small and superficially located [6]. Only 5% of benign soft tissue masses exceed 5 cm and only 1% are seated underneath the superficial fascia [6].

Hung et al. [7] proposed the following diagnostic criteria for malignant superficial masses: rapid clinical growth, known primary tumor, medium-sized to large tumor, moderate to severe intratu-moral hypervascularity and absence of US features recognized as typical of another specific tumor type (e.g. lipoma, nerve sheath tumor) (Figure 17.8).

All soft tissue masses - that appear suddenly, are painful and more than 5 cm or masses, enlarge, and are symptomatic - should be thoroughly investigated [3].

Measuring the diameter of large tumors (exceeding the length of the probe) is tricky; one should put marks on the skin and measure between these marks. If available, panoramic views offer a solution.

As mentioned before, making a specific diagnosis with US is often impossible, because of the lack of specificity of the exam. Therefore, complementary exams are often required. Magnetic resonance imaging (MRI) is usually the first choice for local staging. It helps to show the relation with surrounding structures (muscles, nerves and vessels, bones and joints). Although it is very useful to characterize certain soft tissue masses (e.g. lipoma, liposarcoma, giant cell tumor of the tendon sheath), other tumors (e.g. fibrosarcoma, leiomyosarcoma and even myositis ossificans) can not be always diagnosed correctly with MRI [3]. Radiography and computed tomography can provide information about calcifications and bone changes, origin or consequence of soft tissue abnormality [5].

Still, despite progress in diagnostic imaging, a correct diagnosis in terms of tumor subtype and

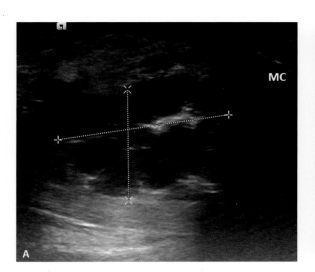 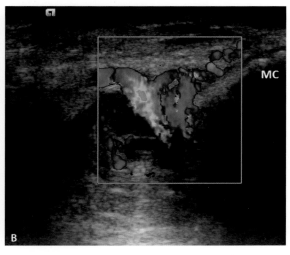

**Figure 17.7** A - A 85-year-old female, operated 6 years before for a chondrosarcoma (amputation of digit and metacarpal 3), pain and swelling in the operated webspace. Hypoechoic lobulated mass: recidive. MC, metacarpal bone. B - Same mass, with color Doppler signal.

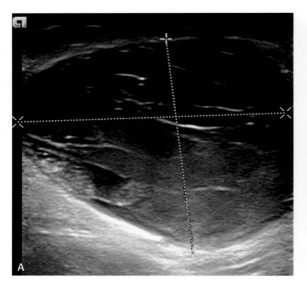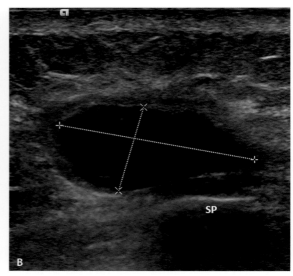

**Figure 17.8** A - A 60-year-old female with known uterine leiomyosarcoma and palpable mass over the spina scapulae: subcutaneous inhomogeneous hypoechoic soft tissue mass, 24x15x12 mm, highly vascularised (not shown): metastasis. B - Three weeks after surgical removal of the metastasis: no detectable mass. Presence of a compressible, anechoic fluid collection 25x23x12 mm, without vascularisation (not shown). SP, spina scapulae.

definition of malignant potential is rarely achieved based on imaging alone [6]. Biopsy taking is the

**Table 17.1**   Use of US in the follow-up of musculoskeletal tumors

**1. Soft tissue tumors**

- Recurrence
- Lymph nodes
- Complications?:
    - fluid collections
    - aspect of muscles

**2. Orthopedic hardware, including prostheses**

- Recurrence/cortical abnormalities
- Metastasis - skip lesions
- Lymph nodes
- Complications?:
    - fluid (loosening, metallosis, infection)
    - mechanical problems

**3. Amputation stump**

- Recurrent mass/cortical abnormalities
- Metastasis
- Lymph nodes
- Complications?:
    - fluid (abscess)
    - orthotopic ossification/ calcification
    - neuroma

final step. Nevertheless, a biopsy should never be done before MRI. It should always be done after consulting the radiologist (in active tumor, not in a necrotic or reactive zone). If there is no neurovascular invasion, excision biopsy is possible. If there is neurovascular invasion or a very big lesion, incision biopsy is performed. Ultrasound might also be an indicator in guiding diagnostic biopsy.

## 17.3  ULTRASOUND IN FOLLOW-UP

Either due to the presence of metal implants or patient related conditions (e.g. renal insufficiency, allergy, claustrophobia) imaging may be quite challenging in patients with tumoral lesions. As such, owing to its several advantages, US seems to be a good alternative for assessing recurrence, regional lymph nodes and remnant tissues (i.e. amputee stump) or pertinent complications [8, 9] (Table 17.1).

### 17.3.1  Soft Tissue Tumors

US is very convenient (especially in children) for local follow-up for recurrence after surgery. In the region of the scar, because of inhomogeneous appearance of postoperative fibrosis, detecting small masses can be difficult [5] (Figure 17.9). It is interesting to start serial follow-up soon after the healing of the skin and to save and compare images. For evaluation of lymph nodes, early start of serial follow-up is also important. There is not one characteristic property helping to differentiate definitely benign vs. malignant changes in the lymph nodes.

It is often progressive changing that is indicative. Evaluation of lymph nodes has more implications in case of presence of orthopedic hardware and will be described there.

For rehabilitation specialists, looking for complications such as fluid collections, muscle atrophy can be helpful to evaluate pain or poor function.

## 17.3.2 Presence of Orthopedic Hardware, including Prostheses

Metal is easily recognized due to reverberation artefact or comet tail behind it. The presence of metal does not preclude the use of US for visualization of the borders of the metal, the surrounding cortex and overlying soft tissues. Recurrence or skip lesions (always evaluate proximally, till reaching the more proximal joint) with cortical abnormalities and overlying soft tissue masses and metastases in the soft tissues can be looked for, even in the presence of extensive hardware (Figures 17.10 and 17.11).

In case of presence of hardware, changes in lymph nodes can happen because of metallosis, infection or neoplasm. Normal lymph nodes are oval, with a hilum and a cortex (normally < half diameter of hilum). They are avascular or have hilar vascularisation [10]. There are three aspects as to the sonographic assessment of abnormal lymph nodes [10]:
- differentiating lymph nodes from other masses;
- deciding whether the node is normal or abnormal;
- determining whether the abnormal appearance is caused by inflammation or neoplasm. There is not one criterion helping to make a definite differentiation. Several parameters are evaluated (number, size, ratio cortex/hilum, shape or longitudinal/transverse diameter ratio, borders, vascularization) and often a serial change during follow-up is indicative for inflammation or neoplasm (Figures 17.12 and 17.13) (Table 17.2).

Ultrasound can be used to look for complications, the most important parameter being fluid. An increasing amount of fluid against the pros-

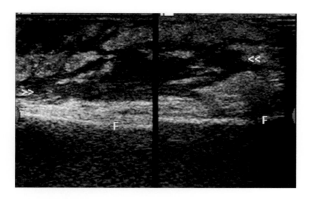

**Figure 17.9** A 72-year-old female in follow-up after resection of a pleiomorphous fibrosarcoma of the thigh. Oval hypoechoic zone (>> <<) within the scar, unsharp borders, highly vascularised (not shown): recidive. Split image with longitudinal reconstruction. F, femur.

thesis can be an alarming sign for loosening, metallosis or infection (Figure 17.14). For hip prosthesis, an intra-articular collection of >3.2 mm at the border of prosthesis/bone and an associated extra-articular collection are suspicious for infection [9]. Around the voluminous tumor-prostheses, there is often fluid; again a serial increase would be much more important. Additionally, the dynamic evaluation with US allows to check for mechanical problems (e.g. metal parts or

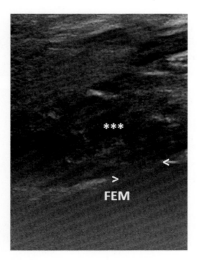

**Figure 17.10** A 16-year-old girl, in follow-up after treatment of an osteosarcoma of the right knee. Painful swelling of the left knee fold. Dorsal vertical view of the left knee: interruption (> <) of the cortex of the femur (FEM). Overlying soft tissue mass, inhomogeneous and hypoechoic (***). New osteosarcoma.

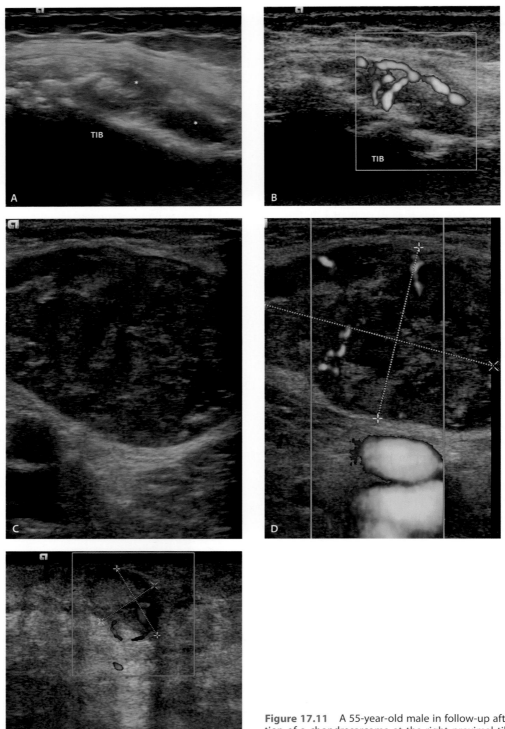

**Figure 17.11** A 55-year-old male in follow-up after resection of a chondrosarcoma at the right proximal tibia (TIB). Irregular bone cortex, with inhomogeneous hypoechoic masses (*) against the bone (A), and high vascularisation: recidive (in B). C and D - Subcutaneous inhomogeneous hypoechoic mass 4x4x3 cm in the thigh: metastasis. E - Rounded pathological lymph node of 12 mm.

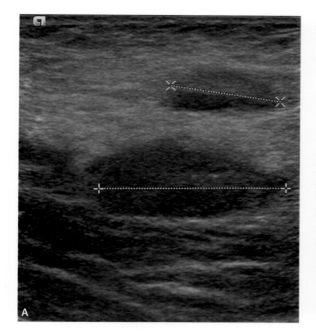

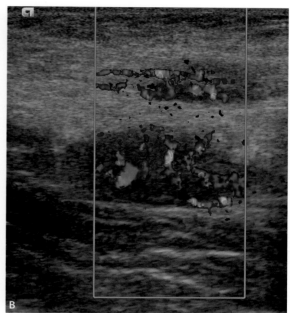

**Figure 17.12**  A - A 15-year-old boy, teleangiectatic osteo-sarcoma of the knee, chronical low grade infection of the prosthesis. Two enlarged lymph nodes (25 and 15 mm) with small hilum and large hypoechoic halo. B - Same lymph nodes, with color Doppler signal. Multiple feeding vessels.

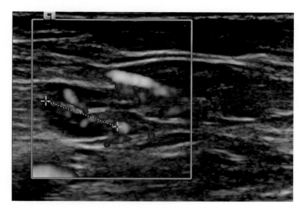

**Figure 17.13**  A 31-year-old female, in follow-up of an os-teosarcoma of the knee. After ending the chemotherapy: multiple bilateral lymph nodes. Diagnosis of mixed-lineage leukemia.

**Table 17.2**  Features of lymph nodes in different health conditions

|  | Normal | Inflammation | Neoplasm |
|---|---|---|---|
| Size | ? | ? | Serial increase |
| Shape | Oval | Oval | Round |
| Hilum | Hyperechoic | Hyperechoic | Thinning/Absent |
| Cortical thickness | <Half transverse diameter of hilum |  | Asymmetric thickening |
| Cortical echogenicity |  | Hypoechoic | Markedly hypoechoic/cystic necrosis |
| Borders |  | Unsharp in tubercolosis | Sharp/ >3 cm extracapsular spread |
| Vascular features | Avascular or hilar | Hilar | Multiple feeding vessels in a centripetal array |

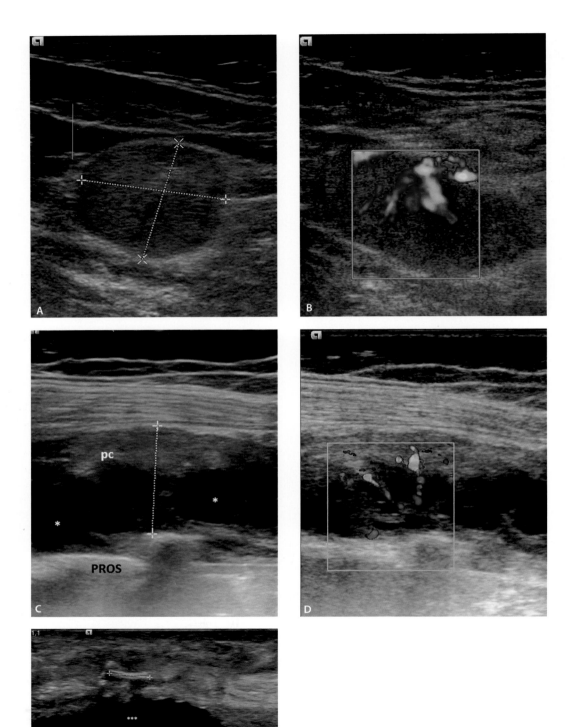

**Figure 17.14**  A and B - A 17-year-old girl in follow-up after resection of a teleangiectatic osteosarcoma of the knee: infection of the tumor prosthesis. Enlarged, hypoechoic lymph node (20 mm), no visible hilum, multiple feeding vessels. C - Fluid (*) against the femoral component of the prosthesis (PROS) and thick pseudocapsule (pc) with vascularisation (in D). E - Fluid (***) against the prosthesis and 6 mm long foreign body (suture) (+ +).

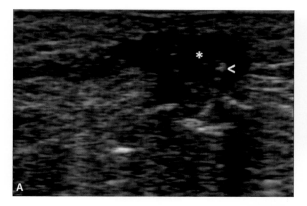

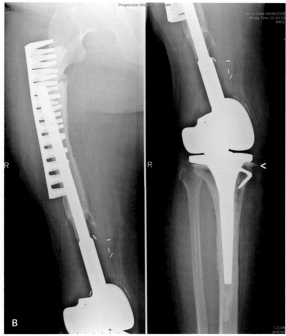

Figure 17.15   A - A 57-year-old female, tumor prosthesis; mechanical pain at the medial aspect of the knee. US shows a small spur (<) with surrounding edema (*). B - Corresponding radiographs confirm a bony spur (<).

bony spurs causing friction against soft tissues) or secondary tendon ruptures (Figure 17.15).

### 17.3.3 Amputation Stumps

Serial US can again be used to examine recurrent mass, cortical abnormalities, metastasis, regional lymph nodes. Complications that can be evaluated are: fluid collections (abscess), orthotopic ossification, calcification, neuromas (rather considered to be pseudotumors than tumors) [5]

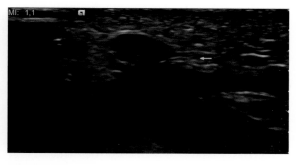

Figure 17.16   Amputation of fifth digit for chondrosarcoma. Asymptomatic neuroma: small hypoechoic mass in continuity with a nerve (arrow).

(Figure 17.16). Overall, it should be emphasized that reliable results can only be achieved if a baseline US is performed, followed by subsequent studies at regular intervals [8].

## 17.4  ANATOMICAL VARIANTS AND FOREIGN BODIES

Anatomical variants can mimic swelling and be the cause of complaints, e.g. prominent fabella bones can irritate the fibular nerve. Muscular variants are not that well known. In the wrist, an extra extensor digitorum brevis manus muscle can cause swelling and pain, e.g. in windsurfers. Langer's axillary arch is a muscle variant between latissimus dorsi and pectoralis major muscles, superficial to the neurovascular bundle. It might be a possible cause of TOS. It is a flat muscle or fibrous band with a length of 7-10 cm and a width 5-15 mm [11] (Figure 17.17). On the thoracic wall,

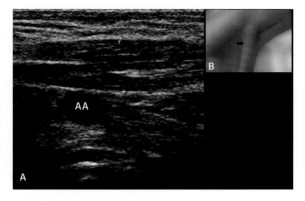

Figure 17.17   A - Transverse view of the axilla: longitudinal view of the superficial, 9.5 mm thick, muscular arch. B - "Swelling" in the axilla: Langer's arch (arrow) (by courtesy of dr. Van Hoof T). AA, axillary artery.

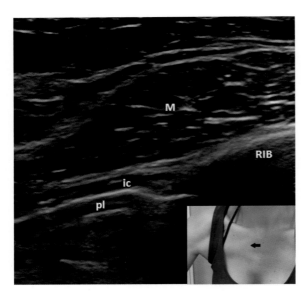

**Figure 17.18** "Swelling" on the chest wall: sternalis muscle. Vertical view of the chest wall: during contraction swelling of the sternal muscle (M). RIB, rib; pl, pleura; ic, intercostal muscles.

sternalis and pectoralis quartus muscles can cause alarming "masses" (Figure 17.18).

Certainly, in children foreign bodies can be present without a typical anamnesis.

## 17.5 TECHNICAL LIMITATIONS

In general, everything covered by bone can not be evaluated. Obesity can be a problem, even when using lower frequency probes.

A specific problem for oncological patients and amputation stumps can be the presence of open wounds. Using self-adhesive plastic dressings to cover the skin (taking care not to leave to many air bubbles in between) offers a practical solution. Because of radiotherapy and the presence of flaps or lymphedema, soft tissues can become very dense (hyperechoic), making visualization of deeper structures difficult.

## 17.6 NEW DEVELOPMENTS

Panoramic views allow to depict all the margins of large masses. By the use of microbubble contrast, detection of low-volume blood flow becomes possible (contrast-enhanced US). Sonoelastography, measurement of tissue displacement in terms of tissue stiffness changes, can offer extra information while assessing mass lesions or lymph nodes (see Chapter 19 - "Developing New Technologies in Musculoskelatal Ultrasound"). The use of three-dimensional imaging and software tools might allow quantification of altered tissue. Fusion or superimposed image data sets can further help guide interventions [5, 12, 13].

In conclusion, in parallel with the technological developments, ultrasound imaging is of mounting importance in the diagnosis, management and follow-up of musculoskeletal tumors.

# REFERENCES

1) Czechowski JJ. Static ultrasound examination in the diagnosis of soft tissue masses. Acta Orthop Belg. 1986; 52: 717-31.

2) Ilaslan H, Sundaram M. Advances in musculo-skeletal tumor imaging. Orthop Clin North Am. 2006; 37: 375-91.

3) Widmann G, Riedl A, Schoepf D, Glodny B, Peer S, Gruber H. State-of-the-art HR-US imaging findings of the most frequent musculoskeletal soft-tissue tumors. Skeletal Radiol. 2009; 38: 637-49.

4) Lee MH, Kim NR, Ryu JA. Cyst-like solid tumors of the musculoskeletal system: an analysis of ultrasound findings. Skeletal Radiol. 2010; 39: 981-6.

5) Pierucci A, Teixeira P, Zimmermann V, Sirveaux F, Rios M, Verhaegue JL, et al. Tumours and pseudotumours of the soft tissue in adults: perspectives and current role of sonography. Diagn Interv Imaging. 2013; 94: 238-54.

6) Loizides A, Peer S, Plaikner M, Djurdjevic T, Gruber H. Perfusion pattern of musculoskeletal masses using contrast-enhanced ultrasound: a helpful tool for characterisation? Eur Radiol. 2012; 22: 1803-11.

7) Hung EH, Griffith JF, Hung Ng AW, Lee RK, Lau DT, Leung JC. Ultrasound of musculoskeletal soft-tissue tumors superficial to the investing fascia. AJR Am J Roentgenol. 2014; 202: 532-40.

8) Sys G, De Muynck M, Poffyn B, Uyttendaele D, Vanderstraeten G. Follow-up of sarcoma by ultrasound. J Bone Joint Surg (Br). 2010; 92-B Supp III: 456.

9) Van der Woude H, Vanderschueren G. Ultrasound in musculoskeletal tumors with emphasis on its role in tumor follow-up. Radiol Clin North Am. 1999; 37: 753-66.

10) Esen G. Ultrasound of superficial lymph nodes. Eur J Radiol. 2006; 58: 345-59.

11) Van Hoof T, Vangestel C, Forward M, Verhaeghe B, Van Thilborg L, Plasschaert F, et al. The impact of muscular variation on the neurodynamic test for the median nerve in healthy population with Langer's axillary arch. J Manipulative Physiol Ther. 2008; 31: 474-83.

12) Klauser A, Peetrons P. Developments in musculoskeletal ultrasound and clinical applications. Skeletal Radiol. 2010; 39: 1061-71.

13) Hwang S, Panicek D. The evolution of musculoskeletal tumor imaging. Radiol Clin N Am. 2009; 47: 435-53.

# Ultrasound Imaging for Musculoskeletal Interventions

Ke-Vin CHANG, Chueh-Hung WU, Tyng-Guey WANG

18

## 18.1 INTRODUCTION

The use of ultrasound (US) guided interventions to diagnose and manage musculoskeletal disorders has become a common skill in clinical practice [1-3]. US-guided interventions include sono-guided operations, tissue biopsy, aspiration and injections. It is believed that the use of US-guided injections has better accuracy and effects of pain relief when compared with blinded approaches [4-6]. Several studies showed that the accuracy of blind injections to the glenohumeral joint varied between 28 to 96 % [4, 5, 7], while US and fluoroscopy guided injections had the accuracy of 94% and 74%, respectively [6]. It has been also reported that US-guided injection to the subdeltoid bursa resulted in better symptom relief [8, 9]. A cadaver study showed that US-guided injection to the distal radioulnar joint had a 100 % of accuracy [10].

The US-guided injection can avoid unnecessary injury to the surrounding tissues through real time visualization. Further, the procedure has the advantages of zero radiation, portability, and real time multiplanar monitoring compared with computed tomography or fluoroscopy guided approaches. The other benefit would be the possibility to simultaneously identify the pain generator; simply by visualization or with a small amount of local anesthetic injection. The US-guided technique is also useful for deeply situated structures e.g. in case of piriformis syndrome or sacroiliac joint disorders [11, 12].

Is US-guided injection always better or more effective than a blind or palpation guided approach? Some skillful specialists debate the necessity of US-guided procedures for musculoskeletal pain [13], but we believe that the use of US guidance can accelerate the learning curve of injection techniques as well. Herewith, an extensive review of US-guided interventions is beyond the scope of this chapter.

This chapter will briefly discuss the indications, contraindications, cautions, medications and potential adverse events pertaining to US-guided injections and focus on the skills of needle placement at individual joints.

## 18.2 TECHNICAL CONSIDERATIONS

US-guided interventions can help the operator in two aspects. Before the procedure, US facilitates the recognition of the lesion, planning the route of intervention, and identification of the surrounding neurovascular structures. During the procedure, it can ensure localization of the needle tip and distribution of injected medication.

### 18.2.1 Probe Selection and Common Settings of the Ultrasound Machine

For deeper structures such as the hip joint, a curvilinear probe with lower frequency (5-8 MHz) is selected for better penetration of the echo beams. For superficial structures such as the shoulder joint, a linear probe with higher frequency (10-15 MHz) is preferred. For smaller structures such as the finger joints, a hockey stick probe with much higher frequencies (15-20 MHz) offers superior resolution and greater dexterity [1].

### 18.2.2 Needle Selection

Selection of the needle depends on the purpose of the procedure. A larger-gauge needle (e.g. 18-gauge) may be required for aspiration, especially when the fluid appears turbid and less compressible. Regarding interventions for deep structures such as the hip joints and spine, a spinal needle with a length of at least 3.5 inches is need-

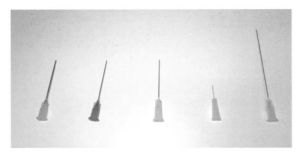

**Figure 18.1** Needles for aspiration or injection. From left to right: 18G × 1.5" (for aspiration of abscess or sticky fluid), 22G × 1.5" (for calcification puncturing and aspiration of synovial fluid), 25G × 1.5" (for most injection conditions), 30G × 0.5" (for small joints injection), 23G × 2.75" (for hip joint injection or caudal epidural injection).

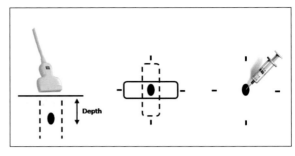

**Figure 18.2** Indirect approach. After locating the lesion and measuring the depth, the probe is moved and the needle is introduced without real-time visualization.

ed. For small and superficial joints, a needle sized 25-27 gauge causes less discomfort and can also be visible under US. It is noteworthy that a longer needle is more likely to deviate from the planned trajectory, making the targeting more difficult. The shortest needle route should be planned prior to the injection and this may vary in different subjects (Figure 18.1) [2].

### 18.2.3 Sterile Technique

The procedural site should be disinfected with a bactericidal solution (for example, those containing povidone iodine or chlorhexidine) and shaved if the area is furry. The puncture spot should be kept away from the probe, if the physician decides not to use a sterile cover or aseptic gel. In some cases that need the approximation of the needle tip to the probe for approaching small superficial structures, a sterile probe cover or aseptic gel is mandatory to reduce the risk of contamination. The sterile technique can be conducted more easily by having another assistant to adjust the machine and deliver the instruments [3, 14].

### 18.2.4 Indirect Approach versus Direct Approach

The indirect approach indicates a pre-intervention US scan to locate the lesion and measure the depth whereby real time imaging is not performed thereafter during the procedure (Figure 18.2). The skin is marked at both sites of the probe when the target is clearly visualized in the center of the screen. Then the probe is rotated 90 degrees to

repeat the same marking process. After removal of the transducer, connecting the marks at both sides forms a crosshair. The needle is inserted vertically to the skin at the center of the crosshair and is supposed to hit the target at the pre-defined depth. Of note, the amount of skin compression

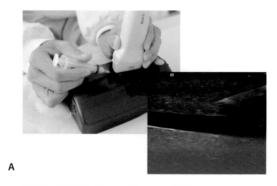

A

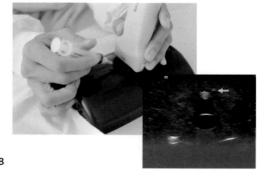

B

**Figure 18.3** A - Direct approach (In-plane). Whole needle length can be visualized. B - Direct approach (out-of-plane). Only a hyperechoic spot (yellow arrow) is visible. Exact location of the needle tip is difficult to determine.

during the measurements should be taken into account and likewise applied during the procedure as well [1, 2, 14].

The direct approach allows the simultaneous visualization of the target and the needle tract. This technique requires a longer period of training for the coordination of needle handling and probe adjustment. When using the direct approach, the axes of the needle can be parallel (in-plane) or perpendicular (out-of-plane) to the probe (Figure 18.3). The in-plane approach is usually preferred because the entire course of the needle can be visualized during the whole procedure. Adjusting the probe as parallel as possible to the needle will enhance its visualization. This maneuver may not be easy for deep structures and some US machines have softwares to intensify the needle reflection by angling the sound beams more perpendicular to the needle. Regarding the direct approach, a needle guide mounted on the probe grants the operator to guide the needle along a predetermined tract on the monitor. But in most situations, the needle advancement is done freehandedly. But, while this allows the operator maximal flexibility to manipulate the needle, the technique requires more training and practice.

In the out-of-plane approach, the investigator only visualizes a small echogenic dot when the tip or shaft of the needle passes through the scan plane. The exact location of the needle tip is hard to be seen on US, causing a higher risk of unwanted injuries. Nevertheless, the out-plane approach is often applied to inject small and distal structures, such as hands, since a regular-length probe is difficult to accommodate the in-plane approach at such a limited area [1, 2, 14].

## 18.3 COMMON MEDICATIONS ADMINISTERED BY ULTRASOUND GUIDANCE

### 18.3.1 Corticosteroids

Corticosteroids are the most commonly used agents for US-guided injections and its clinical effect consists of reduction of synovial blood flow, modulation of inflammatory response and alternation of collagen synthesis [15]. Methylprednisolone acetate and triamcinolone acetonide are corticosteroids commonly injected for musculoskel-

etal disorders. Compared with triamcinolone acetate, methylprednisolone has less risk to develop post-injection skin atrophy and is preferred for superficial lesions [16, 17]. Triamcinolone acetonide, which has lower solubility but longer duration of action, is favored for injections to deep structures or joints. The major concern is increased risk of post-injection synovitis flare reaction, which is rarely severe and usually subsides spontaneously [15]. The combination with local anesthetics increases the volume for injection, facilitating the distribution of corticosteroids in the target region. Additional benefits are rapid relief of symptoms before corticosteroids come into effect and reduction of immediate post-injection pain. Lidocaine 2% (Xylocaine) is the preferred agent based on its prompt onset (1-2 minutes after injection) and duration of action (for at least one hour) [15].

### 18.3.2 Hyaluronic Acid

Hyaluronic acid -a non-sulfated, naturally occurring glycosaminoglycan- exists in the normal joint fluid. Its administration may restore viscoelasticity through the replenishment of dysfunctional synovial fluid and possibly has an anagelsic effect by modifying the inflammatory response. The application of hyaluronic acid is extensively studied in knee osteoarthritis. Although most meta-analyses favored the use of hyaluronic acid over corticosteroids for the treatment of knee osteoarthritis (based on longer efficacy and less cartilage degradable effects), a large scaled meta-analysis discouraged hyaluronic acid injection due to a clinically irrelevant advantage and more post-injection adverse events [18-20]. Regarding ankle osteoarthritis, a meta-analysis indicated that hyaluronic acid injection was associated with significantly improved outcome when compared with the condition prior to treatment, and a non-significant advantage over the reference treatment (saline, exercise and arthroscopy) [21]. In terms of osteoarthritis in the metatarsophalangeal, hip, sacroiliac joint, facet, carpometacarpal and temporo-mandibular joints, there is no strong evidence to show the superiority of hyaluronic acid over corticosteroid and physical therapy [22]. Although hyaluronic acid is effective in improving chronic shoulder pain, the effectiveness varies according to different shoulder pathology.

### 18.3.3 Hypertonic Dextrose Prolotherapy

Hypertonic dextrose is the mostly used agent in the field of prolotherapy, a therapy using some stimulants to induce inflammatory reactions and subsequent tissue regeneration. The exact mechanism for symptomatic improvement after dextrose injection remains unknown. Current evidence suggests that dextrose prolotherapy can effectively reduce pain in chronic tendinopathy and lateral epicondylitis, and probably improves function in patients with knee osteoarthritis [23-26].

### 18.3.4 Platelet Rich Plasma

Platelet rich plasma (PRP) is a blood derivative with high concentration of platelets. Several meta-analyses demonstrated that PRP was not superior to placebo in improving shoulder function and decreasing re-tear rates in overall patients following arthroscopic rotator cuff repair, but benefited the subgroup with small to medium-sized tear [27]. A meta-analysis was conducted to determine the efficacy of PRP for the treatment of various bone and soft-tissue injuries at sites like the acromion, rotator cuff, lateral humeral epicondyle, anterior cruciate ligament, patella, tibia, and spine and suggested a non-significant trend favoring PRP [28]. Current evidence based research indicated better effectiveness of PRP than placebo against lateral epicondylitis, although there was no consensus regarding doses and numbers of injections [23]. Regarding knee cartilage degenerative pathology, PRP was shown to improve function from basal evaluations and tend to be more effective than hyaluronic acid administration [29]. Discrepancy in the degenerative severity modified the treatment responses, leading to participants with lower degrees of degeneration benefiting more from PRP injections.

### 18.3.5 Botulinum Toxin

Botulinum toxin, a neurotoxin produced by the bacterium Clostridium botulinum, can block neuromuscular transmission through the inhibition of acetylcholine release. The common indications for botulinum toxin injection comprise dystonia, blepharospasm, tremor, hyperhydrosis and focal spasticity resulting from cerebral disorders. Current evidence indicated that botulinum toxin injection reduced upper extremity spasticity with improved arm function in post-stroke victims as well as increased gait speeds following injection for lower extremities [30, 31]. A recent application of botulinum toxin in the musculoskeletal field is pain management, such as treatment for lateral epicondylitis and hemiplegic shoulder pain and the potential mechanism might involve modulation of nociceptive substance release [32].

### 18.3.6 Phenol

Phenol, as well as alcohol, is a chemical agent commonly used for nerve block. Phenol destructs peripheral nerves through the induction of precipitation, resulting in axonal edema and subsequent separation of the myelin sheath from the axon. The neurolytic effect reaches the maximum in two weeks and may gradually decline in four months after the regeneration or sprouting of the axons. Phenol can be injected perinerually or near the motor points to reduce focal spasticity but the patients should be informed about the risk of post-injection dysesthaesia. Phenol can be used to relieve spasticity of a large muscle group (the adductor muscle) by blocking the nerve truck (the obturator nerve), whereas botulinum toxin can be selectively administered for spasticity of smaller muscles [33-35].

## 18.4 COMMON ULTRASOUND GUIDED THERAPEUTIC APPLICATIONS

### 18.4.1 Pain Management

Ultrasound guidance enables the injection of medication to a selected structure such as tendons, ligaments, bursas and joints. With precise drug delivery, treatment success of a certain musculoskeletal disorder will be focused on the indication and regimen of injected medication and patients' individual response. Several randomized controlled trials and quasi-experimental studies have compared the effectiveness of US-guided injection techniques with those using palpation or surface landmarks. One meta-analysis indicated that US-guided steroid injection was better than the landmark guided approach in pain relief for patients with shoulder pain [36]. Likewise, another meta-analysis demonstrated more pain reduction and longer effectiveness after US-guided steroid injection than the palpation-guided method regarding plantar fasciitis [37]. Therefore, using US guidance for drug delivery is highly suggested based on its better efficacy on symptomatic relief and lower risks of injury to surrounding structures.

## 18.4.2 Diagnostic/Therapeutic Aspirations

Under US, most fluid appears an-/hypo-echoic and may display posterior acoustic enhancement. Dynamic compression together with color/power Doppler imaging helps the differentiation of fluid from other hypoechoic tissues e.g. hypertrophic synovium. The above mentioned step is crucial for avoiding the puncture of solid or hypervascular structures. In most conditions, US is incapable of discriminating the content of fluid whereby aspiration would be required for prompt diagnosis. However, the investigator can speculate about the nature of fluid. For example, when seeing fluid accumulating between the torn medial gastrocnemius and soleus muscles, the lesion may be interpreted as fresh blood or liquefaction of an antecedent hematoma. Likewise, if visualizing a hypoechoic fluid collection with hyperechoic sediments, septa, loculations and gas bubbles inside, a liquefied abscess caused by an anaerobic infection is highly indicated.

Besides the diagnostic purpose, aspiration of fluid can lead to significant pain relief. Patients with severe knee osteoarthritis usually suffer from pain due to large effusion, which can be easily drawn out from the supra-patellar pouch under US guidance. A large ganglion cyst on the wrist can impede the movement of tendons or irritate adjacent neurovascular structures and aspiration with a subsequent bandage can effectively relieve the compressive symptoms. A huge intramuscular hematoma may result in compartment syndrome and US guidance is helpful to localize the deeply-lying hematoma and to aspirate the most serous part. For sure, a thicker needle sized 18 gauge is usually necessary for aspiration to prevent the debris or clots from blocking the needle.

A similar condition would be the extraction of calcific materials from the tendons. For a calcific supraspinatus tendinopathy, the procedure is started with injection of local anesthetics into the subdeltoid bursa and followed by fenestration of the calcific spot with a 16-gauge needle under US monitoring. Normal saline (200 to 400 ml) is injected through one needle and aspiration of the fluid con-

taining the calcific deposits is performed by another needle. The treatment leads to shoulder function recovery and pain relief at least for one year [38].

## 18.4.3 Ultrasound Guided Nerve Block

Peripheral nerves can be well depicted by high resolution US as multiple hypoechoic bands in the longitudinal view and as a honeycomb appearance in the transverse view. The specific pattern derives from hypoechoic fascicular nerve bundles and hyperechoic surrounding epineurium. Compared with fluoroscopic guidance which mainly demonstrates the nearby bony structures, US guidance allows direct visualization of the peripheral nerve, reducing the risk of injury. In addition, some nerves have accompanying vessels and the use of power or color doppler US can be beneficial for easier localization of the nerves and avoiding vessel damage. Another advantage of US guidance is to reduce the volume of local anesthetics, which improves the selectiveness of the nerve block. Under US guidance, 2 to 4 ml of lidocaine is effective for upper limb nerve blockade [39].

## 18.4.4 Ultrasound Guided Injection for Anti-Spasticity Treatment

Botulinum toxin is the most commonly used medication against spasticity. It can be injected into big and superficial muscles, such as the gastrocnemius, through the recognition of the surface landmarks. For smaller and deeper muscles, like the forearm flexors, guidance by electric stimulation or US are required to selectively infiltrate the toxin. The use of electric needles to target wanted muscles is time-consuming, especially in limbs with contracture or deformity. The patients suffer from pain due to repetitively introduction and withdrawal of the needles and subsequent electrical stimulation. Another concern is the injury to adjacent neuromuscular structures during the probing of the motor branch [1].

High resolution US enables the visualization of the wanted muscle. While the indirect approach does not need the use of sterile gel and can ensure better sterilization, the major drawback is the difficulty in precisely targeting thin muscles where their thicknesses vary significantly due to self contraction or compression from adjacent structures. The direct approach (in-plane technique) is preferable due to the benefit of monitoring the exact course of needle advancement. However, for deep muscles, the out-of-plane technique may be better because it can better/clearly demonstrate the depth of the needle tip [1].

Compared with the injection through surface landmarks, current evidence suggests that US guidance resulted in more decrease in spasticity over upper and lower extremities [40-42]. Regarding the comparison with electrical stimulation, some randomized controlled trials found that US guidance had similar effectiveness against spasticity and a small but significantly better improvement in ankle range of motion for patients with lower extremity spasticity [41, 42].

### 18.4.5 Ultrasound Guided Percutaneous Surgery and Biopsy

The most common surgery performed on the wrist and hand is for carpal tunnel syndrome. The key element of a successful surgery derives from complete release of the transverse carpal ligament, a strong fibrous band arching the carpal tunnel. Sonographically guided percutaneous needle release can be conducted by using an 18-gauge spinal needle without any customized device. A retrospective study reported the feasibility of this procedure and a symptom-relief effect for patients with lower severity. The US-guided percutaneous surgery requires specific surgical instruments and can be approached from the palmar or antebrachial side by using either pulling (retrograde) or pushing (antegrade) cutting methods [43, 44]. Besides carpal tunnel syndrome, the surgical release for A1 pulley can be guided by US for patients with finger stenosing tenosynovitis.

Synovial hypertrophy is the hallmark of inflammatory arthritis and is associated with many autoimmune disorders. Biopsy for synovial histology is crucial for a correct diagnosis. Guidance by arthroscopy is less applicable on small and distal joints, whereas the blind approach often misses the pathological region. US-guided synovial biopsy has been proposed as a feasible method for sampling of synovium and the procedure can be performed percutaneously by techniques like "Tru-Cut needles" and "portal and forceps". Current studies proved that US-guided synovial biopsy was a reliable tool to assess histopathology of synovium in joints with rheumatoid arthritis [45, 46].

## 18.5 REGION-SPECIFIC ULTRASOUND GUIDED TECHNIQUES

### 18.5.1 Biceps Long Head Tendon

The patient is in the supine position with the shoulder slightly externally rotated. The transducer is placed along the long axis of the biceps long head tendon. The needle is inserted at an angle of 30 degrees through the in-plane approach from the proximal end of the biceps tendon. If the patient is in the seated posture, the transducer is suggested to be placed perpendicular to the biceps long head tendon (Figure 18.4 A). In the short axis view, the needle is inserted at an angle of 0-15 degrees through the in-plane approach from the lateral edge of the biceps tendon. The injected fluid can be seen to run into the sheath (Figure 18.4 B).

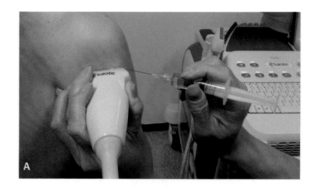
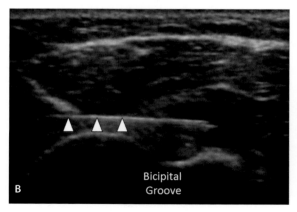

**Figure 18.4** Biceps tendon. A - Illustration of the posture and transducer placement for injection of the long head biceps tendon at its short axis. B - Introduction of the needle (arrowhead) at an angle of 0-15 degrees from the lateral side until targeting the tendon sheath.

## 18.5.2 Subacrominal-subdeltoid Bursa

The patient is in the seated posture with the hand placed behind the buttock to expose the supraspinatus tendon. The subacrominal-subdeltoid bursa is a synovial space located between the supraspinatus tendon, acromion and the deltoid muscle. Injection to the bursa can be easily performed by the lateral to medial approach. The probe is placed perpendicular to the supraspinatus tendon (Figure 18.5 A). In the short axis view, the needle is introduced laterally to the probe through the in-plane approach at an angle of 30 degrees until it reaches the bursa. A small amount of fluid can be injected first to observe the distension of the bursa and to confirm the correct position of the needle tip (Figure 18.5 B).

## 18.5.3 Acromioclavicular Joint

The patient is in the seated posture with the hand lying on the thigh. The probe is placed between the lateral clavicle end and the medial edge of the acromion to obtain the coronal view of the acromioclavicular joint (Figure 18.6 A). The joint capsule may bulge out in case of synovitis or increased articular joint effusion. The needle is introduced laterally to the probe through the in-

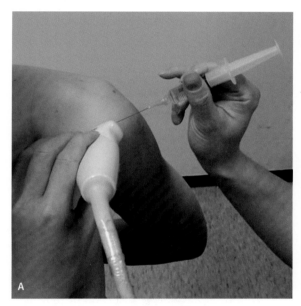

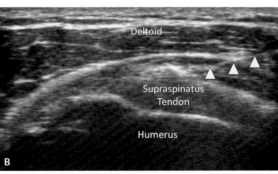

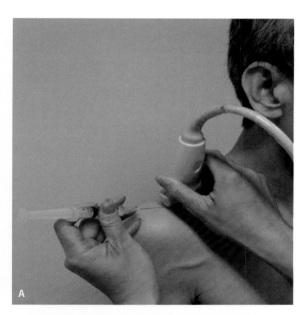

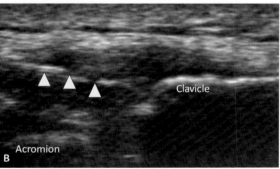

**Figure 18.5**  Subacrominal-Subdeltoid bursa. A - Illustration of the posture and transducer placement for injection of the subdeltoid bursa through the lateral to medial approach. B - Introduction of the needle (arrowhead) laterally to the probe at an angle of 30 degree until targeting the bursa.

**Figure 18.6**  Acromioclavicular joint. A - Illustration of the posture and transducer placement for injection of the acromioclavicular joint. B - Introduction of the needle (arrowhead) laterally to the probe at an angle of 30 degree until puncturing the capsule of the acromioclavicular joint.

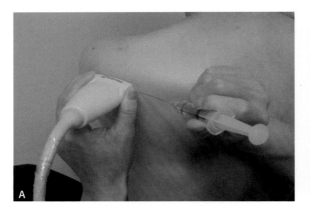
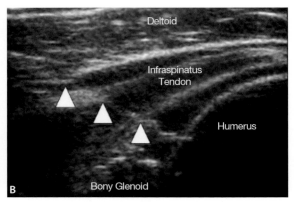

**Figure 18.7** Glenohumeral joint. A - Illustration of the posture and transducer placement for injection of the glenohumeral joint. B - Introduction of the needle (arrowhead) medially to the probe at an angle of 45 degrees until it reaches the area between the humeral head and bony glenoid of the scapulae.

plane approach at an angle of 30 degrees until it punctures through the joint capsule (Figure 18.6 B). A feeling of loss of resistance can be appreciated when the joint capsule is passed.

### 18.5.4 Glenohumeral Joint

The glenohumeral joint is usually approached through the posterior aspect. The patient is in the seated posture with the hand of the affected shoulder put over the shoulder at the opposite site. The probe is placed below the spine of the scapula and parallel to the long axis of the infraspinatus tendon (Figure 18.7 A). In this view, the overlying intraspinatus tendon, triangular-shaped posterior labrum, humeral head and bony glenoid can be clearly identified. The needle is introduced laterally to the probe through the in-plane approach at

an angle of 45 degrees until it reaches the area between the humeral head and bony glenoid of the scapula (Figure 18.7 B). With the correct needle placement, the medication should flow into the joint smoothly without any resistance.

### 18.5.5 Common Extensor Tendon and its Insertion on the Lateral Epicondyle

The patient is in the seated position with the elbow in flexion and pronation. The probe is placed along the long axis of the forearm to visualize the common extensor tendon and its insertion on the lateral epicondyle (Figure 18.8 A). The needle is introduced proximal to the probe through an in-plane approach at an angle of 10 degrees until it reaches the insertion of the com-

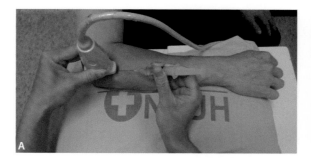
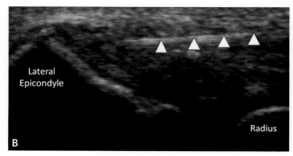

**Figure 18.8** Common extensor tendon and its insertion on the lateral epicondyle. A - Illustration of the posture and transducer placement for injection of the insertion of the common extensor tendon of the wrist. B - Introduction of the needle (arrowhead) proximally to the probe at an angle of 10 degrees until its arrival at the insertion of the common extensor tendon of the wrist.

Musculoskeletal Ultrasound in Physical and Rehabilitation Medicine

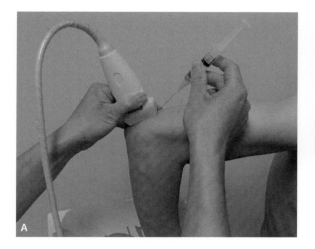

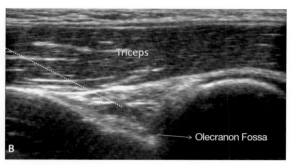

**Figure 18.9** Olecranon fossa. A - Illustration of the posture and transducer placement for injection of the olecranon fossa. B - Introduction of the needle (dash line) proximally to the probe at an angle of 45 degrees until its arrival at the concave olecranon fossa.

mon extensor tendon. The medication is usually distributed at the superficial part of the tendon and strong resistance will be encountered while performing the intra-tendinous injection (Figure 18.8 B).

### 18.5.6 Olecranon Fossa

The patient is in the supine or seated position with the elbow flexed and the hand put on the shoulder at the opposite site (Figure 18.9 A). The probe is placed between the olecranon and the distal humerus along its long axis. In the longitudinal view, the triceps tendon, proximal pole of the olecranon, posterior fat pad and olecranon fossa are visualized. The needle is introduced proximally to the probe through an in-plane approach at an angle of 45 degrees until it reaches

the concave olecranon fossa (Figure 18.9 B). The procedure is the mostly used technique for injection to the elbow joint.

### 18.5.7 First Compartment of the Wrist Extensor Tendons

De Quervain disease is the tenosynovitis of the abductor pollicis longus and extensor pollicis brevis, two tendons inside the first compartment of the wrist. A meta-analysis has demonstrated the effectiveness of corticosteroid injection against De Quervain disease [47]. A clinical trial suggested that US-guided injection was more effective than manual injection, especially in patients with separations inside the first compartment [48]. The injection can be performed by an out-of-plane or in-plane approach. We prefer the

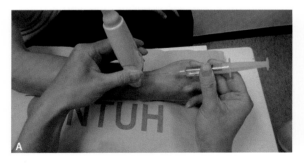

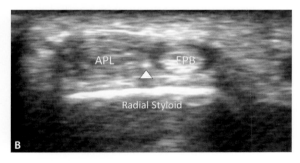

**Figure 18.10** First compartment of the wrist extensor tendon. A - Illustration of the posture and transducer placement for injection of the first compartment of the wrist extensor tendon. B - Introduction of the needle (arrowhead) distally to the probe through an out-of-plane approach at an angle of 10 degrees until targeting the tendon sheath. APL, abductor pollicis longus; EPB, extensor pollicis brevis.

out-of-plane approach because it is easier to maintain a sterile zone between the needle insertion point and the probe. In case of sub-compartmentalization, an additional benefit is to precisely target each sub-compartment in only one view. The first compartment can be visualized in the transverse plane by placing the probe near the radial styloid (Figure 18.10 A). The needle is introduced distally to the probe through an out-of-plane approach at an angle of 10 degrees until the needle tip, a bright spot, is seen inside the tendon sheath (Figure 18.10 B).

### 18.5.8 Carpal Tunnel

Corticosteroid injection into the carpal tunnel has been proven to relieve clinical symptoms in patients with carpal tunnel syndrome. A randomized controlled trial suggested that US-guided corticosteroid injection had an earlier onset and better response than the palpation guided technique [49]. The injection can be performed by placing the probe on the wrist crease to obtain the proximal carpal tunnel in the short axis view. The needle is introduced from the ulnar side with a shallow angle, permitting the needle to skip the ulnar nerve and artery. After the needle tip passes the flexor retinaculum and reaches the border of the median nerve, the mixture of corticosteroid and local anesthetics can be gradually injected and results in the effect of hydrodissection [50].

### 18.5.9 First Annual Pulley Injection for Stenosing Tenosynovitis

Stenosing tenosynovitis (trigger finger) is a common painful condition of the hand, causing the hand or thumb to catch or lock in a bend position. The pathology is known to be an entrapment of tendon gliding due to a mismatch between the size of the first annular pulley (A1) and the corresponding flexor tendon sheath. Current evidence suggests that intra-tendon sheath corticosteroid injection has a short term better effect for trigger fingers than local anesthetics alone [51]. Injection into the tendon sheath is usually through the out-of-plane approach. The probe is placed on the metacarpal phalangeal joint in the short axis view to visualize the A1 pulley and the finger flexor tendon (Figure 18.11 A). The needle is introduced distally to the probe at an angle of 20 degrees until the needle tip hit the circular area

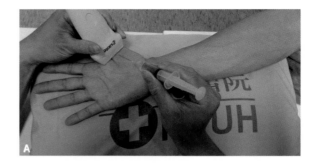

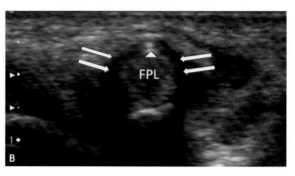

**Figure 18.11** First annual pulley injection. A. Illustration of the posture and transducer placement for injection of the first annual pulley of the finger. B. Introduction of the needle distally to the transducer at an angle of 20 degrees until the needle tip (arrowhead) hit the circular area (arrow) between the A1 pulley and the finger flexor tendon.

between the A1 pulley and the finger flexor tendon (Figure 18.11 B). The resistance of flow is usually high during the initial injection but will drop after the pulley is distended.

### 18.5.10 Sacroiliac Joint

The patient is lying prone with the feet hanging over the examination bed. The probe is placed between the posterior superior iliac spine (laterally) and the spinous process of the fifth lumbar vertebra (medially) (Figure 18.12 A). The probe is moved caudally to depict the dorsal surface of the sacrum, the medial and lateral sacral crest, the gluteal surface of the ilium, and the first posterior sacral foramen. A hypoechoic cleft between the surface of the sacrum and the medial border of the ilium indicates the upper compartment of the sacroiliac joint. Then the probe is placed caudally to scan the median and lateral sacral crest at the dorsal surface of the sacrum and the gluteal surface of the ilium until the second posterior sacral foramen is visualized. A hypoechoic cleft between

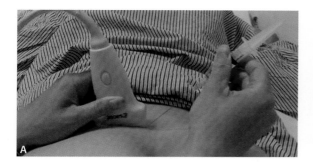

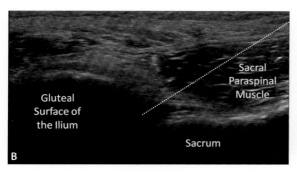

Figure 18.12    Sacroiliac joint. A - Illustration of the posture and transducer placement for injection of the upper compartment of the left sacroiliac joint. B - Introduction of the needle medially to the transducer at an angle of 40 degrees until the needle tip hits the sacroiliac joint.

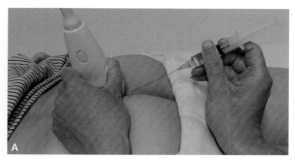

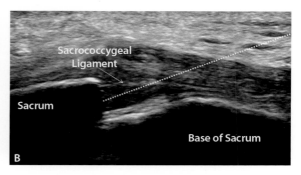

Figure 18.13    Caudal epidural injection. A. Illustration of the posture and transducer placement for caudal epidural injection. B - Introduction of the needle caudally to the transducer at an angle of 30 degrees until the needle tip hits the caudal epidural space.

the sacrum and the ilium indicates the lower compartment of the sacroiliac joint [52]. The upper compartment is a fibrous joint, whereas the lower compartment is a synovial joint. The selection of injection sites depends on patient's symptoms. The needle is advanced from medial to lateral (Figure 18.12 B). The angle between the needle and the probe is usually steep, making the needle difficult to be visualized. Injection of a small amount of fluid can help identify the location of the needle tip.

### 18.5.11  Caudal Epidural Injection

The patient is lying prone with the pelvis supported by a pillow. The probe is placed transversely just proximal to the anus and then is moved cranially until two hyperechoic reversed U-shaped structures (bony prominences of sacral cornua) are seen. The sacral hiatus is the hypoechoic region observed between the two hyperechoic band-like structures. For caudal epidural injection, the probe is rotated 90° to check the longitudinal view of the sacral hiatus (Figure

18.13 A). A 21-gauge spinal needle is punctured through the sacrococcygeal ligament with a feeling of "pop" and enters the epidural space of the sacral canal in the caudal-cranial direction [53]. When the needle pierces the sacrococcygeal ligament, the portion of the needle inside the caudal epidural space is less visible under sonography (Figure 18.13 B). The needle should not be advanced further and injection is performed when the needle tip is partly seen.

### 18.5.12  Coxofemoral Joint

The patient is lying supine, with the hip in the neutral position. The upper pole of the probe is placed on the lateral third of the inguinal ligament in an oblique longitudinal plane over the anterior femoral neck (Figure 18.14 A). At this level, the anterior synovial recess is identified. When the probe is moved cranially, the anterior hip labrum can be recognized. The injection site is usually caudal to the probe and the target is the anterior recess because the acetabulum and the labrum may block the way into the joint space itself [54].

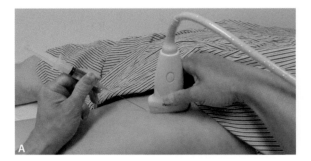

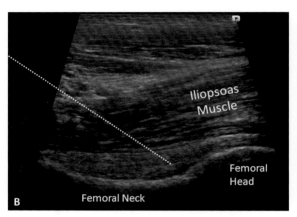

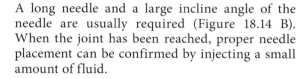

Figure 18.14 Coxofemoral joint. A - Illustration of the posture and transducer placement for injection of the left coxofemoral joint. B - Introduction of the needle caudally to the transducer at an angle of 45 degrees until the needle tip hits the anterior recess.

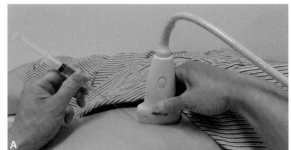

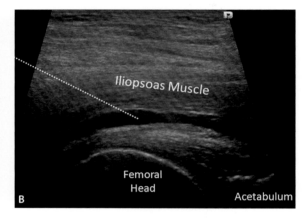

Figure 18.15 Iliopsoas bursa. A - Illustration of the posture and transducer placement for injection of the left iliopsoas bursa. B - Introduction of the needle caudally to the transducer at an angle of 45 degrees until the needle tip hits the potential space or the bursa.

A long needle and a large incline angle of the needle are usually required (Figure 18.14 B). When the joint has been reached, proper needle placement can be confirmed by injecting a small amount of fluid.

### 18.5.13 Iliopsoas Bursa

The patient is lying supine, with the hip in the neutral position. After drawing a line between the anterior superior iliac spine and the pubic symphysis, placing the probe at the upper one-third level depicts the transverse section of the iliopsoas muscle. In this view the iliopsoas bursa can be identified medial or lateral to the iliopsoas muscle if distended. For US-guided intervention the probe is usually positioned longitudinally along the iliopsoas muscle (Figure 18.15 A). The needle is introduced in the same way (in the caudal-cranial direction) as for the coxofemoral joint injection, while the needle is introduced more crani-

ally (Figure 18.15 B). Injection should stay below the iliofemoral ligament to avoid injury to the intestines and also lateral to the neurovascular bundles to prevent the femoral nerve, artery and vein from damages.

### 18.5.14 Piriformis Muscle Injection

Because it is a deep structure, a curvilinear probe with lower frequency (for example, 5-7 MHz) is recommended. The patient is lying prone with the feet hanging over the examination bed. The probe is placed between the posterior inferior iliac spine and the upper margin of the greater trochanter. At the greater sciatic notch, the piriformis muscle is seen above the curved hyperechoic shadow representing the ilium (Figure 18.16 A). Passively rotating the hip can confirm the piriformis moving relative to the gluteus maximus. The course of the sciatic nerve should be identified before the procedure since

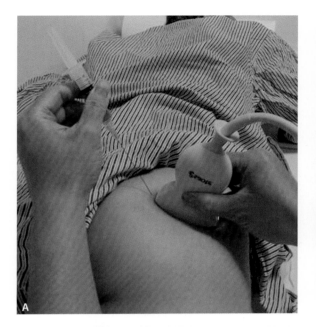

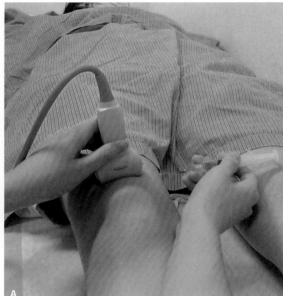

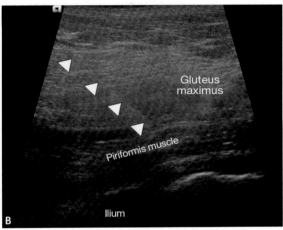

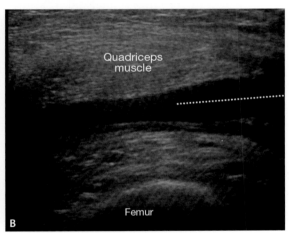

**Figure 18.16** Piriformis muscle injection. A - Illustration of the posture and transducer placement for injection of the right piriformis muscle. B - Introduction of the needle medially to the transducer at an angle of 45 degrees until the needle tip hits the piriformis muscle. Introduce some medication between the gluteus maximus muscle and the piriformis muscle, and then inject into the piriformis muscle (arrowheads: needle).

**Figure 18.17** Suprapatellar recess. A - Illustration of the posture and transducer placement for injection of the right suprapatellar recess. B - Introduction of the needle medially and parallel to the transducer until the needle tip enters the recess.

the nerve is close to the piriformis muscle. The sciatic nerve can be identified superficial to the quadratus femoris, lateral to the ischial tuberosity and deep to the gluteus maximus [11]. A 23-gauge spinal needle is advanced under direct US guidance in the medial to lateral approach (Figure 18.16 B).

## 18.5.15 Suprapatellar Recess

The patient lies supine on the examination bed with the knee extended or slightly flexed. The probe is placed transversely proximal to the patella (Figure 18.17 A). The needle can be inserted from the medial or lateral side and advanced parallel to the probe (Figure 18.17 B). US guidance is helpful especially when the amount of effusion is minimal. An assistant may compress the recess opposite to the needle insertion site to converge the fluid in a limited area.

## 18.5.16 Tibiotalar Joint Injection

Before the procedure, it is important to document the location of the dorsalis pedis artery, which usually courses lateral to the tibialis anterior tendon. The patient is placed supine on the examination bed, with the knee flexed and the foot in plantar flexion. The probe is placed parallel and medial to the tibialis anterior tendon (Figure 18.18 A). After the anterior recess of the joint is identified, the needle can be advanced from distal to proximal towards the distal tibia (Figure 18.18 B). It may be difficult to see the needle due to its steep angle. The needle tip can be confirmed by injecting some fluid. If aspiration is planned, it should be noticed that a joint

effusion is compressible, whereas hypertrophic synovium is incompressible or abundant in vascularity, which can be differentiated by using probe compression and Doppler imaging, respectively.

## 18.5.17 Posterior Talocalcaneal Joint Injection

The patient is placed in the prone position with the foot dorsi-flexed and the toes resting on the examination bed. The probe is placed on a sagittal plane, parallel and slightly lateral to the Achilles tendon (Figure 18.19 A). The following structures can be visualized (from cranial to caudal): the peroneal tendons, posterior talus and posterior calcaneus. The posterior articular recess can be seen between the last two structures when it is distended. The needle is inserted anteriorly to the probe (out-of-plane approach) and advanced to the recess through the Kager's fat (Figure 18.19 B). The posterolateral approach is favored by the au-

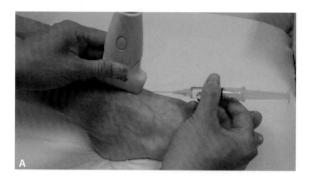

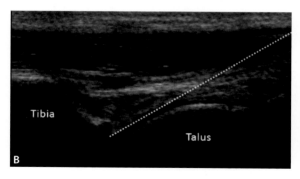

**Figure 18.18** Tibiotalar joint injection. A - Illustration of the posture and transducer placement for injection of the right tibiotalar joint. B - Introduction of the needle caudally to the transducer at an angle of 30 degrees until the needle tip enters the recess.

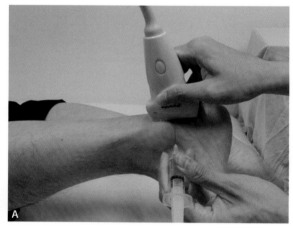

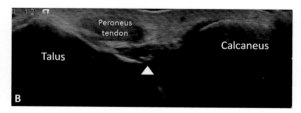

**Figure 18.19** Posterior talocalcaneal joint injection. A - Illustration of the posture and transducer placement for injection of the left posterior talocalcaneal joint. B - Introduction of the needle anteriorly and perpendicular to the transducer (out-of-plane approach) until the needle tip (arrowhead) hits the talocalcaneal joint.

thors because the route does not cross neurovascular structures.

### 18.5.18 Plantar Fascia Injection

The patient is placed prone on the examination bed, with the feet hanging over the edge of the bed. The probe is placed near the insertion of the proximal plantar fascia at the calcaneus, showing the longitudinal view of the plantar fascia (Figure 18.20 A). Debate exists as to whether the injection should be within or around the plantar fascia, and as to whether it should be performed medially (from medial to lateral) or longitudinally (from posterior to anterior) to the plane of the plantar fascia. Injection within the plantar fascia may result in rupture and injection around the plantar fascia may cause plantar fat pad atrophy or necrosis. The medial-to-lateral approach may cause less pain and the medication can be administered deep to the plantar fascia, avoiding plantar fat pad atrophy. On the other hand, the posterior-to-anterior approach allows the injections to a larger area [55] (Figure 18.20 B). A meta-analysis suggested that US-guided injection of corticosteroid tends to be more effective than palpation-guided injection [37].

## 18.6 CONCLUSION

Musculoskeletal US not only facilitates recognition of the pathology, but also guides the treatment to the predetermined structures. Various techniques and medications can be used and should actually be chosen based on the pathology, its anatomical location and the physician's expertise. For sure, sterility is a prerequisite.

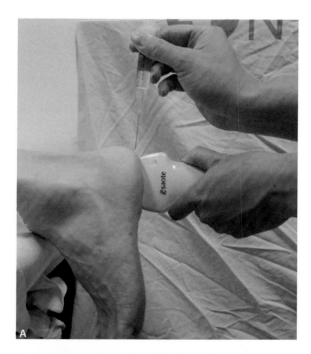

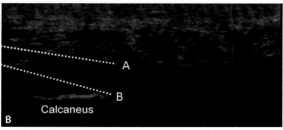

**Figure 18.20** Plantar fascia injection. A - Illustration of the posture and transducer placement for injection of the left plantar fascia. B - Introduction of the needle posteriorly to the transducer at an angle of 20 degrees until the needle tip hits the plantar fascia. It is difficult to inject within the fascia, so the authors suggest inject some medication superficial to the fascia (dot line A) and some deep to the fascia (dot line B).

# REFERENCES

1) De Muynck M, Parlevliet T, De Cock K, Vanden Bossche L, Vanderstraeten G, Ozcakar L. Musculoskeletal ultrasound for interventional physiatry. Eur J Phys Rehabil Med. 2012; 48: 675-87.

2) Louis LJ. Musculoskeletal ultrasound intervention: principles and advances. Radiol Clin North Am. 2008; 46: 515-33, vi.

3) Robotti G, Canepa MG, Bortolotto C, Draghi F. Interventional musculoskeletal US: an update on materials and methods. J Ultrasound. 2013; 16: 45-55.

4) Hsieh LF, Hsu WC, Lin YJ, Wu SH, Chang KC, Chang HL. Is ultrasound-guided injection more effective in chronic subacromial bursitis? Med Sci Sports Exerc. 2013; 45: 2205-13.

5) Hashiuchi T, Sakurai G, Sakamoto Y, Takakura Y, Tanaka Y. Comparative survey of pain-alleviating effects between ultrasound-guided injection and blind injection of lidocaine alone in patients with painful shoulder. Arch Orthop Trauma Surg. 2010; 130: 847-52.

6) Rutten MJ, Collins JM, Maresch BJ, Smeets JH, Janssen CM, Kiemeney LA, et al. Glenohumeral joint injection: a comparative study of ultrasound and fluoroscopically guided techniques before MR arthrography. Eur Radiol. 2009; 19: 722-30.

7) Sethi PM, Kingston S, Elattrache N. Accuracy of anterior intra-articular injection of the glenohumeral joint. Arthroscopy. 2005; 21: 77-80.

8) Chen MJ, Lew HL, Hsu TC, Tsai WC, Lin WC, Tang SF, et al. Ultrasound-guided shoulder injections in the treatment of subacromial bursitis. Am J Phys Med Rehabil. 2006; 85: 31-5.

9) Lee HJ, Lim KB, Kim DY, Lee KT. Randomized controlled trial for efficacy of intra-articular injection for adhesive capsulitis: ultrasonography-guided versus blind technique. Arch Phys Med Rehabil. 2009; 90: 1997-2002.

10) Smith J, Rizzo M, Sayeed YA, Finnoff JT. Sonographically guided distal radioulnar joint injection: technique and validation in a cadaveric model. J Ultrasound Med. 2011; 30: 1587-92.

11) Smith J, Hurdle MF, Locketz AJ, Wisniewski SJ. Ultrasound-guided piriformis injection: technique description and verification. Arch Phys Med Rehabil. 2006; 87: 1664-7.

12) Jee H, Lee JH, Park KD, Ahn J, Park Y. Ultrasound-guided versus fluoroscopy-guided sacroiliac joint intra-articular injections in the noninflammatory sacroiliac joint dysfunction: a prospective, randomized, single-blinded study. Arch Phys Med Rehabil. 2014; 95: 330-7.

13) Taras JS, Raphael JS, Pan WT, Movagharnia F, Sotereanos DG. Corticosteroid injections for trigger digits: is intrasheath injection necessary? J Hand Surg. 1998; 23: 717-22.

14) Bruyn GA, Schmidt WA. How to perform ultrasound-guided injections. Best Pract Res Clin Rheumatol. 2009; 23: 269-79.

15) Stephens MB, Beutler AI, O'Connor FG. Musculoskeletal injections: a review of the evidence. Am Fam Physician. 2008; 78: 971-6.

16) Dean BJ, Lostis E, Oakley T, Rombach I, Morrey ME, Carr AJ. The risks and benefits of glucocorticoid treatment for tendinopathy: A systematic review of the effects of local glucocorticoid on tendon. Semin Arthritis Rheum. 2013; 43: 570-6.

17) Berthelot JM, Le Goff B, Maugars Y. Side effects of corticosteroid injections: what's new? Joint Bone Spine. 2013; 80: 363-7.

18) Rutjes AW, Juni P, da Costa BR, Trelle S, Nuesch E, Reichenbach S. Viscosupplementation for osteoarthritis of the knee: a systematic review and meta-analysis. Ann Intern Med. 2012; 157: 180-91.

19) Lo GH, LaValley M, McAlindon T, Felson DT. Intra-articular hyaluronic acid in treatment of knee osteoarthritis: a meta-analysis. JAMA. 2003; 290: 3115-21.

20) Bellamy N, Campbell J, Robinson V, Gee T, Bourne R, Wells G. Viscosupplementation for the treatment of osteoarthritis of the knee. Cochrane Database Syst Rev. 2006(2): CD005321.

21) Chang KV, Hsiao MY, Chen WS, Wang TG, Chien KL. Effectiveness of intra-articular hyaluronic acid for ankle osteoarthritis treatment: a systematic review and meta-analysis. Arch Phys Med Rehabil. 2013; 94: 951-60.

22) Colen S, Haverkamp D, Mulier M, van den Bekerom MP. Hyaluronic acid for the treatment of osteoarthritis in all joints except the knee: what is the current evidence? BioDrugs. 2012; 26: 101-12.

23) Krogh TP, Bartels EM, Ellingsen T, Stengaard-Pedersen K, Buchbinder R, Fredberg U, et al. Comparative effectiveness of injection therapies in lateral epicondylitis: a systematic review and network meta-analysis of randomized controlled trials. Am J Sports Med. 2013; 41: 1435-46.

24) Rabago D, Patterson JJ. Prolotherapy: an effective adjunctive therapy for knee osteoarthritis. J Am Osteopath Assoc. 2013; 113: 122-3.

25) Carayannopoulos A, Borg-Stein J, Sokolof J, Meleger A, Rosenberg D. Prolotherapy versus corticosteroid injections for the treatment of lateral epicondylosis: a randomized controlled trial. PM R. 2011; 3: 706-15.

26) Rabago D, Best TM, Beamsley M, Patterson J. A systematic review of prolotherapy for chronic

musculoskeletal pain. Clin J Sport Med. 2005; 15: 376-80.

27) Zhang Q, Ge H, Zhou J, Cheng B. Are platelet-rich products necessary during the arthroscopic repair of full-thickness rotator cuff tears: a meta-analysis. PLoS One. 2013; 8(7): e69731.

28) Sheth U, Simunovic N, Klein G, Fu F, Einhorn TA, Schemitsch E, et al. Efficacy of autologous platelet-rich plasma use for orthopaedic indications: a meta-analysis. J Bone Joint Surg Am. 2012; 94: 298-307.

29) Chang KV, Hung CY, Aliwarga F, Wang TG, Han DS, Chen WS. Comparative effectiveness of platelet-rich plasma injections for treating knee joint cartilage degenerative pathology: a systematic review and meta-analysis. Arch Phys Med Rehabil. 2014; 95: 562-75.

30) Ozcakir S, Sivrioglu K. Botulinum toxin in post-stroke spasticity. Clin Med Res. 2007; 5: 132-8.

31) Teasell R, Foley N, Pereira S, Sequeira K, Miller T. Evidence to practice: botulinum toxin in the treatment of spasticity post stroke. Top Stroke Rehabil. 2012; 19: 115-21.

32) Francisco GE, Tan H, Green M. Do botulinum toxins have a role in the management of neuropathic pain?: a focused review. Am J Phys Med Rehabil. 2012; 91: 899-909.

33) Ghai A, Garg N, Hooda S, Gupta T. Spasticity - Pathogenesis, prevention and treatment strategies. Saudi J Anaesth. 2013; 7: 453-60.

34) McIntyre A, Lee T, Janzen S, Mays R, Mehta S, Teasell R. Systematic review of the effectiveness of pharmacological interventions in the treatment of spasticity of the hemiparetic lower extremity more than six months post stroke. Top Stroke Rehabil. 2012; 19: 479-90.

35) Yelnik AP, Simon O, Parratte B, Gracies JM. How to clinically assess and treat muscle overactivity in spastic paresis. J Rehabil Med. 2010; 42: 801-7.

36) Sage W, Pickup L, Smith TO, Denton ER, Toms AP. The clinical and functional outcomes of ultrasound-guided vs landmark-guided injections for adults with shoulder pathology - a systematic review and meta-analysis. Rheumatology (Oxford). 2013; 52: 743-51.

37) Li Z, Xia C, Yu A, Qi B. Ultrasound- versus palpation-guided injection of corticosteroid for plantar fasciitis: a meta-analysis. PLoS One. 2014; 9(3): e92671.

38) Serafini G, Sconfienza LM, Lacelli F, Silvestri E, Aliprandi A, Sardanelli F. Rotator cuff calcific tendonitis: short-term and 10-year outcomes after two-needle us-guided percutaneous treatment-nonrandomized controlled trial. Radiology. 2009; 252: 157-64.

39) Koscielniak-Nielsen ZJ, Dahl JB. Ultrasound-guided peripheral nerve blockade of the upper extremity. Curr Opin Anaesthesiol. 2012; 25: 253-9.

40) Picelli A, Lobba D, Midiri A, Prandi P, Melotti C, Baldessarelli S, et al. Botulinum toxin injection into the forearm muscles for wrist and fingers spastic overactivity in adults with chronic stroke: a randomized controlled trial comparing three injection techniques. Clin Rehabil. 2013; 28: 232-42.

41) Picelli A, Tamburin S, Bonetti P, Fontana C, Barausse M, Dambruoso F, et al. Botulinum toxin type A injection into the gastrocnemius muscle for spastic equinus in adults with stroke: a randomized controlled trial comparing manual needle placement, electrical stimulation and ultrasonography-guided injection techniques. Am J Phys Med Rehabil. 2012; 91: 957-64.

42) Picelli A, Bonetti P, Fontana C, Barausse M, Dambruoso F, Gajofatto F, et al. Accuracy of botulinum toxin type A injection into the gastrocnemius muscle of adults with spastic equinus: manual needle placement and electrical stimulation guidance compared using ultrasonography. J Rehabil Med. 2012; 44: 450-2.

43) Rojo-Manaute JM, Capa-Grasa A, Rodriguez-Maruri GE, Moran LM, Martinez MV, Martin JV. Ultra-minimally invasive sonographically guided carpal tunnel release: anatomic study of a new technique. J Ultrasound Med. 2013; 32: 131-42.

44) McShane JM, Slaff S, Gold JE, Nazarian LN. Sonographically guided percutaneous needle release of the carpal tunnel for treatment of carpal tunnel syndrome: preliminary report. J Ultrasound Med. 2012; 31: 1341-9.

45) Koski JM, Hammer HB. Ultrasound-guided procedures: techniques and usefulness in controlling inflammation and disease progression. Rheumatology (Oxford). 2013; 51 Suppl 7: vii31-5.

46) Scire CA, Epis O, Codullo V, Humby F, Morbini P, Manzo A, et al. Immunohistological assessment of the synovial tissue in small joints in rheumatoid arthritis: validation of a minimally invasive ultrasound-guided synovial biopsy procedure. Arthritis Res Ther. 2007; 9(5): R101.

47) Ashraf MO, Devadoss VG. Systematic review and meta-analysis on steroid injection therapy for de Quervain's tenosynovitis in adults. Eur J Orthop Surg Traumatol. 2013; 24: 149-57.

48) Kume K, Amano K, Yamada S, Kuwaba N, Ohta H. In de Quervain's with a separate EPB compartment, ultrasound-guided steroid injection is more effective than a clinical injection technique: a prospective open-label study. J Hand Surg Eur Vol. 2012; 37: 523-7.

49) Ustun N, Tok F, Yagz AE, Kizil N, Korkmaz I, Karazincir S, et al. Ultrasound-guided vs. blind steroid injections in carpal tunnel syndrome: A

single-blind randomized prospective study. Am J Phys Med Rehabil. 2013; 92: 999-1004.

50) Smith J, Wisniewski SJ, Finnoff JT, Payne JM. Sonographically guided carpal tunnel injections: the ulnar approach. J Ultrasound Med. 2008; 27: 1485-90.

51) Peters-Veluthamaningal C, van der Windt DA, Winters JC, Meyboom-de Jong B. Corticosteroid injection for trigger finger in adults. Cochrane Database Syst Rev. 2009(1): CD005617.

52) Klauser A, De Zordo T, Feuchtner G, Sogner P, Schirmer M, Gruber J, et al. Feasibility of ultrasound-guided sacroiliac joint injection considering sonoanatomic landmarks at two different levels in cadavers and patients. Arthritis Rheum. 2008; 59: 1618-24.

53) Chen CP, Tang SF, Hsu TC, Tsai WC, Liu HP, Chen MJ, et al. Ultrasound guidance in caudal epidural needle placement. Anesthesiology. 2004; 101: 181-4.

54) D'Agostino MA, Schmidt WA. Ultrasound-guided injections in rheumatology: actual knowledge on efficacy and procedures. Best Pract Res Clin Rheumatol. 2013; 27: 283-94.

55) Yablon CM. Ultrasound-guided interventions of the foot and ankle. Semin Musculoskelet Radiol. 2013; 17: 60-8.

# Trends and Research

# Developing New Technologies in Musculoskeletal Ultrasound

## 19

### Alparslan Bayram ÇARLI

The twenty-first century has opened a new era for musculoskeletal ultrasonography (US). Sonographic technology is a very fast-changing process -even when compared to only a decade before. As US is the most frequently used imaging modality in the world, with almost 25% of all imaging studies performed [1], manufacturers invest significant engineering resources to develop the technology and to improve the diagnostic capabilities of US imaging. As a result of strategic partnerships among industry, pharmaceutical companies and academia; along with the advances in electronics and computing, new imaging technologies are constantly being introduced to the clinicians.

New technologies in US can be covered in three main categories: i) developments in transducers, ii) developments in image enhancement techniques and imaging algorithms, and iii) other technologies.

## 19.1 DEVELOPMENTS IN TRANSDUCERS

As the performance of the transducer determines the sensitivity, resolution and quality of the information coming out of the human body, transducer technology may be considered as the most critical part of US imaging. As such, various most important advances in the field of US imaging emerge with the developments in transducer technology. In the last 30 years, piezoelectric materials have been developed to produce high sensitive and efficient probes that have a wide dynamic range and frequency bandwidth [2]. Broadband technology has led the way towards the development of non-linear and harmonic imaging [3].

Superficial and tiny anatomical structures could be visualized with smaller and higher frequency transducers. Likewise, the development of

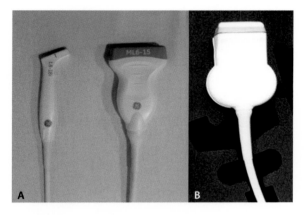

**Figure 19.1**  A - 5-18 MHz, 25 mm footprint linear hockey stick probe (left) and 5-15 MHz, 50 mm footprint linear matrix probe (right). B - Linear volume (3D) probe.

the hockey stick or pen probes have facilitated the examination of smaller joints that are otherwise quite difficult to be scanned especially in the presence of deformities (Figure 19.1).

Newer transducers are already equipped with biopsy guiding systems and needle tracking facilities to improve needle visualization [4]. Array configurations, transducer materials, higher frequency probes, higher element densities, innovative geometries, advances in beam forming and improved ferroelectrics that are still in research phase will determine future transducer developments.

## 19.2 DEVELOPMENTS IN IMAGE ENHANCEMENT TECHNIQUES AND IMAGING ALGORITHMS

### 19.2.1 Tissue Harmonic Imaging

While conventional US transmits/receives at the same frequency and forms the image from echoes of the transmitted frequency; tissue harmonic imaging (THI) uses the tissue-generated echoes and the second harmonic signal is used to form the image by separating it from the fundamental echoes using filters [4, 5]. However, as the waves from superficial structures have less time to distort, this has less impact in musculoskeletal conditions [6]. Better spatial and contrast resolutions are obtained with the images generated with THI [7].

THI improves the 'good' artifacts (distal acoustic shadowing and enhanced through transmission) and reduces the 'bad' artifacts (lobe, ringdown, and volume averaging) [8]. THI has often been highlighted as working best in obese patients [9] and every manufacturer by now has THI on majority of their probes/systems (Figure 19.2).

## 19.2.2 Compound Imaging

This is a technique that reduces artifacts and improves resolution by combining images acquired from different angles or aperture positions, or using multiple frequencies. There are three types of compounding; spatial compounding, frequency compounding and strain compounding [7]. The technique that has received most attention is real time spatial compounding, which has already been implemented by several manufacturers. It produces a single real-time image from multiple fused frames that are acquired at different imaging angles [10]. Spatial compounding uses software enhancements to make better use of reflected echoes especially from superficial tissues [6] (Figure 19.3).

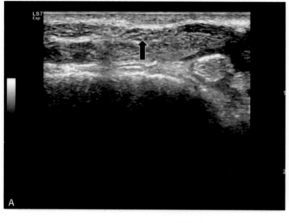

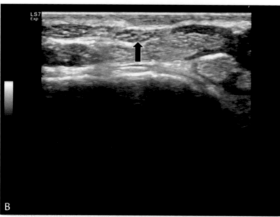

**Figure 19.2** Axial sonogram of the median nerve (arrows) without (A) and with (B) tissue harmonic imaging (note the enhancement of the image in B).

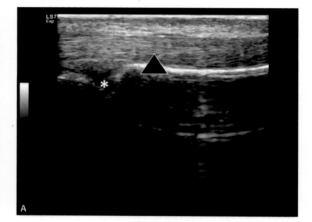

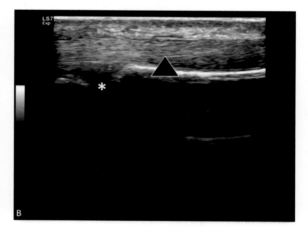

**Figure 19.3** Longitudinal sonogram of the metacarpophalangeal joint (asterisks) and the flexor tendons (arrowheads) without (A) and with (B) Compound Imaging (note the enhancement of the image in B).

Musculoskeletal Ultrasound in Physical and Rehabilitation Medicine

### 19.2.3 Extended Field-of-view

Sometimes, it can be difficult to visualize the lesions that are longer than the length of the transducer footprint. In this case, extended field-of-view technology may be helpful to scan the entire lesion in one image [8]. This method uses amalgamated multiple images obtained in a steady sweep to form an image of a complete tissue structure, providing a more global perspective [11]. Extended field-of-view is most useful for superficial structures such as the musculoskeletal system, neck, scrotum, and breast [4] (Figure 19.4).

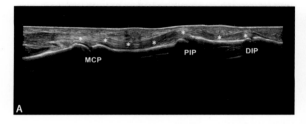

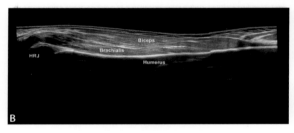

**Figure 19.4** A - Extended Field-of-view image of the third finger (flexor side). Asterisks: Flexor tendons. B - Extended field-of-view image of the biceps muscle from its origin to insertion. HRJ, humero-radial joint. MCP, metacarpophalangeal joint; PIP, proximal interphalangeal joint; DIP, distal interphalangeal joint.

### 19.2.4 Beam Forming

This technique forms the ultrasound beam for improved propagation and provides a better penetration, and thereby a better resolution with decreased artifacts (i.e. side-lobes and speed of sound errors) [7]. Ultrasound beams generated by beam forming are less affected by tissue inhomogeneities and they provide imaging of the same tissue multiple times in different directions. The echoes from these acquisitions are averaged into a single composite image and the probability of the beam encountering a reflector at or closer to 90° is

increased [7]. Newer devices are labeled as having digital beam formers.

### 19.2.5 Photopic Imaging

This is a real-time or post-processing technology which can be considered as an automatic optimization method and utilizing ability of the human eye to separate colors by using an adaptive contrast optimization scheme. It expands the grey scale dynamic range and applies monochromatic color to stimulate photopic vision [11] (Figure 19.5).

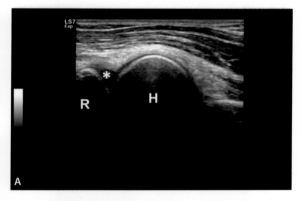

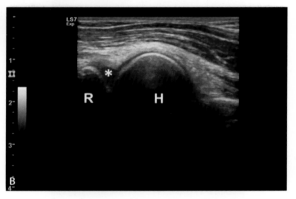

**Figure 19.5** Longitudinal sonogram of the humeroradial joint (asterisks) without (A) and with (B) photopic imaging. R, radius; H, humerus.

### 19.2.6 Fusion Imaging

Combination of high contrast resolution images of computed tomography or magnetic resonance with the high resolution and dynamic properties of US is referred as fusion imaging [6].

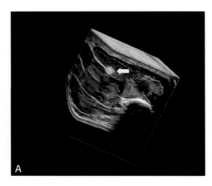

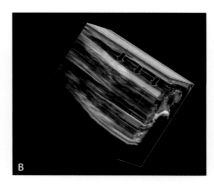

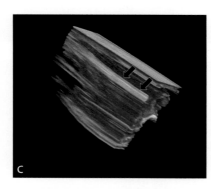

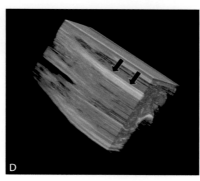

**Figure 19.6** 3D Imaging of the flexor pollicis longus tendon (arrows). A - Anterior view. B - Lateral view. C - Render parameter mixture, Grey surface. D - Render parameter mixture, Grey surface/Texture.

It uses simultaneous mapping of ultrasound images onto a pre-acquired tomographic or magnetic resonance imaging volume dataset. Fusion imaging has been shown useful for the differentiation of anatomical structures or for injection of the sacroiliac joint [12]. For sure, additional research in this area is warranted.

### 19.2.7 3D/4D Imaging

In recent years, three-dimensional (3D) US has become one of the most fascinating new tools with its potential of changing the traditional approach to musculoskeletal US. 3D imaging uses stored sets of adjacent 2D slices to create an ultrasound volume. 2D slices are captured either with a 2D probe sweeping over the tissue volume by the operator or with placing a bulky 3D probe (Figure 19.1 B) over the tissue volume and holding it there while the probe obtains multiple side-by-side 2D slices. 4D probes are actually 3D probes collecting volumes rapidly, the fourth dimension referring to time [6] (Figure 19.6).

A unique advantage of 3D US is that it can improve operator reliability. Yet, it is an operator-independent method; unskilled personnel can acquire/save data which can later be reviewed by skilled physicians if necessary [6, 12].

3D US imaging has already found its place as a clinically useful tool in obstetrics; particularly for the diagnosis of facial abnormalities [11]. On the other hand, having been applied to musculoskeletal imaging only recently, the clinical relevance of this promising technology still needs to be ascertained with future studies.

## 19.3 OTHER TECHNOLOGIES

### 19.3.1 Sonoelastography

Sonoelastography (SE) is a very exciting new area of research and it is probably the most important technical development in the field of US, except Doppler imaging. This technique pertains practically to tissue stiffness imaging with the use of US. The main principle of SE is simple: when pressure is applied, soft tissues will deform more and hard tissues will deform less. SE uses the elastic characteristics of the tissues; when pressure is applied tissues deform and move away from the US probe. This amount of displacement is called

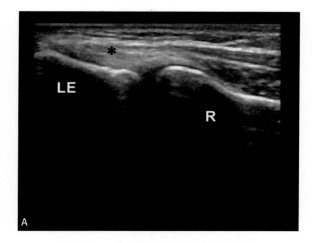

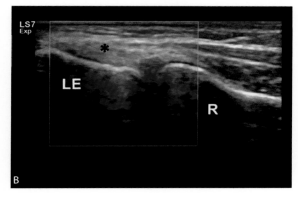

**Figure 19.7** Sonoelastogram of the common extensor tendons (asterisks) at the level of lateral epicondyle (LE). B - mode image (A) and sonoelastogram of the same area (B). R, radius.

strain [13]. The software detects and calculates the strain and converts the values to color codes that represent different degrees of stiffness superimposed on the conventional B-mode images. In most devices, red is often used for encoding soft tissues, blue for hard tissues and yellow/green for intermediate tissues. By this way, lesions in tissues can be distinguished as altered areas of stiffness; but, of note, the information of elasticity obtained with this method is qualitative or semi-quantitative [13].

There are four main SE techniques based on the type of stress applied and the method used to detect tissue displacement: strain SE, shear wave SE, transient SE and acoustic radiation force SE [14]. Strain SE, also called compression SE, free-hand SE or real-time SE, is the most commonly used approach. This technique uses compression applied manually via the hand-held ultrasound transducer to generate tissue deformation. Strain SE actually measures the relative strain of one area vs another, and displays it as a map. On the other hand, shear wave SE uses an impulse generated by the ultrasound probe for tissue excitation [15] (Figure 19.7).

SE is not widely used in routine musculoskeletal clinical practice but its usefulness has been well proven for breast, thyroid, liver, lymph node, prostate, atheromatous plaque imaging [16]. SE can actually be used for almost every musculoskeletal tissue including muscles, tendons, ligaments, fluid collections and nerves. Likewise, there are growing reports on musculoskeletal applications of SE in the literature as regards plantar fasciitis [17], Achilles tendon degeneration/injury [18], lateral epicondylitis [19], trigger finger [20], carpal tunnel syndrome [21], fibromyalgia [22], systemic sclerosis [23], congenital muscular dystrophy [24], myositis [25] and lymphedema [26]. SE has also been reported helpful for guiding myofascial trigger point treatment [27], for detecting the optimal site for botulinum toxin injection [28] and for predicting treatment outcomes in congenital muscular torticollis [29]. On the other hand, further research for proper technical standardization is still warranted before SE can be adopted into daily musculoskeletal practice.

## 19.3.2 Tissue Velocity Imaging and Speckle Tracking

Tissue Velocity Imaging (TVI) is a technique used for the analysis of mechanical parameters and functionality of tissues such as velocity and deformation in real-time [30]. US images include many small particles which move together with the tissue. Actually they are natural acoustic markers called speckles. The main idea of TVI comprises the identification and tracking of these speckles during sequential frames [31, 32]. By analyzing the motion of these speckles; the system calculates displacement, the rate of displacement (velocity), deformation (strain), and the rate of deformation (strain rate) of the selected tissue segment [32]. The speckle tracking method can be described as displacement maps showing tissue motion in real time [33]. This technique was firstly developed for evaluation of the segmental movement and velocity of the myocardium [30]. For instance, different patterns of dyskinesia due to cardiac infarction or ischemia can easily be evaluated with this method [34].

Speckle tracking technology has recently become commercially available as a software. As the TVI aims to study the tissue dynamics, the technique can also be applied to evaluate various musculoskeletal disorders [34, 35]. Owing to the possibility to evaluate deeply located muscles non-invasively, this technology can also serve as a complementary method to electromyography [30]. Again, future studies will better demonstrate how these can be applied reliably/effectively in musculoskeletal medicine.

### 19.3.3 Contrast-enhanced Ultrasound

Contrast-enhanced US (CEUS) technology refers to the use of intravenous ultrasound contrast agents (UCAs) -that are actually microbubbles-during imaging [36]. The main idea is to improve the visualization of blood flow. All UCAs have some common characteristics: i) a core containing a non-diffusible and acoustically reflective gas, ii) stabilized by a thin protective outer shell (phospholipid or albumin), and iii) a diameter range of 0.5–10 μm allowing them to pass through the systemic capillary beds [36, 37].

While CEUS imaging can be applied for any structure, currently, the only FDA-approved clinical applications are cardiac and hepatic imaging [36,37]. Studies have demonstrated that microbubbles are phagocytosed by neutrophils and monocytes, which can thus be assessed by ultrasound imaging [38]. In this sense, CEUS imaging may potentially be useful for the diagnosis and follow up of different inflammatory conditions of the musculoskeletal system.

### 19.3.4 Endoluminal Ultrasound

Endoluminal US uses nano-probes that can be inserted through a 21 G needle or catheter. This technique is used for the imaging of the gastro-intestinal tract, biliary system, urogenital tract, tracheobronchial tree and the cardio-vascular system. Intravascular US has been applied to the coronary and carotid arteries for plaque characterization, or to guide/monitor angioplasty [4].

### 19.3.5 Acoustic Microscopy

Acoustic microscopy uses ultra-high frequency (30-100 MHz) micro-probes. Although this in-situ histological tool is yet not commonplace in daily practice, dermatology and ophthalmology seem to be the potential areas for its application [4].

### 19.3.6 Ultrasonographic Drug and Gene Delivery

It is known that US increases cell membrane permeability in a process called sonoporation. With this technique, tissues can be targeted to improve the cellular uptake of a drug or a gene. Sonoporation needs high acoustic powers (beyond the diagnostic range), but this power is reduced in the presence of microbubbles (similar with those used for contrast enhanced US). A drug or gene vector is implemented in or on the surface of a microbubble and tracked in the vascular circulation. In case of high power US exposure, microbubbles rupture and release the agent (drug/gene) inside the target tissue. There are encouraging studies in the field of US-directed, site-specific delivery systems using UCAs in the literature [4].

### 19.3.7 High Intensity Focused US

This is actually not a new technique [39]; but recent advances in transducers and imaging algorithms made it possible for clinical applications. High intensity focused US (HIFU) uses a highly focused US beam to destroy a defined volume of tissue by inducing a rapid increase in temperature to greater than 50° C. It is a non-invasive technique that is used in the treatment of malignant tumors via percutaneous/transrectal approach or even intra-operatively [4].

# REFERENCES

1) Goldberg BB. International arena of ultrasound education. J Ultrasound Med. 2003; 22: 549-51.

2) Kollmann C. New sonographic techniques for harmonic imaging - Underlying physical principles. Eur J Radiol. 2007; 64: 164-72.

3) Whittingham TA. Broadband transducers. Eur Radiol. 1999; 9: 298-303.

4) Harvey CJ, Pilcher JM, Eckersley RJ, Blomley MJ, Cosgrove DO. Advances in ultrasound. Clin Radiol. 2002; 57: 157-77.

5) Desser TS, Jeffrey RB. Tissue harmonic imaging techniques: physical principles and clinical applications. Semin Ultrasound CT MR. 2001; 22: 1-10.

6) McNally EG. The development and clinical applications of musculoskeletal ultrasound. Skeletal Radiol. 2011; 40: 1223-31.

7) Ortiz SHC, Chiua T, Fox MD. Ultrasound image enhancement: A review. Biomed Signal Proces. 2012; 7: 419-28.

8) O'Brien RT, Holmes SP. Recent advances in ultrasound technology. Clin Tech Small Anim Pract. 2007; 22: 93-103.

9) Tanaka S, Oshikawa O, Sasaki T. Evaluation of tissue harmonic imaging for the diagnosis of focal liver lesions. Ultrasound Med Biol. 2000; 26: 183-7.

10) Oktar SO, Yücel C, Özdemir H, Ulutürk A, Işik S. Comparison of conventional sonography, real-time compound sonography, tissue harmonic sonography, and tissue harmonic compound sonography of abdominal and pelvic lesions. Am J Roentgenol. 2003; 181: 1341-7.

11) Forsberg F. Ultrasonic biomedical technology; marketing versus clinical reality. Ultrasonics. 2004; 42: 17-27.

12) Kang T, Lanni S, Nam J, Emery P, Wakefield RJ. The evolution of ultrasound in rheumatology. Ther Adv Musculoskelet Dis. 2012; 4: 399-411.

13) Li Y, Snedeker JG. Elastography: modality-specific approaches, clinical applications, and research horizons. Skeletal Radiol. 2011; 40: 389-97.

14) Garra BS. Elastography: current status, future prospects, and making it work for you. Ultrasound Q. 2011; 27: 177-86.

15) Drakonaki EE, Allen GM, Wilson DJ. Ultrasound elastography for musculoskeletal applications. Br J Radiol. 2012; 85: 1435-45.

16) Kuo WH, Jian D, Wang TG, Wang YC. Neck muscle stiffness quantified by sonoelastography is correlated with body mass index and chronic neck pain symptoms. Ultrasound Med Biol. 2013; 39: 1356-61.

17) Wu CH, Chang KV, Mio S, Chen WS, Wang TG. Sonoelastography of the plantar fascia. Radiology. 2011; 259: 502-7.

18) Klauser AS, Myamoto H, Tamegger M, Faschingbauer R, Moriggi B, Klima G. Achilles tendon assessed with sonoelastography: histologic agreement. Radiology. 2013; 267: 837-42.

19) De Zordo T, Lill SR, Fink C, Feuchtner GM, Jaschke W, Bellmann-Weiler R. Real-time sonoelastography of lateral epicondylitis: comparison of findings between patients and healthy volunteers. AJR Am J Roentgenol. 2009; 193: 180-5.

20) Miyamoto H, Miura T, Isayama H. Stiffness of the first annular pulley in normal and trigger fingers. J Hand Surg Am. 2011; 36: 1486-91.

21) Orman G, Özben S, Hüseyinoğlu N, Duymus M, Orman KG. Ultrasound elastographic evaluation in the diagnosis of carpal tunnel syndrome: initial findings. Ultrasound Med Biol. 2013; 39: 1184-9.

22) Muro-Culebras A, Cuesta-Vargas AI. Sono-myography and sono-myoelastography of the tender points of women with fibromyalgia. Ultrasound Med Biol. 2013; 39: 1951-7.

23) Iagnocco A, Kaloudi O, Perella C, Bandinelli F, Riccieri V, Vasile M. Ultrasound elastography assessment of skin involvement in systemic sclerosis: lights and shadows. J Rheumatol. 2010; 37: 1688-91.

24) Drakonaki EE, Allen GM. Magnetic resonance imaging, ultrasound and real-time ultrasound elastography of the thigh muscles in congenital muscle dystrophy. Skeletal Radiol. 2010; 39: 391-6.

25) Botar-Jid C, Damian L, Dudea SM, Vasilescu D, Rednic S, Badea R. The contribution of ultrasonography and sonoelastography in assessment of myositis. Med Ultrason. 2010; 12: 120-6.

26) Tsubai M, Fukuda O, Ueno N, Horie T, Muraki S. Development of an ultrasound system for measuring tissue strain of lymphedema. Conf Proc IEEE Eng Med Biol Soc. 2008; 2008: 5294-7.

27) Sikdar S, Shah JP, Gebreab T, Yen RH, Gilliams E, Danoff J. Novel applications of ultrasound technology to visualize and characterize myofascial trigger points and surrounding soft tissue. Arch Phys Med Rehabil. 2009; 90: 1829-38.

28) Park GY, Kwon DR. Sonoelastographic evaluation of medial gastrocnemius muscles intrinsic stiffness after rehabilitation therapy with botulinum toxin a injection in spastic cerebral palsy. Arch Phys Med Rehabil. 2012; 93: 2085-9.

29) Kwon DR, Park GY. Diagnostic value of real-time sonoelastography in congenital muscular torticollis. J Ultrasound Med. 2012; 31: 721-7.

30) Lindberg F, Martensson M, Grönlund C, Brodin LÅ. Evaluation of ultrasound Tissue Velocity Imaging: a phantom study of velocity estimation in skeletal muscle low-level contractions. BMC Med

Imaging. 2013; 13: 16.

31) Reisner SA, Lysyansky P, Agmon Y, Mutlak D, Lessich J, Friedman Z. Global longitudinal strain: A novel index of left ventricular systolic function. J Am Soc Echocardogr. 2004; 17: 630-3.

32) Leitman M, Lysyansky P, Sidenko S, Shir V, Peleg E, Binenbaum M. Two-dimensional strain-a novel software for real-time quantitative echocardiographic assessment of myocardial function. J Am Soc Echocardiogr. 2004; 17: 1021-9.

33) Nordez A, Gallot T, Catheline S, Guével A, Cornu C, Hug F. Electromechanical delay revisited using very high frame rate ultrasound. J Appl Physiol. 2009; 106: 1970-5.

34) Peolsson M, Larsson B, Brodin LA, Gerdle B. A pilot study using Tissue Velocity Ultrasound Imaging (TVI) to assess muscle activity pattern in patients with chronic trapezius myalgia. BMC Musculoskelet Disord. 2008; 9: 127.

35) Arndt A, Bengtsson AS, Peolsson M, Thorstensson A, Movin T. Non-uniform displacement within the Achilles tendon during passive ankle joint motion. Knee Surg Sports Traumatol Arthrosc. 2012; 20: 1868-74.

36) Castle J, Butts M, Healey A, Kent K Marino M, Feinstein SB. Ultrasound-mediated targeted drug delivery: recent success and remaining challenges. Am J Physiol Heart Circ Physiol. 2013; 304: 350-7.

37) Liu JB, Wansaicheong G, Merton DA, Forsberg F, Golberg BB. Contrast-enhanced ultrasound imaging: State of the art. J Med Ultrasound. 2005; 13: 109-26.

38) Shohet RV, Chen S, Zhou YT, Wang Z, Meidell RS, Unger RH. Echocardiographic destruction of albumin microbubbles directs gene delivery to the myocardium. Circulation. 2000; 101: 2554-6.

39) Ter Haar G. Intervention and therapy. Ultrasound Med Biol. 2000; 26: 51-4.

# Musculoskeletal Ultrasound in Research

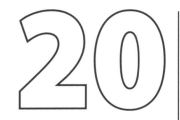

Levent ÖZÇAKAR, Wen-Shiang CHEN, Franco FRANCHIGNONI

The general concept regarding the use of musculoskeletal ultrasound (US) is "to see in order to believe". Naturally, the next two steps would be "if you see, you can quantify it" and "if you see, you can have access to that structure/pathology". The former has built up the rationale why/how US can be used for research in musculoskeletal medicine. Yet, while imaging structures, you can make quantitative (measurement), semi-quantitative (grading) or qualitative assessments (presence/absence, echogenicity). Likewise, as one starts to acquire data as regards the musculoskeletal system, those can naturally be converted into analysis and used in research, aside from daily clinical practice. Additionally, the acquisition of certain data is unique to US and cannot be provided with other imaging tools (Figure 20.1). For sure, the advances in US technology over years, the industrial evolution of new-generation machines, and probe quality have made a great contribution in that sense.

Being aware of this issue, we have previously evaluated the actual use of US in research in Physical and Rehabilitation Medicine (PRM) [1, 2]. Our results have clearly shown that publications of physiatrists are increasing in parallel with their mounting interest in musculoskeletal US [1, 2]. Importantly, the percentage of those research papers published in PRM journals also shows a tendency to increase, i.e. 44% in 2011 [1] and 46% in 2013 [2]. Being "the egg or chicken", several projects or working groups on musculoskeletal US (e.g. TURK-MUSKULUS, EURO-MUSCULUS, USPRM, WORLD-MUSCULUS) have been founded in the meantime [3-6].

A snapshot on the more recent analyses shows that physiatrists use musculoskeletal US in their research mainly to study knee-shoulder (as region/joint), muscle-tendon (as tissue type), and more human beings rather than cadavers or ani-

mals [2]. In addition, orthopedic or peripheral nerve problems seemed to be the mostly studied topics (diagnostic more than interventional US) [2]. There were no quantitative or semi-quantitative assessments in 40.7% of the papers; however, 8.6% comprised semi-quantitative, 38.8% quantitative evaluations, and 11.9% included both [2]. While 8.2% of the papers were validity/reliability studies for US, 8.6% were intra-observer and/or inter-observer testing studies. A few studies (13.4%) had used at least one other imaging modality for comparison, whereas most of the studies had used only US.

On the other hand, keeping in mind the user-dependency of US, care and vigilance should always remain as the prerequisite concerning the different types of sonographic measurements/evaluations. It has been previously shown that novice sonographers tend to measure erroneously and that the difference between their measurements and those of an expert decreases in line with the number of patients they evaluate with US

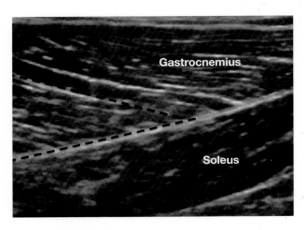

**Figure 20.1** Longitudinal ultrasound imaging on the medial head of the gastrocnemius muscle exemplifies pennation angle and fascicle length measurements.

[7, 8]. Moreover, similar to the role during the lengthy US training, the effect of supervision by a mentor is again noteworthy [9]. In this sense, it is suggested that the sonographer takes an average of several measurements should the US assessment entail any quantification.

As for exemplary topics, there is growing interest for physiatrists in using US to guide interventions such as injection, biopsy or aspiration [10]. US allows real-time visualization of the needle and target to avoid injuries to the surrounding vulnerable structures and increase success rate. New US-guidance techniques are increasingly being proposed in the literature. However, when compared with blind injections, whether US-guidance affects the treatment outcome remains to be further elucidated. Another popular US-related topic for physiatrists is sonoelastography. It allows the assessment of mechanical properties of soft tissues and can be used to detect musculoskeletal disorders and to follow-up treatment re-sponse (see also Chapter 19 - "Developing New Technologies in Musculosckeletal Ultrasound"). For instance, softer plantar fasciae were found in patients with plantar fasciitis on elastography [11].

Another interesting topic would be speckle tracking whereby precise movements of various tissues can be quantified [12]. Although the relevant research is still in its infancy, the technique -which is frequently used in echocardiography- seems to be promising for several musculoskeletal pathologies. Lastly, the addition of contrast materials might significantly add further data to the already existing body of literature.

In short, physiatrists are progressing with respect to the use of US in musculoskeletal research [13]. However, there is a long way to go; and there is need to enrich the academic applicability of US and to ameliorate/optimize its training alike. Yet, the importance of prompt imaging in the diagnosis and therapeutic follow-up of patients in the daily/academic life of physiatrists is ever-increasing.

## REFERENCES

1) Ulaşli AM, Kara M, Özçakar L. Publications of physical and rehabilitation medicine physicians concerning musculoskeletal ultrasonography: an overview. J Rehabil Med. 2011; 43: 681-3.
2) Akkaya N, Ulaşli AM, Özçakar L. Use of musculoskeletal ultrasound in clinical studies in physiatry: the "stethoscope" is also becoming the "pen". J Rehabil Med. 2013; 45: 701-2.
3) Özçakar L, Tunç H, Öken Ö, Ünlü Z, Durmuş B, Baysal Ö, et al. Femoral cartilage thickness measurements in healthy individuals: learning, practicing and publishing with TURK-MUSCULUS. J Back Musculoskelet Rehabil. 2014; 27: 117-24.
4) Özçakar L, De Muynck M, Imamura M, Vanderstraeten G. Musculoskeletal ultrasound in PRM. From EURO-MUSCULUS towards WORLD-MUSCULUS. Eur J Phys Rehabil Med. 2012; 48: 649-50.
5) Özçakar L, Kara M, Chang KV, Carl AB, Akkaya N, Tok F, et al. Nineteen reasons why physiatrists should do musculoskeletal ultrasound: EURO-MUSCULUS/USPRM recommendations. Am J Phys Med Rehabil. 2014 Oct 8 [Epub ahead of print].
6) Imamura M, Özçakar L, Fregni F, Hsing WT, Battistella LR. Exploring a long-term global approach for musculoskeletal ultrasound training: WORLD-MUSCULUS. J Rehabil Med. 2012; 44: 991-2.
7) Özçakar L, Palamar D, Çarli AB, Aksakal FN. Precision of novice sonographers concerning median nerve and Achilles tendon measurements. Am J Phys Med Rehabil. 2011; 90: 913-6.
8) Tekin L, Kara M, Türker T, Özçakar L. Shoulder measurements in the early period of ultrasound learning: chasing the butterfly? J Rehabil Med. 2011; 43: 961-2.

9) Özçakar L, Kara M, Tekin L, Karanfil Y, Esen E, Utku B, et al. Effect of supervision on ultrasonographic measurements. A blinded randomized cross-over study. Eur J Phys Rehabil Med. 2013; 49: 527-31.

10) De Muynck M, Parlevliet T, De Cock K, Vanden Bossche L, Vanderstraeten G, Özçakar L. Musculoskeletal ultrasound for interventional physiatry. Eur J Phys Rehabil Med. 2012; 48: 675-87.

11) Klauser AS, Miyamoto H, Bellmann-Weiler R, Feuchtner GM, Wick MC, Jaschke WR. Sonoelastography: musculoskeletal applications. Radiology. 2014; 272: 622-33.

12) Korstanje JW, Selles RW, Stam HJ, Hovius SE, Bosch JG. Development and validation of ultrasound speckle tracking to quantify tendon displacement. J Biomech. 2010; 43: 1373-9.

13) Deimel GW, Jelsing EJ, Hall MM. Musculoskeletal ultrasound in physical medicine and rehabilitation. Curr Phys Med Rehabil Rep. 2013; 1: 38-47.